AMBIENT DIAGNOSTICS

AMBIENT DIAGNOSTICS

Yang Cai

Carnegie Mellon University
Pittsburgh, Pennsylvania, USA

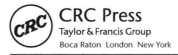

CRC Press
Taylor & Francis Group
Boca Raton London New York

CRC Press is an imprint of the
Taylor & Francis Group, an **informa** business

CRC Press
Taylor & Francis Group
6000 Broken Sound Parkway NW, Suite 300
Boca Raton, FL 33487-2742

First issued in paperback 2019

© 2015 by Taylor & Francis Group, LLC
CRC Press is an imprint of Taylor & Francis Group, an Informa business

No claim to original U.S. Government works

ISBN-13: 978-1-4665-1041-8 (hbk)
ISBN-13: 978-0-367-37808-0 (pbk)

Library of Congress Cataloging-in-Publication Data

Cai, Yang, 1961- author.
    Ambient diagnostics / Yang Cai.
    p. ; cm.
    Includes bibliographical references and index.
    ISBN 978-1-4665-1041-8 (hbk. : alk. paper)
    I. Title.
    [DNLM: 1. Diagnosis, Computer-Assisted--methods. 2. Computing Methodologies. 3. Diagnosis, Computer-Assisted--instrumentation. 4. Diagnostic Equipment. WB 141]

R857.O6
610.28--dc23   2013031006

Visit the Taylor & Francis Web site at
http://www.taylorandfrancis.com

and the CRC Press Web site at
http://www.crcpress.com

To my parents.

Contents

SECTION 1   *Fundamentals*

SECTION 3   Pervasive Sensors

SECTION 4   Crowdsourcing

SECTION 5   Appendices

Preface

Our instinctual senses behave like a diagnostic system. We sense smell, color, sound, motion, and balance in order to maintain critical situation awareness. Knowledge about our bodies and our environment has been condensed and passed on for generations after generations as an important tool for our survival. Like humans, modern electronic devices such as mobile phones are also equipped with abundant sensors. They extend our natural capacities to see what is invisible to us, such as microwaves, bacteria, and chemical compounds. A new kind of market is arising from these simple, slick, and affordable products. In turn, a new kind of science is needed to interpret this multimedia data and to bridge the gap between pixels, words, and—most importantly—reasoning with intuition and knowledge. The convergence of computational diagnostics and emerging device economics catalyzed the creation of this book. *Ambient Diagnostics* is a systematic way of seeing diagnostic patterns using free or affordable alternatives to high-end diagnostic equipment. A single physician visit produces a diagnosis. Multiple visits become diagnoses. When we have millions of people sharing their diagnostic knowledge, it forms the diagnostics.

The history of diagnostic tools is the history of hackers who could think outside the box. This book presents how Willem Einthoven, René-Théophile-Hyacinthe Laënnec, and Richard Bernstein invented the stethoscope, microscope, and personal use of the glucose meter, respectively. It is worth noting that René-Théophile-Hyacinthe Laënnec was an "amateur" from today's point of view. However, he was an expert in making lenses, enabling him to discover bacteria with simple handmade microscopes.

The best way to learn ambient diagnostics is to do simple experiments. Aristotle proclaimed that women have fewer teeth than men. To prove his point, he could have simply counted Mrs. Aristotle's teeth.

This book contains several cognitively inspired algorithms, such as artificial synesthesia, peak shift, and proportion models. It presents simple but elegant solutions to complex problems, such as how to see sound and smell patterns and detect anomalous shapes from three-dimensional body surfaces in microwaves.

This book also has a high dose of multimedia analytics to reflect the rapid technical changes in our lives. This creates not only new opportunities for brave developers but also potential barriers to folks who have never been exposed to this field. To ease the learning curve, this book provides rudimentary models and graphical examples.

Numerous real-world case studies and historical stories are presented in this book to illustrate that the concepts presented are not a fantasy but a reality. The challenge is that ambient diagnostics is a constantly growing area. It encompasses a variety of different sciences and engineering disciplines, such as computer science, electrical and computer engineering, biomedical engineering, design, chemistry, and mechanical engineering. In order to present a lot of related technologies within a finite volume, the topics in the book are limited to those areas that emphasize diagnostic applications with mobile phones, webcams, and Kinect sensors.

THE STRUCTURE OF THE BOOK

This book is divided into five sections: fundamentals, multimedia intelligence, pervasive sensors, crowdsourcing, and appendices. The fundamentals section covers the background of ambient diagnostics, basic data transformation, and pattern recognition methods. The multimedia intelligence section covers sound, color, Kinect, video analysis, and a case study for fatigue detection. The section on pervasive sensors contains overviews about sensors on mobile phones and do-it-yourself devices such as microscopes and spectrometers. The crowdsourcing section reflects the rapidly growing platforms for remote sensing, gaming, and social networking, including potential technologies and case studies.

Each chapter contains main concepts, case studies, and exercise problems. All the references are listed in the footnotes so that they are easier to find. The appendices include the sample code and further readings.

THE ON-LINE RESOURCES OF THE BOOK

The downloadable source code, color images, and updates of the book can be found on the publisher's web site: http://www.crcpress/product/isbn/9781466510418/.

TO READERS

I anticipate that readers from biomedical, healthcare, business, management, psychology, public policy, and other areas will be able to learn to explore the significant potential of ambient diagnostics. If the reader is not technically inclined but simply interested in this subject, then I suggest just to read the introduction in Chapter 1 and Chapters 14 and 15 about gaming for diagnoses and social media, respectively. It may also be helpful to browse the rest of the chapters for figures, stories, and further readings in the appendices. It is hoped that this book is timely and useful for inventors, engineers, researchers, and entrepreneurs, as well as students in engineering, computer science, and life sciences.

This book is based on the lecture notes and assignments for my graduate courses "Cognitive Video" and "Image, Video and Multimedia" at Carnegie Mellon University in Pittsburgh, Pennsylvania. The courses have attracted students from multiple disciplines, such as electrical and computer engineering, computer science, biomedical engineering, mechanical engineering, physics, and information management. The majority of students are graduate students and seniors with a technical background. The prerequisites include knowledge of at least one programming language and calculus. The courses were one semester long and included 15–20 lectures, one term project, a poster and demo session, and a final report at the end of the semester.

For the term project, I recommend small teams. As the African proverb says: "If you want to walk fast, walk alone; if you want to walk longer, walk with others." The key is to simplify the project tasks so that even one person can do them.

The best practice for term projects so far has been "virtual teams," in which individuals work independently but can share ideas and tools with others, especially people outside their disciplines. For example, an electrical engineering student collaborated with a materials science professor to use a 3D printer to build a nanometer structural model, which was novel and relevant.

I benefited greatly from the help of teaching assistants (TAs) while I taught the related courses. The TAs helped to give tutorials about particular hardware and software and helped students solve problems instead of just grading homework. Due to the broader coverage of contents such as vision algorithms, Kinect, and mobile phones, it is desirable to have two TAs to cover the full spectrum of the knowledge and skill sets.

ACKNOWLEDGMENTS

I would like to thank many researchers and organizations for the remarkable images and cases used in this book: Kenneth S. Suslick from the University of Illinois at Urbana-Champaign, Jennifer A. Lewis from Harvard University, Nicholas Kotov from the University of Michigan, Adrien Treuille of Google, Jonas S.S.G. de Jong and Enno T. van der Velde of the Einthoven Foundation, Tirza L. Derflinger of the Breast Health and Preventive Education Center, John Rogers, Kevin Dowling, Conor Rafferty and Elyse Kabinoff from MC10, Inc., and Amany Qassem of Hindawi Publishing. I am also grateful to Zachary J. Smith of the University of California at Sacramento and his coauthors for their inspiration of the cellphone-based biomedical devices.

I benefited greatly from the in-depth conversations with a few medical researchers, educators, and entrepreneurs: Jay Sander of the Global Telemedicine Group and Johns Hopkins University, Piet C. de Groen of Mayo Clinic, Shyam Thakkar of West Penn Health Systems, Alan Russell, Keith E. Lejeune, Lynn Brusco, and Charollte Emig of Disruptive Health Technology Initiative Program of Highmark and Carnegie Mellon University, Jason Hwang, the coauthor of the book *The Innovator's Prescription*, Mark Wiederhold and Brenda K. Wiederhold from Virtual Reality Medical Center, and Larry Miller from Innovation Works.

I have been inspired by my fellow faculty members at Carnegie Mellon University: Herbert Simon taught me about the gap between sequential problem solving and parallel visual processing. William Eddy helped me to understand the beauty of Fourier transformation from the functional magnetic resonance imaging (fMRI) point of view. David Kaufer advised me to look into the connections between images and words. Mel Siegel mentored me through multiple departments. Scott Steven provided his ground breaking video footages from a nursing home. James Hoe and Yu-Li Wang supported the development of graduate courses in Electrical Engineering and Biomedical Engineering. Brian Zeleznik helped with technical writing and refining technical concepts. Margaret Nasta introduced me to the smell sensor article and helped me to test the portable spectrometer. Michael Stroucken provided valuable comments about human color vision and textbook styles. Howard Lipson used his own medical venture to convince me about the life-saving potential of social media. Reed McManigle encouraged me to commercialize the research products.

I appreciate the support from the former dean of the College of Engineering, Pradeep Khosla, who has invested in my ideas and encouraged me to concentrate on research.

Special thanks go to Chen Jin Song, who inspired me to look into the alternative medicine and diagnostic software for heart diseases.

I would like to extend my gratitude to Virtu Calabuif from University of Pittsburgh Medical Center for her help on microscopic imaging and diabetes literatures, and my collaborators: Wencheng Wu, Robert Loce and Lalit K. Mestha from Xerox Research, José Bravo Rodriguez from Castilla-La Mancha University, Julio Abascal from University of Basque Countries, Xavier Alaman, and Manuel Garcia-Herranz del Olmo from Universidad Autonoma de Madrid.

I am grateful to my research assistants and students who implemented and verified many algorithms in the book. It is a long list but I would like to name a few individuals: Aravind Subrnmanian, Tania Ros Codina, Andrew Russell, Daniel Chen, Jian Li, Yufei An, Bahula Gupta, Hao Chen, Shaurya Jagtap, Shengyi Zhang, Joshua Kangas, Bing Yang, Sophoia Shao, Han Lin, Ting Xu, Ajmal Thanikkal, Dev Shah, Ajmal Yashwant Vemuru, Ligen Peng, and Yucheng Wang.

Many thanks go to Jenna Blake and Angela Runge, who edited the book and provided valuable comments and suggestions. I appreciate Mitchell Flaherty's help on the case study of social media. I am also grateful to Caroline Reilly Lesser for her help on illustrations and Dara Krute for her editorial comments.

The work described in this book was supported by several research grants, including Disruptive Health Technology Initiative, Innovation Works, Carnegie Mellon University, West Penn General Hospital, Army Research Office, Air Force Research Lab (Rome, NY), Xerox Research, and Innovation Works. Special thanks goes to the Jewish Health Foundation, which sponsored my first research project on ambient diagnostics using tongue imaging.

Finally, I would like to thank my family and friends for their ultimate support and understanding. I am sure they are happy to see the book finally published.

Yang Cai
Pittsburgh

About the Author

Yang Cai is a Senior Systems Scientist at CyLab and Adjunct Faculty in Electrical and Computer Engineering, College of Engineering, Carnegie Mellon University, Pittsburgh, Pennsylvania. He has taught graduate courses Cognitive Video, Multimedia, Human Algorithms, Creativity, and Innovation Process. Cai is the founder of the Visual Intelligence Studio and Instinctive Computing Lab. He authored the emerging theories of Instinctive Computing, Ambient Diagnostics, and Empathic Computing. He has hosted international workshops on Ambient Intelligence for Scientific Discovery, Instinctive Computing, Digital Human Modeling, Video Intelligence, and Surreal Media. He has been working with the National Science Foundation, NASA, the Air Force Research Lab, and various industries for research projects. Cai also practices rock-carving art and is a volunteer of the international archeological conservation team at the Neolithic rock art site in the Alps for three-dimensional digital conservation work.

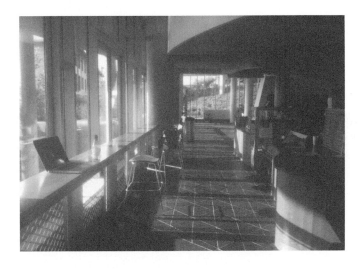

The Gates Building cafeteria at Carnegie Mellon University where the author wrote this book.

Section 1

Fundamentals

1 Introduction

The background in a picture has more information than its foreground.

— An image analyst

1.1 WHAT IS AMBIENT DIAGNOSTICS?

For decades, computers have been built around machines. Calculating for ballistic missiles brought us the first computer ENIAC (Electronic Numerical Integrator and Computer). Sharing printers brought us the Ethernet. Today, the *Internet of things*, such as smartphones, wearable devices, and social media are transforming computing from machine-centric to human-centric. We are seeing a growing demand for affordable, noninvasive, and convenient diagnostic tools to be used anywhere and anytime. In contrast, traditional diagnostic tools are mainly used in clinical environments by professionals. It is often the case that the symptom does not conveniently show up at the clinic office but later at home instead. For example, sleep studies should ideally be conducted at a patient's own home instead of the lab, and heartbeat waves should be monitored and diagnosed at home in addition to during the doctor's visit. Unfortunately, the around-the-clock monitoring is normally expensive and almost impossible unless the patient is hospitalized or has a special prescription.

Ambient diagnosis is an affordable, noninvasive, pervasive, and easy-to-use technology for detecting patterns or abnormities from seemingly disconnected ambient data. The word "ambient" refers to surrounding environments, featuring free, subtle, or subconscious signals. Ambient also pertains to close social contact and communication, enabling intimacy and awareness. The word diagnosis comes from Greek: *dia-* means "to distinguish" and *gno-* means "to perceive" or "to know."

Ambient diagnostics is an emerging subject for the multidisciplinary study of ambient diagnostic systems, from novel sensors and analytical algorithms, to interface design and system optimization. Our vision is to develop future diagnostic tools, such as applications for users to download from the Internet, or products to be purchased from local stores; and three-dimensional (3D) objects that can be printed out from a desktop and carried by a person for use at home, at work, or during leisure time.

To illustrate the concept of ambient diagnostics, let's start with a case study of the smartphone *app*, called iStethoscope. An app is computer program that processes data and interacts with users and sensors.

3

The iStethoscope Case

A registered nurse was pregnant. Although she had professional-grade stethoscopes at home, she also often used the iPhone app iStethoscope to listen to her baby's heartbeat because it was convenient and fun. When she was seven months pregnant, her baby's movements decreased. She used her regular stethoscope to listen to the baby, but she could not hear anything. She then used the iStethoscope app and was able to hear the baby's heartbeat. As the woman was a nurse, she knew that a baby's heartbeat should be much faster than an adult's, so she was not concerned with the fast rate that she heard. She was simply relieved that her baby still had a heartbeat. The next day, she called her obstetrician and went in to have her baby checked out since the baby still was not moving. After the doctor listened for a heartbeat with the ultrasound machine, she was sent to the hospital. Her baby was in distress because its heart rate was well over 260 beats per minute. The mother told the doctors that she had used the phone to listen to her baby's heartbeat the day before, and that the rate was the same as what she had heard the day before. Because of this, the doctors were able to determine that the baby had been in heart failure since at least the previous day. The mother was flown by helicopter to another hospital for an emergency cesarean section. The newborn was saved and had no negative long-term effects from her traumatic birth.

The iStethoscope app costs US$0.99 from the online Apple Store. To date, over one million copies have been downloaded. Cell phones can be used for diagnosing asthma remotely as well. The cell phone can record tracheal breath sounds in asthma patients and can be a noninvasive method to monitor airway diseases. There is no doubt that affordable, noninvasive, pervasive, and easy-to-use technologies will make a difference in diagnoses in our lives. Now, let us take a close look at the process of ambient diagnosis.

Elements of Ambient Diagnostics

Ambient diagnostics contains three essential functions: perception, transformation, and recognition. Figure 1.1 illustrates the connection between the three.

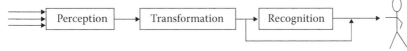

FIGURE 1.1   Basic flowchart of ambient diagnosis.

Perception

Diagnoses start with perception. Since the time of Hippocrates, physicians listened directly to patients' chests to assess cardiac health. In 1816, a young French doctor named René-Théophile-Hyacinthe Laënnec needed to examine an obese young woman. He hesitated to put his head to her chest and came up with the idea for the prototype for a stethoscope. He rolled a stack of paper into a cylinder, pressed one end to the patient's chest, and held his ear to the other end. He was surprised to hear the beating of the heart much more clearly than if he had applied his ear directly to the chest.

Today, professional stethoscopes are still based on a similar principle: two ear-pieces, a rubber tube, an acrylic diaphragm, and metal connectors have replaced the straight paper tube. Electronic stethoscopes are also available commercially; however, they are more expensive than regular stethoscopes. The microphone on a mobile phone has been optimized for human voices and also filters noises, including the low-frequency sounds of heartbeats or breathing. Fortunately, smartphones such as the iPhone and Android phones have been developed to use advanced microelectromechanical system (MEMS) microscopy that is sensitive enough to pick up heart and lung sounds. The application software enables amplification over 100 times digitally with high acoustic fidelity (Figure 1.2).

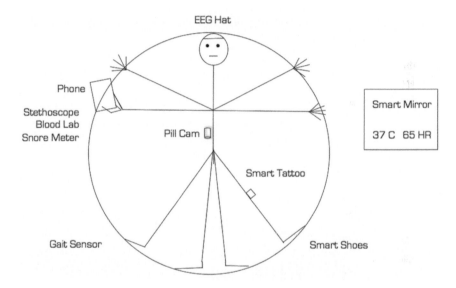

FIGURE 1.2 Ambient perception cloud includes wearable sensors, intelligent funiture, appliances, and networks.

Traditional diagnosis involves two modes of perception: *scanning* and *tracking*. Scanning is a regular checkup without a target. It covers broader exams but does not go in depth. The interval between exams is the essential variable. In the example of the pregnant nurse, this describes how often the pregnant woman checks her baby's motions and how often she checks her baby's heartbeat. *Tracking* is a focused, con-tinuous, and intensive measurement for a period of time. In the case of the pregnant nurse, this type of perception occurred when the woman thoroughly monitored her unborn baby's heart rate using both regular stethoscopes and the iStethoscope. Then, the hospitals continued the tracking task with the ultrasound sensor. The iStetho-scope here just filled the gap in scanning and tracking when a regular stethoscope was unable to detect the heartbeat and other high-end monitoring devices were not available at home. In addition, the recording function of the iStethoscope allowed her doctors to review the past tracking data in order to make important decisions.

The goal of ambient diagnostics is to mimic perceptual intelligence as in nature, the most vital skills to our survival. We smell, listen, look, touch, and feel to characterize a situation by answering questions such as who, what, when, where, and why. Our brain structure also allows us to prioritize perceptual signals; for example, our smell sensors are directly connected to the paleocortex, the prehistorically old area of the brain that is close to the spinal cord, enabling a fast response in case of an emergency.

In contrast to many diagnostics books that are full of ontology and logic, this book is packed with information about state-of-the-art sensors. We will study many perceptual channels throughout the chapters. Many of them are improvised from smartphones or webcams. Perceptual channels we will study include sound (Chapter 4); color (Chapter 5); infrared, gesture, 3D surface, and biometrics (Chapter 6); mobility (Chapter 9); fatigue (Chapter 8); temperature, accelerations, orientations, and proxy (Chapters 9); pill cameras (Chapter 10); light spectrum (Chapter 11); and microscopes (Chapter 12).

Transformation

Signal transformation is a necessary step after collecting sensory data. We have two types of transforms: digital and physical (Figure 1.3). Digital transforms convert one form to another on a computer. On the other hand, physical transforms convert one sensory channel to another. In cognitive science, this is called artificial synesthesia, a cross-channel sensing (e.g., to see smell in color).[1]

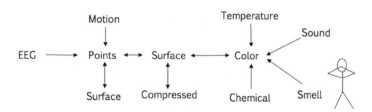

FIGURE 1.3   Transformation in this book.

Chapter 2 reviews basic digital transforms, including conventional transforms (e.g., the Fourier transform, wavelet, and principal component analysis) and nonconventional transforms such as shape to word, word to shape, data to shape, and shape to data.

Furthermore, we introduce physical transforms, including transformations from sound to visual (Chapter 4), smell and chemical component to color (Chapters 5 and 12), and motion to image (Chapters 6 and 7).

---

[1] K. S. Suslick. Synesthesia in science and technology: more than making the unseen visible. *Current Opinion in Chemical Biology* 16:557–563, 2012.

Recognition

Everything that happens around us is driven by physical models, or so-called forward physics. A beating heart creates vibration patterns on the chest wall. Breathing generates flow patterns in the airway. A diagnostic is an inverse physics problem, which means that it is intended to find causes for a phenomenon. Unfortunately, due to the complexities of physics modeling, such as nonlinear mapping, missing data, and noises, inverse physics models are impossible to obtain. In general, we have to use approximate methods to connect patterns to the causes. These methods include machine learning or data mining from historical data, finding correlations to other patterns, or using collective knowledge of user input online. Clustering and classification are essential in diagnostic pattern recognition. Clustering is to group data that has similar attributes. It can significantly reduce the size of information storage. Classification is to detect and categorize objects based on their distances. Clustering and classification are heavily studied in data mining these days to make sense of exponentially growing data.

Chapter 3 provides a review of rudimentary models for clustering and classification. They are useful for preliminary analyses of the collected data, using minimal time and effort.

Ambient diagnostics is pattern recognition from incomplete and fuzzy, yet dynamic information. More rigorous logic and statistical reasoning models are needed. Furthermore, knowledge engineering is needed to incorporate the heuristics and rules into the ambient diagnostics systems. The section that follows provides a brief introduction to related approaches.

1.2   DIAGNOSTIC MODELS

Diagnosis is considered a subfield of Artificial Intelligence (AI). To represent diagnostic knowledge, we need cognitive models.

Diagnostic Trees

A diagnostic tree is a graph model of the logic relations between variables. The goal of a diagnostic tree is to identify all the potential root causes of the problem from the top of the tree to the bottom. A diagnostic tree consists of leaves (nodes) and branches. Each branch represents the connectivity and the order between two leaves (nodes). Figure 1.4 shows an example of a diagnostic tree.

Diagnostic Rules

A diagnostic rule can be represented verbally as an IF-THEN statement, where $R = <A, C>$, consisting of A (antecedent or precondition), a series of tests to be valued as true or false; C (consequent or conclusion), the class or classes that apply to instances covered by rule R. Rules can then be generated from a diagnostic tree, for example:

IF (heart_rate is zero) THEN (distress_call)

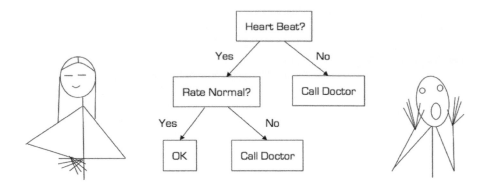

FIGURE 1.4   Diagnostic tree example.

A diagnostic tree can always be used to generate diagnostic rules, but they are not equivalent. The differences between a diagnostic tree and diagnostic rules are as follows: (1) the tree has an implied order in which the splitting is performed, and rules have no order; and (2) a tree is created based on looking at all classes, but only one class must be examined at a time in a diagnostic rule.

Rules can be optimized by generating those that accurately cover a specific class. These technologies are called covering algorithms.[2] A rudimentary pseudocode is

1. Generate a rule on training data
2. Remove the training data covered by the rule
3. Repeat the process until satisfactory

Assume we have a training dataset of normal and distressed cases, including two variables: heart rate and monitoring period. We want to refine our diagnostic rules to cover distress cases accurately. We first cover the distressed area for the heart rate variable only. Then, we cover both the heart rate and the monitoring period variables so that the distressed area on the top right corner is covered completely. Figure 1.5 illustrates the process for the covering algorithm.[3]

From the covering algorithm, we can derive the following rule:

IF (heart_rate > 120) and (day > 1) THEN distress_call

We can also represent the knowledge in the form of the diagnostic tree, shown in Figure 1.6.

[2] S. Pulatova. Covering (rule-based) algorithm. chapter 8, *Data Mining Technology*, 2007. Accessed from: http://www.slideshare.net/totoyou/covering-rulesbased-algorithm
[3] I. H. Witten and E. Frank. *Data Mining*. Morgan Kaufmann, Burlington, MA, 2000.

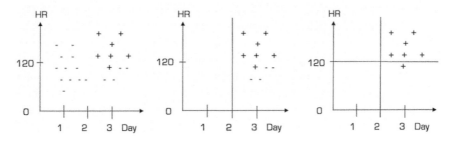

FIGURE 1.5   Covering algorithm.

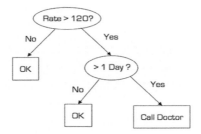

FIGURE 1.6   Diagnostic tree with heart rate and time variables.

Bayesian Reasoning

We can often predict an event from related events. For example, if a mother could not hear her unborn baby's heartbeat, then she won't feel her baby's motion as well. On the other hand, what is the probability of heart failure if the mother couldn't feel the baby's motion? Here we can apply Bayesian reasoning (Figure 1.7).

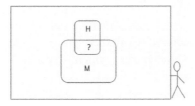

FIGURE 1.7   What is the probability of "no heartbeat" (H), while "no motion" (M) is true?

Assume the mother's sensory channels for sound and motion events are independent. Also, we *assume* the probability of "no motion" (M) of an unborn baby is $P(M)=0.1$; the probability of "no heartbeat" (H) is $P(H)=0.01$; the probability of "no motion" while "no heartbeat" is true is $P(M|H)=0.9$. According to Bayes' rule, the probability of "no heartbeat" in which "no motion" is true equals the joint probability of $P(H)$ and $P(M)$ divided by $P(M)$. Here, we see an asymmetric relationship between H and M:

$$P(H|M) = P(H \cap M) / P(M) = P(M|H) \, P(H) / P(M) = 0.9 \times 0.01 / 0.1 = 0.09.$$

Bayes' rule[4] has been widely used in diagnostic modeling. In the modern era, there are two significant variations. The first is the Bayesian network, or Bayesian belief network (BBN), which uses directed graphs to represent the tree-like conditional probabilities that associate symptoms with diagnostic descriptions.[5] For example, the visual features on the tongue and symptoms can be modeled in a BBN. Another variation is the recursive Bayesian model, which can be used for continuous monitoring and machine learning. Both variations are useful to ambient diagnostics because the field deals with multimedia and continuous data streams. For further reading, please see the excellent textbook Probabilistic Reasoning by J. Pearl,[6] and a list of further readings in Appendix B.

Expert Systems

Expertise in diagnosis is a scarce recourse. For decades, AI researchers have been developing computer programs to emulate the cognitive ability of one or many human experts. Expert systems are developed to solve complex problems, such as diagnosis, by reasoning with knowledge like an expert.[7]

An expert system can be constructed from the following components: (1) the knowledge base, which is the collection of facts and rules that describe all the knowledge about the specific problem domain; (2) the inference engine, which chooses appropriate facts and rules to apply when trying to solve the user's query; and (3) the user interface, which takes in the user's query in a readable form, passes it to the inference engine, and then displays the results to the user.

The first expert system, DENDRAL, was developed in 1965 at Stanford University, led by computer scientists Edward Feigenbaum and Bruce Buchanan and Nobel Laureate molecular biologist Joshua Lederberg in cooperation with chemist Carl Djerassi. DENDRAL was designed to help chemists identify unknown organic molecules.[8] The name DENDRAL is a combination of the term dendritic algorithm. Dendritic means "*tree-like*" in Greek. Dendrites are the branches of a neuron that connect electrical signals received from other neural cells to the cell body. The software was also written in LISP language, which was considered the language of AI because of its symbolic processing abilities.

DENDRAL is a program that uses mass spectra or other experimental data together with a knowledge base of chemistry to produce a set of possible chemical structures that may be responsible for producing the data. Figure 1.8 illustrates an example of the process.

---

[4] T. Bayes. An essay towards solving a problem in the doctrine of chances. *Philosophical Transactions of the Royal Society of London* 53:370–418, 1763.

[5] A. Moore's very good tutorial on Bayes nets for representing and reasoning about uncertainty. Online slides: http://www.cs.cmu.edu/~awm.

[6] J. Pearl. *Probabilistic reasoning in intelligent systems.* Morgan Kaufmann, Burlington, MA, 1988.

[7] http://en.wikipedia.org/wiki/Expert_system.

[8] Robert K. Lindsay, Bruce G. Buchanan, E. A. Feigenbaum, and Joshua Lederberg. DENDRAL: A case study of the first expert system for scientific hypothesis formation. *Artificial Intelligence* 61(2):209–261, 1993.

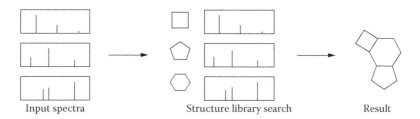

Input spectra   Structure library search   Result

FIGURE 1.8 DENDRAL expert system: mass spectra (left), matching molecular structures with the mass spectra signatures (middle) and the final structure (right).

DENDRAL was also the first expert system that successfully simulated the scientific discovery process (i.e., forming hypotheses, searching for matching structures, optimizing the solution, and so on). In some test cases, the program's performance rivaled that of expert chemists.

MYCIN was the first medical expert system in the early 1970s. It was developed for diagnosing bacteria that caused severe infections. MYCIN was derived from the suffix of antibiotics, "*-mycin.*" In addition, MYCIN was used for the diagnosis of blood-clotting diseases. Like DENDRAL, it was also written in LISP, a list-processing language.

The MYCIN system contained heuristic rules for about 100 causes of bacterial infections, and each rule was coded in an IF-THEN statement. These rules could be combined sequentially or in parallel, forming a rule network. MYCIN used certainty factors (CFs) to represent the credibility of each rule. The result is a modular procedure for determining the certainty of a conclusion, given the credibility of each rule and the certainty of the premises. CFs are useful for solving "conflicting rules" or "parallel rules" problems. With CF calculation, we can select the rule with the highest CF value. Figure 1.9 depicts the combination functions that apply to serial and parallel rules.[8]

After building the rule network, the patient's symptoms, general conditions, medical history, and lab results are put into the system. By taking the data and applying its rules, MYCIN would determine whether a bacterial infection actually

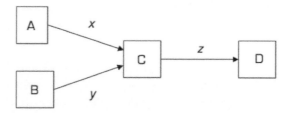

FIGURE 1.9 Certainty combination function used in MYCIN, where x, y, and z denote the certainty factors (CFs). The rules are as follows: IF A THEN C with x; IF B THEN C with y; and IF C THEN D with z. This gives the CF for $C = x + y - xy$.

exists, what type of bacteria is causing the infection, and what the best course of medical treatment is.

Studies found that it diagnosed well in about 69% of cases, which was better than the performance of infectious disease experts.[9]

The early version of MYCIN was used only for bacterial infection diagnoses. To extend the capability of the inference engine, the expert system "shells" E-MYCIN was introduced in the 1980s and supported the development of expert systems in a wide variety of application areas.

Since then, several expert system development tools have been deployed. For example, PROLOG language, developed by a French AI researcher, is a first-order logic-based reasoning engine. Another is CLIPS, an open source language for encoding and reasoning production rules that is written in C.

Unfortunately, the major difficulty in developing expert systems has been the extraction of necessary knowledge from human experts and converting it to the rule base so that it is usable by the inference machine. This is the so-called knowledge acquisition bottleneck. This explains why expert systems are not popular these days: they are too expensive to develop. With the new wave of social media, perhaps we may create crowdsourcing expert systems in the cloud.

1.3 MULTIMEDIA INTELLIGENCE

Perhaps the most exciting progress in ambient diagnostics has been the abundance of multimedia sensors, processors, and display technologies on smartphones and laptops. Multimedia intelligence aims to perceive and recognize symptoms from multimedia data in daily life. Multimedia intelligence is responsible for transforming diagnoses from the lab to the home, from verbal to multimedia, from expensive devices to affordable smartphone applications. It is also transforming data analysis methods, moving from numerical and symbolic analysis to multimedia analysis.

This book covers a significant number of multimedia data analysis models in each chapter. For example, Chapters 2 and 3 review foundations for two-dimensional (2D) transformation and pattern recognition, and Chapters 4 through 15 introduce multimedia algorithms for analyzing color, shape, sound, infrared, tactility, and motion patterns.

This book also presents transformative concepts and sensors for ambient diagnoses. The following sections cover a few examples.

Point and Search

The number of multimedia applications has been growing exponentially since 2008. For example, the song-retrieving app SoundHound[10] allows users to record a few seconds of a song; image-retrieving apps allow users to search for similar images online. These technologies can be applied to ambient diagnoses by searching for asthma sound files and skin disease patterns by uploading the recorded sound or

---

[9] MYCIN WikiPedia page: http://en.wikipedia.org/wiki/Mycin
[10] SoundHound web site: http://www.soundhound.com

images to the search engine, which matches patterns with related diagnostic information. Chapters 2 and 3 provide essential models for distance measurements and basic pattern transformations. Chapter 5 introduces the pattern alignment algorithm for matching multimedia patterns. Furthermore, Chapter 15 discusses cases about how to use social media for sharing and searching for knowledge about rare diseases. Automated multimedia retrieval has transformed the methods for diagnosis in terms of efficiency, scope, and contents.

Miniaturization

Miniaturization is an emerging metaphor in multimedia intelligence. In the science fiction movie Fantastic Voyage, a submarine is shrunk down into a capsule and travels inside a human body. Today, the capsule voyage has become a reality: Pill cameras are the most widely used, patient-friendly tool for directly viewing the small intestine to detect and monitor abnormalities. By simply having a patient swallow a vitamin-size capsule, a physician can detect and monitor lesions, ulcers, tumors, and bleeding within the small intestine—without putting the patient through the lengthy and uncomfortable procedure of an endoscopy, which requires sedation and anesthesia. Furthermore, the pill camera costs a few hundred dollars, while a typical endoscope costs thousands of dollars in the USA.

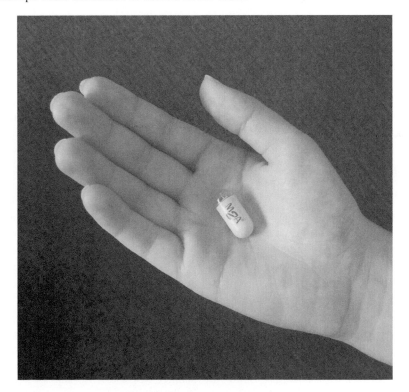

FIGURE 1.10   Pill camera M2A made by Givenimaging.

Chapter 10 gives an overview of state-of-the-art wearable sensors and elaborates on the structure of the pill camera (Figure 1.10) as well as the preliminary algorithm for video processing.

Active Sensing

Listening to the sound of heartbeats through a stethoscope is a passive sensing method in which the sensor receives signals but does not emit any signals. In many cases, low signal strength and noisy conditions prevent us from perceiving signature patterns. Active sensing methods, on the other hand, send out distinguishable physical signals that help reveal signature patterns. Active sensing methods have been widely used in medical diagnoses. For example, ultrasound heart monitors send out ultrasound waves through the chest and receive the echoes from the heart to obtain clearer signals than those from normal stethoscopes.

Chapter 6 introduces a revolutionary active sensor, Kinect, which emits infrared dots from a video camera to reconstruct the 3D surface in front of it.

Digital Human Lab

For centuries, people have obtained diagnostic knowledge through reasoning and experiments. Today, computational simulation is the third scientific method. "Digital humans" provide not only anatomically correct structures but also physiological process models.[11]

Chapter 13 presents a case study about how to design a remote diagnostic system with the digital human and digital device models. This method allows us to study electromagnetic strength distributions and surface properties in the microwave field, making it possible to test new devices on digital humans before the devices are even built.

Negative Spaces

According to the pioneer of AI, Herbert A. Simon, "An ant, viewed as a behaving system, is quite simple. The apparent complexity of its behavior over time is largely a reflection of the environment in which it finds itself. A man, viewed as a behaving system, is quite simple. The apparent complexity of his behavior over time is largely a reflection of the complexity of the environment in which he finds himself."[12] Here, an ant and a human are figures represented in a positive space; their environment is called a negative space or background.

In multimedia, for every figure there is a subtractive function to obtain the negative space or background. In some cases, a complex diagnostic problem can be simplified or even solved by monitoring the surrounding environments. The complex, sparse,

---

[11] Y. Cai (ed.). *Digital human modeling. LNAI 4650.* Springer, New York, 2008. http://www.springer.com/computer/ai/book/978-3-540-89429-2.

[12] H.A. Simon. *The science of artificial.* MIT Press, Cambridge, MA, 1980.

or disconnected patterns in figures can be detected and connected from the negative space around it.

Chapter 4 presents a case study about how to monitor environmental sounds to diagnose health problems in a workspace, and Chapter 7 also describes algorithms for background modeling based on motion features.

Relational Features

Conventional computer algorithms are used more to precise measurements with absolute values. In the diagnostic world, absolute values without context are relatively meaningless. More often, we use relative measurements. For example, the body mass index describes the ratio between height and weight. Relative features, such as proportion, relative speed, relative direction, and relative distance, help to simplify representations and the problem-solving process.

Chapters 4 and 12 describe how to use relative sound and color features to characterize patterns. Chapter 13 presents how proportional features can be used in surface pattern recognition.

Semantic Gap

Medical experts use verbal and visual media for diagnostic reasoning, but mapping between words and features is a great challenge. In many cases, the mapping function is just a black box without an explicit representation. We call this a *semantic gap*.

Let us look at a rudimentary example: assume we have two sample images from the pill camera that represent two symptoms. Each image contains 640 × 480 pixels and 256 grayscale intensity levels. If the intensity of each pixel is a feature, then the direct image-to-word mapping would have 157,286,400 bytes of information, which grow exponentially if we expand the image database to thousands of images and then categorize hundreds of symptoms. Now, if we add a "hidden layer" of intermediate representations between the visual features and words (e.g., edges in the grayscale images, which are in binary values), then the size of the information can be dropped to 614,400 bytes. Note that the number of hidden layers can be more than one; and

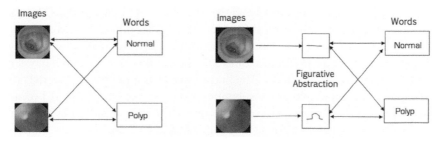

FIGURE 1.11   Direct image-to-verb mapping and the hidden-layer abstract mapping.

the size of the feature space can be smaller for the hidden-layer images. Figure 1.11 illustrates the mapping process for both scenarios.

The hidden-layer representations are important for filling the semantic gap. It can reduce the feature space to a manageable size and represent nonlinear mapping relations (e.g., mixed Gaussian kernel functions).

Chapter 4 describes a case study of asthma sound classification in which the verbal descriptions are represented by spectrum features. Chapter 10 also describes the algorithm that converts a doctor's verbal description into a computer visual model.

1.4   CROWDSOURCING

Social media adds more dimensions to ambient diagnosis. Specifically, it enables several potential applications: collective intelligence for diagnosing rare disease, gaming for diagnostic research, correlation analysis, and recommending systems. Chapters 14 and 15 are devoted to crowdsourcing methods.

Detecting Influenza Epidemics

For over a decade, researchers have been using drugstore sales data and online search engine query data to detect influenza epidemics as well as bioattacks. The assumption is that the spikes in the ambient data have correlation with outbreaks. Machine learning scholars such as Andrew Moore from Carnegie Mellon University (Pittsburgh, PA) and now Google have worked on data mining for biosurveillance, sponsored by the Defense Advanced Research Projects Agency (DARPA). Moore's Auton Lab has developed computational models for collective intelligence for epidemic monitoring and prediction.

Traditional biosurveillance systems, including those employed by the U.S. Centers for Disease Control and Prevention (CDC) and the European Influenza Surveillance Scheme (EISS), rely on both virologic and clinical data (such as that for influenza-like illness, ILI) and physician visits. Unfortunately, the data collection and reporting cycle is not in real time. For example, CDC publishes national and regional data from these surveillance systems on a weekly basis, typically with a 1- to 2-week report lag. Google recently used online web search queries submitted by millions of users each day to monitor health-seeking behavior. Because there is a correlation between the relative frequency of certain queries and the percentage of physician visits about the influenza-like symptoms, the team at Google was able to estimate the current level of weekly influenza activity in the United States with a reporting lag of about one day.

Google used a simple model to estimate the probability that a random physician visit in a region is related to an ILI. The linear model has a single variable: the probability that a random search query submitted from the same region is ILI related. Google scientists then built a linear model using the log odds of an ILI physician visit data and the log odds of an ILI-related online search query data.[13]

[13] J. Ginsberg, M. H. Mohebbi, R. S. Patel, L. Brammer, M. S. Smolinski, and L. Brilliant. Detecting influenza epidemics using search engine query data. *Nature* 457(19), 1012–1015, 2009.

Chapter 15 covers some fundamental models for correlation analysis, including the Pearson correlation coefficient and Spearman rank coefficient. Those are simple statistical methods that in fact work quite well in many real-world analyses. In addition, we emphasize visualization methods such as a scatter plot and heat map throughout the book. Simple and intuitive models win.

Rare Disease Diagnosis

Health diagnosis is a learning process: A doctor's expertise is limited by training, practice, and communication. Social media create additional channels for users to search, share, and track rare diseases for which local doctors may not have expertise. As an example, Facebook enabled the writer Deborah Kogan to diagnose her son's rare disease before the doctors identified it. In her case, the speed of the diagnosis turned out to be crucial because the disease needed to be treated within days of the first symptoms, or else it would be life threatening. Facebook essentially saved her son's life. Chapter 15 provides the "pregnant man" case study to show how online social media have actually saved lives, not by chance, but by the science of network.

Gaming for Diagnoses

Video games can be used for serious diagnoses or disease research. Chapter 14 describes games for infection diagnoses, DNA multiple-sequence alignment and structure analyses, gait analysis, tremor evaluation, and social media for autism patients. Chapter 14 also reviews basic video game development tools from simple utilities to professional packages.

Recommendation Algorithms

Collective intelligence comes from shared knowledge from communities. It can also come from online software, called recommendation algorithms, which use collaborative filtering and content-based filtering. Chapter 3 reviews similarity measurements that enable pattern matching with predefined errors, similar to Google's search results, which come up with recommended results even when the input has some spelling errors.

1.5 SOFT SENSORS

The concept behind soft sensors is to treat sensors like software. In this way, we can make new sensors by combining available sensors or by deriving them from related data. For example, the signal strength of the Bluetooth phone headset as it is received from a television set can be used for deriving the proxy distance of the user.

Early Attempts

Oxygen was an early project for smart environments at the Massachusetts Institute of Technology (MIT) Artificial Intelligence Lab in the early 1980s. Its vision was to bring abundant computation and communication naturally into people's lives so that they could be as pervasive and free as air,[14] similar to the standardization of batteries and power sockets. These infrastructures are embedded in our environments and work everywhere and anytime. It was the early movement that inspired ambient intelligence, ubiquitous computing, the Internet of things, smart environments, and human-centered computing waves.

The ZigBee chip was invented at the MIT Media Lab in 1999 for small, low-cost, low-data-rate, and long-battery-life personal networks.[15] It was intended to be simpler and less expensive than Bluetooth or Wi-Fi. Remarkably, ZigBee is a network with no centralized control or high-power transmitter and receiver capable of reaching all of the networked devices. The decentralized nature of such wireless ad hoc networks makes them suitable for applications where a central node cannot be relied on, such as body sensor networks.

Crossbow's Mote was one of the first commercial sensor network products[16] and included wireless sensors such as magnetic, infrared, sound, and accelerometers, as well as wireless modules. Similar to ZigBee, its low cost, low data rate, and long battery life are suitable for short-distance sensor networking. The Mote project team implemented the University of California at Berkley's open source TinyOS software, which enables ad hoc wireless communication from node to node, creating a decentralized sensor network.

ZigBee, Mote, and similar products have been used in environmental monitoring and home automation, such as for lighting. However, they have not been widely used in the digital healthcare consumer market. There are three reasons for this: limited sensor capacities (e.g., three to five sensors per node), expensive costs, and the lack of hackers who are interested in these applications.

Sensor-Rich Computing

The sensing revolution has finally started with the new generation of smartphones, which are integrated with an abundance of sensors. The general idea behind their development is to design once and grow later. For example, iPhones and Android phones have at least twenty sensors, including accelerometers, magnetic sensors, gyroscopic sensors, light sensors, stereo microphones, two cameras, temperature sensors, moisture sensors, multitouch sensors, GPS sensors, Wi-Fi strength sensors, Bluetooth strength sensors, and near-field communication sensors. Because these sensors are already in the smartphones, it costs almost nothing to develop apps around them. Despite this, many of the available smartphone sensors are underused. Most users are probably not even aware these capacities exist. Similar to smartphones, the Kinect, originally designed for Microsoft's Xbox, is also packed with additional sensors, including four microphones, one color camera, one infrared camera, and three-axis accelerometers.

---

[14] http://oxygen.lcs.mit.edu/Overview.html
[15] http://en.wikipedia.org/wiki/ZigBee
[16] http://bullseye.xbow.com:81/Products/wproductsoverview.aspx

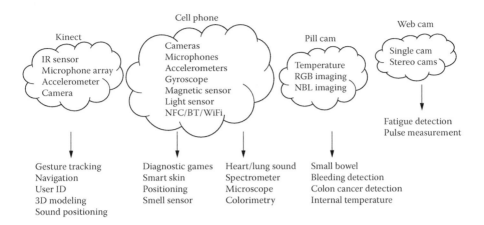

FIGURE 1.12   Clouds of sensors and applications in this book: IR=Infrared; RGB= Red, Green and Blue; NFC=Near-Field Communication; BT=Bluetooth; NBL=Narrow-Bandwidth Lighting.

Ambient diagnostics brings a new paradigm of sensor-rich computing that incorporates more distributed measurements than centralized computing. To illustrate this concept, a modern aircraft requires about six million lines of code, using only a few sensors, to be aware of changing conditions. On the other hand, a fly uses only a few hundred neurons in its brain (about 2%) to do the same job, whereas the other 98% of the neurons are devoted to process nearly one million channels of sensory data. In light of this, we must embrace a similar heuristic to use more distributed sensors to replace heavy-duty centralized computing. This also suggests that there is no need for high-resolution sensors; instead, a large number of coarse-grained sensors could give reasonable results. Most biosensors are transformers that convert one kind of signal into another. For example, a cockroach can feel human motion by sensing the airflow that passes its hairs since it obviously is not capable of solving complex fluid dynamics equations.

Although important research has gone into developing sophisticated diagnostic instruments, many important medical decisions are still based on expert opinions formed by trained professionals on the basis of data gathered via conventional devices, like microscopes, cell counters, and spectrophotometers. Replacing some of these costly and monolithic instruments with cheaper, portable devices that can achieve similar performance is an attractive option for reducing the cost and infrastructure burdens that quality healthcare places on society.

An ad hoc sensor web can generate more data than we can handle (Figure 1.12). Most information today has not been analyzed even though it contains actionable information. For this reason, automation is essential to process, filter, and correct this flood of data and to transform and present it as accurate and actionable information for people. As information from multiple sources flows up to higher levels of awareness, a more complete picture can be created, enabling adjudication at a higher level to correct for erroneous information that arose at lower levels. Adjudication also helps reduce the volume of information that is being pushed up, which can have the effect of overwhelming decision makers.

1.6 SCIENCE OF SIMPLICITY

Leonardo Da Vinci once said, "Simplicity is the ultimate sophistication." Ambient diagnostics is a science of simplicity. It seeks minimal components or descriptive features. Ideally, a diagnostic kit should be so simple that it is nearly impossible for it to make errors. Simplicity has multiple advantages: It is faster, cheaper, easier, and more robust.

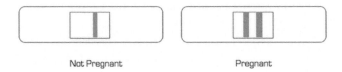

FIGURE 1.13   Pregnancy test kit: one bar indicates the woman is not pregnant and two bars indicate the woman is pregnant.

Pregnancy Test Kit

Perhaps the best example of simplicity in design is pregnancy test kits (Figure 1.13). Beginning in the 1920s, the rabbit test, or Aschheim-Zondek test, was sometimes used to test women for pregnancy. When a woman is pregnant, her body produces the hormone human chorionic gonadotropin (hCG), which shows up in her urine and blood. During the rabbit test, a woman's urine would be injected into a female rabbit, whose ovaries would enlarge and show follicular maturation in response to hCG if it was present in the tested woman. After injection, the rabbit's ovaries would be examined for changes. The test was considered to have less than a 2% error rate. Modern-day pregnancy kits test for the same hormone as that tested in the rabbit test. Women today are able to purchase a kit from a drugstore, which they then urinate on and watch for the appearance of a certain symbol. If the symbol appears, then the woman is probably pregnant.[17]

Reduced Instruction-Set Computing Strategy

In computer development history, reduced instruction-set computing (RISC) is a central processing unit (CPU) design strategy based on the insight that simplified instructions can provide higher performance if the simplicity enables much faster execution of each instruction. Take Berkeley's RISC-I processor in 1982 for example: It reduced transistors from 100,000 to 44,420 and had only 32 instructions. Yet, RISC-I completely outperformed any other single-chip design. In the

---

[17] Pregancy Test Kit website: http://imgur.com/oG492

following year, the RISC-II came with 40,760 transistors and only 39 instructions; it ran over three times as fast as RISC-I. The moral is the fewer components, the faster the hardware.

Simple Algorithms

Simple and rudimentary algorithms perform well on most commonly used datasets.[18] Simple and cheap algorithms often come up with rather good rules for characterizing the structure of data and frequently achieve surprisingly high accuracy. Perhaps this is because the structure underlying many real-world datasets is quite rudimentary.

For example, a comprehensive study of the performance of the classification algorithm 1R procedure reported on sixteen datasets frequently used by machine learning researchers to evaluate their algorithms.[19] Surprisingly, despite its simplicity, 1R did surprisingly well in comparison to state-of-the-art learning schemes. The rules it produced turned out to be just a few percentage points less accurate on almost all of the datasets compared to the more complex decision tree induction scheme.

Naïve Bayes is a simple classification algorithm for representing and learning probabilistic knowledge. It also surprisingly outperforms more sophisticated classifiers on many datasets. The simple classifier K-Nearest Neighbor also showed better performance than Gausian Mixture Model (GMM) in many cases in this book.

The moral is always try the simple things first. Use simple, rudimentary techniques to establish a performance baseline before progressing to more sophisticated learning schemes.

1.7   PERSONAL DIAGNOSES

The future of ambient diagnoses relies on hackers, affordable prices, and personalization. The history of medical instrumentation is a history of hacking in scientific ways. The main contents in this book, Chapters 4 through 15, are inspired by hackers and written for aspiring hackers.

History of the Personal Glucose Meter

Measuring changes to blood sugar, or glucose, throughout the day is vital to the health of diabetic patients. The original glucose test device, the Ames reflectance meter (ARM) was bulky and very expensive, around US$495 in the 1970s, and it was used in clinic offices and labs only. The situation changed dramatically because of a coincidence. Richard Bernstein, a diabetic patient and an engineer, called the glucose meter manufacturer and asked to buy one for his personal use. However, the company had never sold the device to individuals before and told him that he would have to get a prescription. Coincidentally, his wife was a medical doctor, so she

---

[18] Witten, I.H. and Frank, E. *Data mining*. Morgan Kaufman, Burlington, MA, 2002.
[19] Robert C. Holte. Very simple classification rules perform well on most commonly used datasets. *Machine Learning* 11:63–90, 1993.

wrote the prescription for him. After that incident, the idea of testing blood sugar at home came to reality.[20] Companies started to produce glucose meters for home use. Today, handheld glucose meters are widely available in pharmacy stores.

Moore's Law for Sensors

The abundance of computing power largely benefits from Moore's law, named after Gordon E. Moore, who described the trend in his 1965 article on the number of transistors on integrated circuits (ICs) doubling approximately every two years.[21] The capabilities of many digital electronic devices are strongly linked to Moore's law: processing speed, memory capacity, sensors, and even the number and size of pixels in digital cameras and flat-panel displays. All of these are improving at roughly exponential rates. This exponential improvement has dramatically enhanced the impact of digital electronics in nearly every segment of the world economy.

Most miniature sensors greatly benefited from MEMS (microelectromechanical system) technology. The MEMS community borrowed lithography and batch fabrication techniques from IC manufacturing to build precise and inexpensive sensory and mechanical devices. Today, MEMS devices have found their way into our phones, automobiles, and televisions, as well as the data streamed for voice, video, and data communications.

MEMS technology follows Moore's law even further because it not only makes things smaller but also puts multiple devices on a single chip[22] (e.g., live organisms on a chip, which goes beyond the limit of silicon materials).

"Appnomics"

The abundance of sensors on a chip does not automatically warrant exponential growth. Field programmable gate array (FPGA) technology is an example. FPGA integrated a large quantity of gates, a basic component for building a computer, on a single chip. However, it has not been booming as expected because of a lack of open source utilities and enthusiastic hackers.

Smartphone technologies have changed the technical ecology. The emerging apps create new models, called "*appnomics*." Multiple sensors and processors have already been integrated into phones, so the cost of an app (application software) is just a download fee. Google and Apple have provided open source application programming interfaces (APIs) and software development kits (SDKs). The app market has grown exponentially, largely because of the massive number of consumers and affordable prices.

Price elasticity measures how strongly the supply or demand of a good changes when the price of the good changes. It is the ratio of the change of quantity of either

---

[20] T. S. Danowski and J. H. Sunder. Jet injections of insulin during self-monitoring of blood glucose. *Diabetes Care* 1:27–33, 1978.

[21] Gordon E. Moore. Cramming more components onto integrated circuits. *Electronics Magazine*, p. 4, 1965. Retrieved November 11, 2006.

[22] http://www.forbes.com/sites/tedgreenwald/2011/10/21/moores-law-meets-mems-embedded-devices-in-your-smartphone-are-the-next-big-thing/

supply or demand to the change of the price. The greater the elasticity, the greater the change of supply or demand in relation to the price change will be.

According to Distimo's app market survey,[23] a price change of US$3 or under had a significant effect on download volumes. Not surprisingly, download volumes generally went up with a price drop and decreased when a price increased. On average, downloads of applications in the Apple App Store for iPhone react most heavily to any price change as compared to other sorts of changes. Download volumes in this store grew by 1,665% five days after the price drop of an app. On the other hand, the outcome of a price raise is that it negatively affects download volumes. However, the extension of the effect is lower for price raises compared to price drops. Downloads decreased by 46% in the Apple's App Store for iPhone when the price increased.

The study also showed that the most downloaded app in the Apple App Store for iPhone in the United States was Bladeslinger, which cost between US$0.99 and US$2.99. Therefore, what can be learned from the microeconomics study is that the ideal price range for an ambient diagnosis product would be equivalent to a cup of Starbucks coffee; this is called the "Starbucks rule."

Chapters 4, 5, 9, 11, 12, 14, and 15 introduce personal diagnostic devices that meet the Starbucks rule.

3D Printing

In the science fiction franchise Star Trek, a replicator is a machine capable of creating objects. Replicators were originally used to synthesize meals on demand, but in later series, they took on many other uses. Today, the replicator is a reality in the form of 3D printing, enabling people to make objects at home. Currently, the mainstream 3D printed materials are plastic, which makes it possible for a user to make a snap-on phone adaptor for a microscope or a spectrometer to personalize the sensor to match the phone model or diagnostic features.

Figure 1.14 shows a 3D printed lithium battery that is smaller than a grain of sand (200 µm). This is a technical breakthrough. For decades, Moore's law has

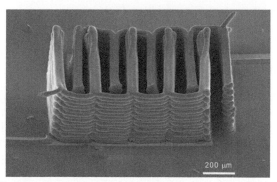

FIGURE 1.14   The 3D printed battery that is smaller than a grain of sand (200 µm). (Courtesy of Professor Jennifer A. Lewis, Harvard University.)

---

[23] Tiuri van Agten. *The impact of price changes*. Distimo, Utrecht, the Netherlands, 2013.

correctly predicted the exponential growth of the transistors and MEMS on a chip. Unfortunately, batteries did not follow Moore's law.[24] They grew linearly. This miniature battery can be printed for personal diagnostic devices (e.g., pill cameras, implantable sensors, and printable smart skins).

Chapters 11 and 12 explore some do-it-yourself (DIY) approaches for building personalized microscopes and spectrometers for a smartphone.

1.8   BASIC ALGORITHMS

To implement ambient diagnostic systems, it is inevitable to use algorithms to filter, visualize, cluster, and classify data and recognize patterns. The algorithms in this book cover a broad spectrum of multimedia analysis (Chapters 4–14), physical modeling (Chapters 9–14), and rudimentary data mining (Chapters 2–3). As we discussed in the section on the science of simplicity, rudimentary algorithms are essential to many applications, and they are often more robust than complicated ones. Chapters 2 and 3 provide an overview of the basic sensory data representation, feature extraction, and pattern clustering and classification method with pseudocode.

1.9   BASIC TOOLS

The old Chinese proverb says: "Tell me, and I will forget. Show me, and I will remember. Involve me, and I will understand." It is recommended that one use the basic tools discussed next for assignments and projects.

MATLAB is the programming language developed by the MathWorks. It comes with Computer Vision Toolbox and Image Processing Toolbox, which contain necessary libraries for multimedia data processing, such as sound, image, and video. Its code is usually compact and portable to common platforms such as Mac and PC. MATLAB is normally available in colleges and research institutions.[25]

Android phone Soft Development Kit (SDK) is recommended for application development on Android phones. The SDK is open source and has a large developer community.

Other specific tools such as Kinect API or SDK and game engines are introduced in individual chapters, such as Chapters 6 and 14.

1.10   SUMMARY

This chapter discussed the definition of ambient diagnostics and its processes: perception, transformation, and recognition. Then, we reviewed diagnostic models for knowledge representation and reasoning, including diagnostic trees, diagnostic rules, the Bayesian reasoning model, and expert systems such as DENDRAL and MYCIN. The significance of DENDRAL involves not only that it was the first expert

---

[24] F. Schlacter. No Moore's law for batteries. *PNAS* 110(14): 5273, 2013. http://www.pnas.org/content/110/14/5273.full

[25] OpenCV is an open source for computer vision hosted by Intel. It is written in C/C++.

system but also its epic effort to convert the 2D chemical structural knowledge into symbolic representations in LIPS language in 1965, when the graphical user interface was not available.

This book covers multimedia intelligence extensively, including innovative concepts for ambient diagnoses such as point and search, the pill camera, active sensing with Kinect, digital human labs, negative and relative feature spaces, and semantic gaps. The book also introduces crowdsourcing methods for collective intelligence from online video games and social media.

Here, we also discuss design strategies for ambient diagnoses, including soft sensors for reconfigurable abundant sensory systems, simplicity, and personalization.

PROBLEMS

1. In the case study of the iStethoscope, what if the nurse had not used the iPhone app iStethoscope? Discuss the risk scenarios. Summarize suggested improvements for the phone apps in the report.
2. The pregnant kit in Figure 1.13 shows two bars if the woman is pregnant and one bar if she is not. Why does the kit show one bar for not pregnant instead of nothing?
3. In Figure 1.3, which transforms are synesthesia?
4. The flu is a common disease in everyone's life. List flu-related diagnostic rules. Draw a diagnostic tree based on those rules.
5. Add a CF to the diagnostic rules in Problem 4. Analyze the possible diagnostic cases with the CF values.
6. Study the open source tool CLIPS (http://clipsrules.sourceforge.net/) for building rule-based expert systems. Enter the diagnostic rules in Problem 4, and analyze the test results.
7. Implement the diagnostic rules from Problem 4 in PROLOG language (http://gprolog. univ-paris1.fr/) and analyze the test results.
8. Temperature and ventilation are two factors in an air-conditioned environment. Unfortunately, ventilation depends on temperature settings. For example, in the summer, if the room temperature is lower than the targeted value or outdoor temperature, the fan would stop working in auto mode, leaving the room without ventilation until the room temperature is hotter than the setting. Redesign the system so that it takes care of ventilation for health. Design the rules for the control system. Collect data from experiments or simulations. Use the covering algorithm to refine the rules. Test the design in experiments or simulations. Summarize the findings in a report.
9. Download the SoundHound app for Android[26] and search for the song link by pointing the phone to the television or the computer. Assess the retrieval rate and performance. Discuss the potential in ambient diagnoses in your report.
10. Download twenty celebrity portraits and describe their facial features with words but without names. Randomize the order of the descriptions and images. Let a second person read the descriptions and pair the descriptions to the images. Let a third person guess the names from the descriptions but without looking at the images. Discuss the semantic gap in the process and summarize findings in the report.

---

[26] http://www.soundhound.com/

2 Data Transformation

> The purpose of computing is not just numbers but insight.
>
> —Richard Hamming

2.1 INTRODUCTION

The key mission of ambient diagnostics is to record, convert, compress, and discover patterns from massive continuous data streams. This chapter focuses on data transformation, which includes general feature descriptions and visualization of patterns. We discuss such key questions as

- How can we represent sequential features in a vector?
- How can we transform spatiotemporal features to a matrix?
- How can we transform features to a shape?
- How can we convert a shape into numbers?
- How can we represent features in a frequency domain?
- How can we decompose an image into tiny self-similar features?
- How can we reduce the dimensions of a feature space?
- How can we automatically measure image quality?

2.2 EARLY DISCOVERIES OF HEARTBEAT PATTERNS

Learning and recognizing patterns are essential to modern diagnostics. In the 1800s, the signals of the transatlantic telegraphy were very weak. The receiving end was required to pay close attention so characters in Morse code were not missed. Clearly, a system that could record the signal would be better. In 1867, Sir William Thompson, professor of natural philosophy at Glasgow University, invented a siphon recorder with the first inkjet printer to improve transatlantic telegraphy. The siphon recorder not only could detect electrical currents but also could record them onto paper. The recorder was a fine coil suspended in a strong magnetic field. Attached to the coil but isolated from it by an insulator was a siphon of ink. The siphon was charged with high voltage so that the ink was sprayed onto the paper that moved over a grounded metal surface; this is basically the same principle of the inkjet printer today. As a result, it required only one ordinary clerk at the receiving end instead of a reader and a writer. Any ambiguities could be checked later by examining the tape in detail (Figure 2.1).

In 1887, Alexander Muirhead, a British electrical engineer and pioneer of the fax machine, attached a siphon recorder to a patient's wrist to obtain a record of

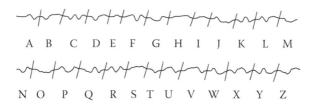

FIGURE 2.1   Thompson siphon recorder's alphabetic patterns of Morse code.

the patient's heartbeat, creating the first human electrocardiogram (ECG).[27] The fully systematic study of the ECG started when Augustus Waller, a British physiologist, first published a paper about an ECG of a human heart in 1891. Waller used a Lippmann capillary electrometer fixed to a projector. The trace from the heartbeat was projected onto a photographic plate that was attached to a toy train, allowing a heartbeat to be recorded in real time (Figure 2.2).

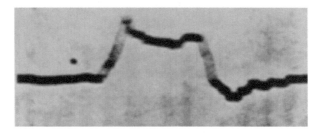

FIGURE 2.2   First published human electrocardiogram (ECG) pattern by Augustus Waller in 1891. He used a Lippmann capillary electrometer projected onto a photographic plate on a toy train.

Willem Einthoven, a Dutch physiologist, invented a new string galvanometer for producing one thousand times more sensitive ECGs than capillary electrometers and previous string galvanometers. However, the original machine required water cooling for the powerful electromagnets needed five operators and weighed 600 pounds. Rather than using today's self-adhesive electrodes, subjects would immerse each of their limbs into containers of salt solutions, from which the ECG was recorded (Figure 2.3).[28]

Einthoven invented not only a powerful sensor but also a pattern annotation system. He assigned the letters P, Q, R, S, and T to the various deflections and described the electrocardiographic features of a number of cardiovascular disorders (Figure 2.4). In 1924, he was awarded the Nobel Prize in Medicine for his discovery.

Einthoven also pioneered the telecardiogram. In 1905, he transmitted and recorded ECGs from the hospital to his laboratory, 1.5 km away, via telephone

---

[27] A. D. Waller. A demonstration on man of electromotive changes accompanying the heart's beat. *Journal of Physiology (London)* 8:229–234, 1887. http://www.ecglibrary.com/ecghist.html

[28] George Edward Burch and Nicholas P. Depasquales. *The history of electrocardiography.* Norman, Norman, OK, 1990.

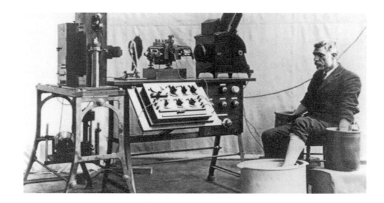

FIGURE 2.3 Early electrocardiograms (ECGs) required five operators and weighed 600 pounds. Subjects would immerse each of their limbs into tanks of salt solutions. (Permission to use this image courtesy of Einthoven Foundation, the Netherlands.)

cables. Today, the bulky devices are replaced with portable ones, and the analogical signals are replaced with digital for telecommunication. Despite the technical advances, the principles behind the ECG systems remain the same. For example, we still need to transform the signal to patterns for analysis, compression, communication, and visualization. The following sections are an overview of the basic methods for turning data into patterns that humans and computers can understand.

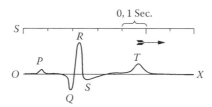

FIGURE 2.4 Einthoven's PQRST system for articulating patterns in an electrocardiogram (ECG).

2.3   TRANSFORMS, FEATURES, AND ATTRIBUTES

Raw sensory data can be converted from one representational form to another. The conversion process is called *transformation*, or *transform* for short. For example, when we make a call from a cell phone, the phone actually transforms the sound wave to a series of coefficients of frequency descriptions over the wireless channel. The sound data is reconstructed through the inverse transform on the receiving phone. The term *transformation* in this book covers a fairly broad area, including not only mathematical transforms but also physical transforms such as from sound to color. The transforms in this chapter focus on two-dimensional (2D) imagery transforms rather than traditional one-dimensional (1D) signal processing.

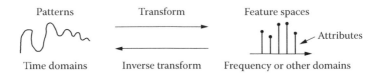

FIGURE 2.5   Patterns of transformation, features, and attributes.

Features are the elements for describing a pattern. For example, the intensity of pixels in an image is a feature, and the speed of walking gestures is a feature. A raw dataset can be represented in many forms of features based on the need of an analysis. Here, we elaborate the feature representations in a variety of forms, including time series, multichannel time series, spatiotemporal, shape, image, frequency domain, and multiresolution.

Attributes are measurements of a feature. Attributes allow us to specify different variants of a feature. For example, if we have a *feature vector* to describe a face, then the *attributes* would be the parameters of the biometric measurements in the vector, such as the distance between eyes, nose length, lip width, and so on. Normally, features are qualitative descriptions, but attributes are more quantitative descriptions (Figure 2.5).

2.4 SEQUENTIAL FEATURES

Most sensory data contain temporal patterns such as those for sound, temperature, blood pressure, glucose, ECG, and electroencephalography (EEG) (Figure 2.6).

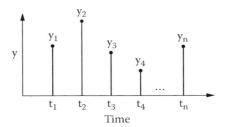

FIGURE 2.6   A temporal profile.

They can be represented as a one-dimensional vector if the sampling intervals are uniform:

$$F = \left[y_1, y_2, \ldots, y_n \right]^T$$

where y_i is the amplitude of the profile at the time i.

In many cases, multiple sensors record data simultaneously, creating multichannel temporal profiles (e.g., a 12-lead ECG cardiograph or 32-lead EEG brainwaves).

The temporal features can be represented in multidimensional vectors, which can be processed in DSP (digital signal processing) chips or computers.

Sequential patterns can primarily be measured by durations, amplitudes, positions, and areas. The following section explores more analytical models for sequential pattern analysis, such as Fourier transform and wavelets.

2.5   SPATIOTEMPORAL FEATURES

Spatiotemporal features, such as eye gaze motion on the screen, can be articulated as a vector with time t_i and location attributes (x_i, y_i) in 2D cases (Figure 2.7).

$$F = \begin{bmatrix} x_1 & y_1 & t_1 \\ x_2 & y_2 & t_2 \\ \vdots & \vdots & \vdots \\ x_n & y_n & t_n \end{bmatrix}$$

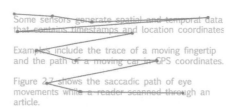

Some sensors generate spatial and temporal data that contains timestamps and location coordinates

Examples include the trace of a moving fingertip and the path of a moving car in GPS coordinates.

Figure 2.7 shows the saccadic path of eye movements while a reader scanned through an article.

FIGURE 2.7   The saccadic path of eye movements while a reader scanned through an article.

Human gestures involve three-dimensional (3D) spatiotemporal dynamics. Motion capture data can be represented by a vector of 3D points, skeletons, or polygons over time.[29] Figure 2.8 is a sequence of skeleton data captured by the Kinect sensor (read Chapter 6 for more details).

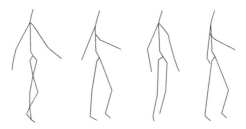

FIGURE 2.8   Motion capture data contains a vector of spatiotemporal features.

---

[29] http://joe-clarke.blogspot.com/

The raw motion capture data consists of a set of joints (points), and each has its x, y, and z coordinates and time stamp.

$$F = \begin{bmatrix} x_{11} & y_{11} & z_{11} & \cdots & x_{1n} & y_{1n} & z_{1n} & t_1 \\ x_{21} & y_{21} & z_{21} & \cdots & x_{2n} & y_{2n} & z_{2n} & t_2 \\ \vdots & \vdots & \vdots & \vdots & & & & \\ x_{n1} & y_{n1} & z_{n1} & \cdots & x_{nn} & y_{nn} & z_{nn} & t_n \end{bmatrix}$$

Clearly, the size of the motion capture dataset is big. New sensors such as Kinect create their own APIs (application programming interfaces) to handle the captured data. There are also some apps to convert the Kinect data to BVH (biovision hierarchical data), a more advanced format for motion capture data.[30,31] The BVH format is mainly used as a standard representation of movements in the animation of a humanoid structure. It is one of the most popular motion data formats and has been widely adopted by computer graphics software such as 3DS MAX, MAYA, Poser, Second Life, and Lightwave 3D.

2.6   SHAPE FEATURES

A *polygon* is a simplification of a shape. If we can sample points along the edge, we can approximate it with a polygon by connecting points in an order. To qualify as a polygon, a shape's starting point must connect with its ending point. However, in many cases, an open-ended contour line is enough to describe the principal features (e.g., the contour of fingers, the profile of a face, and the roof of a building). A polygon can be articulated with a set of orderly connected points in a 2D vector if the polygon is in 2D space. Polygon features include number of corners, point coordinates, and the start point and end point (which must be the same) (Figure 2.9).

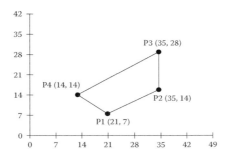

FIGURE 2.9   Polygon features.

---

[30] http://en.wikipedia.org/wiki/List_of_motion_and_gesture_file_formats#BVA_and_BVH_file_formats.
[31] http://www.cgchannel.com/2011/01/new-app-exports-kinect-motion-data-as-bvh-files/

Concavity is a feature in shape representation. A convex shape can be visualized as the shape formed by a rubber band stretched around all the data points (Figure 2.10). The convex shape has lines that curve outward. As soon as any of the lines form an inward curve, or form a dent, the shape is considered to be concave. Concavity is an important feature in many applications, such as the collision detection algorithms in game engines discussed in detail in Chapter 14.

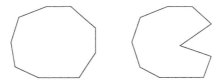

FIGURE 2.10   Convex and concave shapes.

How can we test whether a shape is convex or concave? We can use the simple line test method (Figure 2.11). On any convex shape, no matter where you draw a line that passes through the shape, it will always pass through only two of the lines or polygons making up the shape. On a concave shape, it can pass through more than two of the lines.[32]

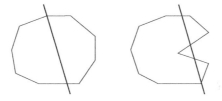

FIGURE 2.11   The line test method.

The line test is intuitive for humans but not efficient for computers. The angle test method is better here (Figure 2.12). A concave shape has lines or segments that form an angle between them that is less than 180 degrees. If any of the angles is smaller than 180 degrees, the shape is concave.

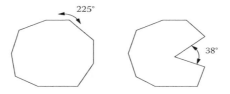

FIGURE 2.12   The angle test method.

---

[32] http://www.rustycode.com/tutorials/convex.html

The *polar coordinate system* uses radial distances and angles to represent a shape, given a centroid (Figure 2.13). The coordinates of a polygon in the Cartesian coordinate system can be converted to the coordinates in a polar coordinate system. Given the fixed angular interval and the rotating cycle from 0 to 360 degrees, the polygon vector can be simplified from a 2D vector to a 1D vector.

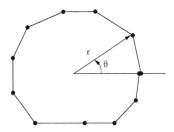

FIGURE 2.13   Polar coordinates.

Chain code converts a shape to a sequence of numbers, which represent lines on a regular grid. Each line segment in a chain code is represented by its length and a unique code. This transforms 2D features to 1D features. Chain code can be defined as either four direction or eight direction. Figure 2.14 shows an illustration of an eight-direction chain code and an example of how the curve shape is coded in numbers. However, chain code has its weaknesses. It reduces the angular resolution to limited numbers, and it is neither rotation-invariant nor scale-invariant.

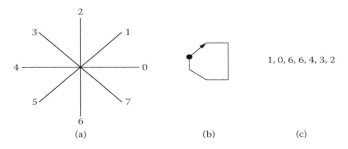

FIGURE 2.14   Chain code lines: (a) eight-directional chain codes; (b) original lines; and (c) chain codes for lines.

Glyph (also known as star plot or radar plot) is a visualization method. It converts a set of multiple-dimensional feature data into a shape (Figure 2.15). Given m-dimensional features, we can evenly divide the angle to $360/m$ from its origin, where the skeletal radials are proportional to the values that are normalized between 0 and 1. The ends of skeletal radials can be sealed or left open.

Chernoff face is also a visualization technique to illustrate patterns in multidimensional data. Chernoff faces were especially effective because they related the data to

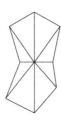
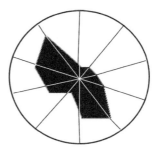

FIGURE 2.15   Glyph turns multidimensional features into shapes.

facial features, something that we are used to differentiating between. Different data dimensions can be mapped to different facial features (e.g., face width, level of the ears, radius of the ears, length or curvature of the mouth, length of the nose, etc.). Chernoff faces are described by facial characteristic parameters: head eccentricity, eye eccentricity, pupil size, eyebrow slant, nose size, mouth shape, eye spacing, eye size, mouth length, and degree of mouth opening. Each parameter is represented by a number between 0 and 1.

We can use facial features to represent trends in the values of the data instead of the values themselves. Knowledge of the trends in the data could help to determine which sections of the data were of particular interest or the overall trend of the health condition. Let us try to use Chernoff faces to monitor the glucose measurements for a diabetic patient. We can map the five variables to five facial parameters (Table 2.1).[33]

TABLE 2.1 Chernoff Parameters for Glucose Data

Chernoff Features	Measurement
Size of face	Pre_Break.
Vertical position of eyes	Pre_Bed
Height of eyes	Overall
Length of nose	OVOF
Mouth arc length	OTBG

Figure 2.16 shows the seven-day log data of the patient. Chernoff faces are able to show a high condensation of data with an interesting way of presentation. Chernoff faces can potentially improve data digestion.

However, current Chernoff faces are still images. Perhaps, with the advance of computer technology, animated Chernoff faces may be worthy of experimentation in the future.[34] Besides, the subjective assignment of facial expressions to variables

[33] G. Phillipou. Geographical display of capillary blood glucose data using Chernoff faces. *Diabetic Medicine* 9(3):293–294, 1992

[34] D. W. Turner and F. E. Tidmore. FACES-A FORTRAN program for generating Chernoff-type faces on a line printer. *American Statisticians* 34:187, 1980

affects the shape of the face.[35] It takes time and training for users to understand the meaning the faces conveyed. The assignment of features may cause errors. It means that classifying two faces as "fairly similar" is greatly influenced by the assignment of variables to specific features.[36]

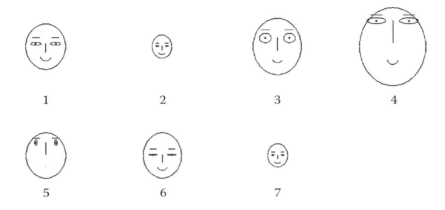

1   2   3   4

5   6   7

FIGURE 2.16   Examples of Chernoff faces for the seven-day log data of the diabetic patient.

2.7 IMAGERY FEATURES

Imagery features become increasingly important because of growing images, videos from sensors and social media, as well as growing needs for visualizing data in the form of images and videos. The MathWorks' handbook for the Image Processing Toolbox is a concise, aspiring tutorial about basic signal processing for images. The book also has many short examples for practice.[37]

Intensity Features

Imagery features can be described in a matrix. For an intensity image or a gray-scale image, the feature matrix is a 2D matrix, where the intensity value of each pixel is indexed by coordinates in terms of rows and columns (Figure 2.17). For a multi-channel image, such as a color image, each pixel value is represented by its color attributes (R, G, B for red, green, blue, respectively) and indexed by its coordinates in a row and column.

[35] D. W. Scott. *Multivariate density estimation: theory, practice, and visualization.* Wiley, New York, 1992.
[36] H. Chernoff and M. H. Rizvi. Effect on classification error or random permutations of features in representing multivariate data by faces. *Journal of American Statistical Association* 70, 548–554, 1975.
[37] MathWorks. *Image Processing Toolbox for Using with MATLAB.* User Guide Version 2. http://amath.colorado.edu/computing/Matlab/OldTechDocs/images_tb.pdf

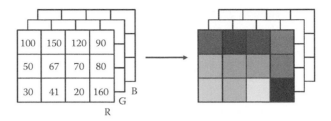

FIGURE 2.17   Pixel values in an intensity map.

Heat Map

We can convert a matrix data into a synthetic image called a heat map to visualize features in the dataset. It is a reverse process of intensity map feature extraction. To generate a heat map, we need to map data values to visible intensity display values using a lookup table that maps data to 255 grayscale levels. Figure 2.18 shows Facebook peak traffic times, indicated by the darker blocks near the center of the map, and the lighter blocks represent less traffic. The data was gathered over a 24-hour period, which is calculated based on the number of clicks on links they posted.

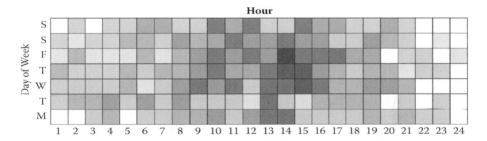

FIGURE 2.18   Heat map of Facebook traffic in 24 hours.

We can display a heat map in color using a color map lookup table. In engineering, it is common to use pseudocolor maps that intuitively map the data values to temperatures, such as minimum values to blue (cold) and maximum to white (hot).

2.8   FREQUENCY DOMAIN FEATURES

Any spatial, time domain, or sequential data can be written as a sum of periodic functions, called Fourier functions. For example, when you talk on your cell phone, the processor inside converts the time domain sound waveforms to features in a frequency domain and sends those compressed features through a microwave. At the receiving end, the processor transforms the frequency domain features back to the time domain sound waveforms. This time-frequency domain data transform enables signal filtering, compression, and reconstruction.

According to Fourier, everything in the world is composed of waves. Heat is a wave; light is a wave; an electromagnetic field is a wave. In the 1D case, we can decompose any signal waveform into many simple periodic waves. The more we add periodic waves, the more subtle details we have. This process works in reverse as well: We can create a wave with a complicated shape by adding periodic waves of different frequency together. Figure 2.19 shows an example of the two-way transformation between a square wave, its synthesized waveform, and the periodic waves A, B, C, D, E, and F.

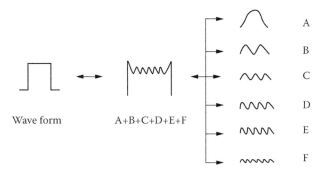

FIGURE 2.19 Decomposition of a waveform from a square form to an infinite number of periodic waves.

We call the process that decomposes a waveform into periodic waves a Fourier transform. Normally, it consists of sinusoid and cosine waves within time from $-\infty$ to $+\infty$. We call the reversal process an Inverse Fourier Transform. For each different frequency component, we need to know the amplitude and the phase to construct a unique wave. Figure 2.20 illustrates how amplitude and phase affect a waveform. Assume we change the amplitude and phase on the period wave C in Figure 2.19. We can see the changes of the synthetic waveforms. In general, amplitude change alters the shape proportionally. Phase change, on the other hand, alters the shape more drastically.

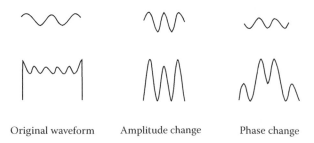

FIGURE 2.20 Effects of amplitude change and phase change on the waveform.

The discrete Fourier transform (DFT) converts a finite amount of sequential data to a matrix of coefficients of a finite combination of complex sinusoids. It can be implemented in computers by numerical algorithms or even dedicated hardware such as Digital Signal Processing (DSP) chips in cell phones. These implementations usually employ efficient fast Fourier transform (FFT) algorithms, so the terms FFT and DFT are often used interchangeably.[38]

In DSP courses, DFT is often introduced in 1D signal processing such as audio signals. Here, 2D data such as an intensity image is introduced. Assume we have a matrix $A(M, N)$. We can have the DCT coefficient matrix $F(m, n)$ of the FFT.[39]

$$F(m,n) = \sum_{y=0}^{N-1}\left(\sum_{x=0}^{M-1} A(x,y) \cdot e^{-j\frac{2\pi mx}{M}} \right) \cdot e^{-j\frac{2\pi ny}{N}} \qquad (2.1)$$

where $0 \leq m \leq M - 1$ and $0 \leq n \leq N - 1$.

The inverse DFT is also available.[40]

$$A(x,y) = \frac{1}{M \cdot N} \sum_{m=0}^{M-1}\left(\sum_{n=0}^{N-1} F(m,n) \cdot e^{-j\frac{2\pi mx}{M}} \right) \cdot e^{-j\frac{2\pi ny}{N}} \qquad (2.2)$$

where $0 \leq m \leq M - 1$ and $0 \leq n \leq N - 1$.

The DFT coefficients produced by the 2D DFT can be displayed in a 2D image. See Figure 2.21.

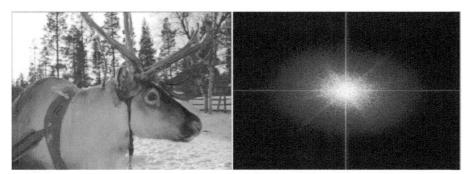

FIGURE 2.21   Original image (left) and the DFT coefficient data image after using the phase shift function to have the low-frequency content in the center of the image and the high-frequency content on the outside of the image (right).

---

[38] For more detailed equations for DFT and FFT in two dimensions, please read MathWorks' tutorial and examples at http://www.mathworks.com/help/images/fourier-transform.html
[39] In MATLAB, the 2D FFT is $y = fft2(A)$, where A is the 2D image matrix.
[40] In MATLAB, the 2D IFFT is $y = ifft2(F)$, where F is the 2D Fourier coefficient matrix. IFFF = Inverse Fast Fourier Transform.

A Fourier transform can be used to efficiently implement filters in a frequency domain. Such operations are usually called spatial frequency filtering.

Assume we have an input image, and F is its Fourier transform. A filter H can be represented by a matrix H. The Fourier transform of the filter output after an image has been convoluted with the filter can be computed in the frequency domain.[41,42]

$$G(m,n) = F(m,n) \cdot H(n,n) \tag{2.3}$$

Note that the equation represents element-by-element multiplication, not matrix multiplication. The filtered image can be obtained by applying the inverse Fourier transform to G. Figure 2.22 shows the result of a low-pass filter applied to the image.

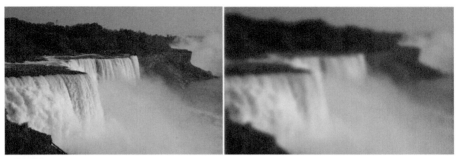

FIGURE 2.22 Low-pass filtering result.

The DFT involves imaginary components and real components. In many cases, we may just use the real components. For this, we have discrete cosine transfer (DCT), which is popular in image and video processing.[43] Similar to 2D FFT, assume we have an M by N matrix $A(x, y)$; the DCT algorithm can be represented as

$$F(m,n) = \frac{2}{\sqrt{MN}} C(m) \cdot C(n) \sum_{y=0}^{N-1} \sum_{x=0}^{M-1} A(x,y) \cdot \cos\frac{(2x+1)m\pi}{2M} \cdot \cos\frac{(2y+1)n\pi}{2N} \tag{2.4}$$

where $C(m)$, $C(n) = 1/\sqrt{2}$ for m, $n = 0$; and $C(m)$, $C(n) = 1$ otherwise. M and N are the row and column of the matrix $A(M, N)$ respectively.

The inverse DCT is

$$A(x,y) = \frac{2}{\sqrt{MN}} \sum_{m=0}^{M-1} \sum_{n=0}^{N-1} C(m) \cdot C(n) \cdot F(m,n) \cdot \cos\frac{(2x+1)m\pi}{2M} \cdot \cos\frac{(2y+1)n\pi}{2N} \tag{2.5}$$

---

[41] For more information about the image filter design, please read the online tutorial at http://www.eletel.p.lodz.pl/mstrzel/imageproc/filter.PDF

[42] M. Sonka, V. Hlavac, and R. Boyle. *Image processing analysis, and machine vision.* PWS, Boston, 1999, pp. 604–606

[43] For more detailed equations and examples, please read Mathworks' tutorial at http://www.mathworks.com/help/images/discrete-cosine-transform.html

where $F(m, n)$ is the DCT of the signal $A(x, y)$ and $C(m)$, $C(n) = 1/\sqrt{2}$ for m, $n = 0$, and $C(m)$, $C(n) = 1$, otherwise.

What do the DCT coefficients tell us? Let us take a look at the coefficient matrix. The top left is the DC component, which is a content value. The value in the second column of the first row represents the first-order horizontal frequency, the variation of pixel values horizontally. The value at the far right corner represents the highest horizontal variation frequency component.

Now, let us look at the values of the DCT coefficients. Few larger values are located at the left top corner (Figure 2.23), and many small values are spread out around the rest of the matrix. Here, we have an idea: How about we set the small values to zero and only keep the left top corner coefficients? Now, we have an image-compression algorithm. Figure 2.24 shows the original image and the compressed image when we set all the DCT coefficients to zero if their absolute values are less than ten.

FIGURE 2.23   There are many small values in the DCT coefficient matrix, visualized as light intensity

Here is the pseudocode for DCT image compression. The sample MATLAB code is in Appendix A:

1. Read an image
2. Compute DCT of the image
3. Set DCT coefficients to zero if less than the threshold
4. Compute inverse DCT

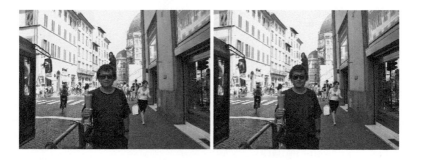

FIGURE 2.24   Original image (left) and DCT compressed image (right).

A DCT image is the fundamental algorithm for well-known image and video compression algorithms such as JPEG, MPEG-1, MPEG-2, MPEG-4, and H.264. If a dictator ordered us to stop using the DCT algorithm, we would lose over 70% of the Internet data traffic.

2.9 MULTIRESOLUTION FEATURES

The tangram is a dissection puzzle game consisting of seven flat shapes that are put together to form millions of shapes (Figure 2.25).[44] The puzzle originated in the Song dynasty (960–1279 AC) of China.

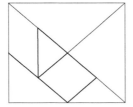 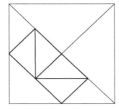

FIGURE 2.25 Ancient tangram in seven pieces of three sizes (left) and the modified tangram in nine pieces and three sizes.

Let us further dissect the diamond and square shapes into four triangular shapes. Now, we have "invented" a nine-piece tangram. The advantage of the nine-piece tangram is that all pieces are triangular in shape but are different sizes and orientations. Similar to its ancestor, the nine-piece tangram can produce millions of different shapes (Figure 2.26). If we dissect the triangular shape to even smaller pieces, we can then compose figures or objects with even finer details. If the number of the small pieces is infinite, we can obtain the exact contour of any shape.

FIGURE 2.26 A tangram can generate millions of shapes from a simple shape in multiple scales and orientations.

Similarly, all the signals can be represented by small waves, called "wavelets," consisting of mother wavelets and their children. The advantages include multi-resolution representation that is good for images and videos, unlimited mother wavelet shapes, and self-similarity.

---

[44] http://commons.wikimedia.org/wiki/File:Tangram-4.JPG

In a 1-D case, the mother wavelet can be described by the wavelet function:

$$\varphi(t) = \frac{1}{\sqrt{a}} \Psi\left(\frac{t-b}{a}\right) \tag{2.6}$$

where a is the scaling parameter, and b is the shifting parameter.

Consider the simplest form Haar wavelet as the mother wavelet, shown in Figure 2.27. We can derive her daughter wavelets by scaling and shifting as shown in Figure 2.28.

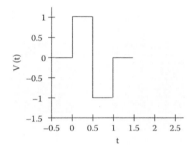

FIGURE 2.27   One-dimensional mother wavelet in the simplest form: Haar wavelet.

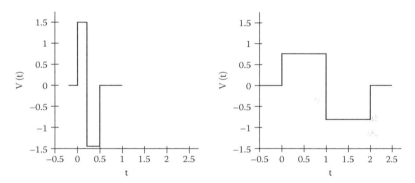

FIGURE 2.28   Daughter wavelets derived from the mother wavelet by scaling and shifting.

The wavelet analysis is to multiply a signal with a wavelet function and then compute the transform for each segment generated. The wavelet transform uses wavelets of finite energy.

The Haar transform can be described as follows:

$$T = H \cdot F \cdot H^T \tag{2.7}$$

where F is the image matrix, H is the transformation matrix, and T is the resulting transform. If image F is not in a square size, we can add zeros to make it in $n \times n$ dimensions. Note that H is the orthogonal matrix where

$$H^{-1} = H^{T} \tag{2.8}$$

For $n = 2$, the Haar transform matrix is

$$H_2 = \frac{1}{\sqrt{2}}\begin{bmatrix} 1 & 1 \\ 1 & -1 \end{bmatrix} \tag{2.9}$$

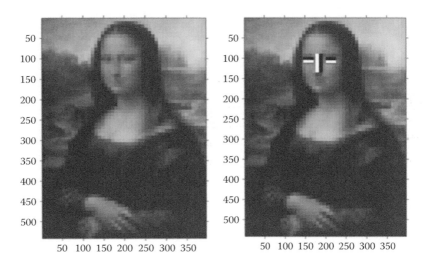

FIGURE 2.29 Haar-like features for face detection.

One important application of DWT in ambient diagnosis is visual feature representation (e.g., face detection). A face image can be represented in the Haar-like features (Figure 2.29). Chapter 7 discusses how to use the Haar-like features for face tracking and object detection.

A discrete wavelet transform (DWT) is any wavelet transform for which the wavelets are discretely sampled.[45] As with other wavelet transforms, a key advantage it has over Fourier transforms is temporal resolution: It captures both frequency and location information (location in time). A general description of a DWT[46] of a matrix A is

$$C = DWT\{A\} \tag{2.10}$$

---

[45] For more details, please read http://www.mathworks.com/help/wavelet/ref/dwt2.html
[46] Use DWT2 for 2D DWT in MATLAB.

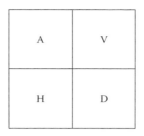

FIGURE 2.30   The typical layout of DWT coefficients in the output matrix.

A typical 2D DWT output matrix C consists of four vectors A, H, V, and D, where A is approximation coefficients, H is horizontal detail coefficients, V is vertical detail coefficients, and D is diagonal detail coefficients (Figure 2.30). The inverse of DWT is

$$B = IDWT\{C\} \tag{2.11}$$

Similar to DCT, DWT can also be used for image compression. The compression can be implemented by setting a large number of nonessential DWT coefficients to zero. The pseudocode for image compression with DWT follows. The MATLAB sample code is in Appendix A.

1.   Input energy retention rate e
2.   Read image
3.   Compute Haar transform
4.   Get the length of the DWT coefficient vector k
5.   Retain $e*k$ coefficients and set the rest to zero
6.   Inverse DWT

The JPEG-2000 compression standard is based on DWT. Compared to DCT, DWT has advantages: it has higher compression ratios, and it avoids block artifacts of DCT. DWT works extremely well in sharp-contrast areas, especially in binary images such as fingerprints. However, DWT's computational cost is higher than DCT's. Compression time is longer. At low compression rates, DWT does not produce better quality than DCT (Figure 2.31).

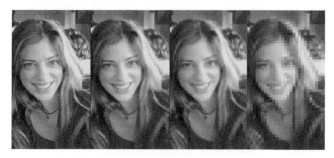

FIGURE 2.31   The wavelet-based compression, from left to right: raw, energy retention 10%, 5%, and 2%.

Peak Signal-to-Noise Ratio

You may have noticed that DCT and DWT are lossy data compression algorithms. After the data transformation, the image quality may be reduced. For visual quality measurement, human subjects are always used but very expensive. Engineers finally came up with a method to evaluate the image quality that is similar to humans but can be done by a machine. This measurement is called the peak signal-to-noise ratio (PSNR):

$$PSNR = 10 \cdot \log_{10} \left(\frac{MAX^2}{MSE} \right) \qquad (2.12)$$

where MAX is the maximum possible pixel value of the image; MSE is the mean squared error.

Generally, when the PSNR is 40 dB or greater, then the original and the reconstructed images are virtually indistinguishable by human observers.

Principal Component Analysis

Johann Sebastian Bach had twenty children with his two wives, Maria Barbara Bach and Anna Magdalena Bach. It could be challenging for someone outside the family to differentiate each child from the others. Assume the facial biometrics contain fifty features, such as eye distance and nose length. Then, we have to deal with a fifty-dimensional feature space. Fortunately, children's faces often resemble their parents' facial features. We can use the father and two mothers' faces as 3D coordinates to represent all the faces in the family. For example, the eldest son is 70% similar to his father, 30% similar to his mother, and 0% similar to his stepmother. In this way, we can reduce the feature space from fifty to three. Here we introduce principle component analysis (PCA) to transform a multidimensional feature space into a more compact representation.

PCA was invented in 1901 by English mathematician Karl Person. It is a linear data transformation that has been widely used to reduce the dimension of the data.

PCA transforms an $n \times n$ matrix M to eigenvectors V and eigenvalues $n \times n$. An eigenvector of a matrix is a vector such that, if multiplied with the matrix, the resulting vector is a scaled version of the original one. The scaling factor is a corresponding eigenvalue of the eigenvector. Their relationship can be described by the equation

$$MV = \lambda V \qquad (2.13)$$

Eigenvectors possess the following properties:

- They can be determined only for square matrices.
- There are n eigenvectors and corresponding eigenvalues in an $n \times n$ matrix.
- All eigenvectors are perpendicular (i.e., at a right angle with each other).

There are many computational libraries and packages for solving PCA problems. MATLAB has the function "eig" for calculating eigenvectors and eigenvalues. Here, let us look at a rudimentary problem. Assume we have a matrix:

$$M = \begin{bmatrix} 4 & 0 & 1 \\ -2 & 1 & 0 \\ -2 & 0 & 1 \end{bmatrix}$$

Call the eig function from MATLAB prompt, just like a "calculator":

$$[V,U] = eig(M)$$

We have eigenvector V and eigenvalue U:

$$V = \begin{bmatrix} 0 & -0.5774 & -0.3333 \\ 1.0000 & -0.5774 & 0.6667 \\ 0 & -0.5774 & 0.6667 \end{bmatrix}$$

$$U = \begin{bmatrix} 1 & 0 & 0 \\ 0 & 3 & 0 \\ 0 & 0 & 2 \end{bmatrix}$$

Now, let us see whether Equation 2.13 is true:

$$V*U = \begin{bmatrix} 0 & 1.7321 & -0.6667 \\ 1.0000 & -1.7321 & 1.3333 \\ 0 & -1.7321 & 1.3333 \end{bmatrix}$$

$$M*V = \begin{bmatrix} 0 & 1.7321 & -0.6667 \\ 1.0000 & -1.7321 & 1.3333 \\ 0 & -1.7321 & 1.3333 \end{bmatrix}$$

It works! We can see that the relationship is true for M*V = U*V.

2.10   SUMMARY

Data transformation extracts important features for computers to perform pattern recognition or for humans to visualize patterns. All sensory data are sequential time series. They can be represented in vectors with features or attributes. Transformation converts data from one feature space to another. The motion capture data can be represented in a spatiotemporal matrix and projected to shapes or images. On the other hand, shapes can be converted to a string of letters via chain code or polar coordinates. DCT and DWT filters compress imagery data and reconstruct images. DWT also can be used for fast object detection. PCA can reduce the dimensions of a feature space so that the first principal component carries the most significant feature. Finally, PSNR enables a computer to measure the image quality in a similar perceptual response as humans. Data transformation is the first step to represent, extract, and compress patterns for ambient diagnoses. In many cases, a diagnostic decision can be reached if the patterns are visibly significant, such as the pregnancy test kit and pH test paper. The next chapter further discusses computational pattern recognition models.

PROBLEMS

1. Plot the following 5-day log data for a diabetes patient using Chernoff faces:

Day	Pre_Break.	Pre_Bed	Overall	OVOF	OTBG
1	110	125	117	135.0277	117.5
2	100	120	110	135.0277	110
3	130	110	120	135.0277	120
4	140	135	137	135.0277	137.5
5	125	130	127	135.0277	127.5

2. The DFT is often used for filtering signals. For image processing, low-pass filters make the image blurred. On the other hand, high-pass filters enhance edges. Build a high-pass filter to be an edge detector.
3. Leonardo da Vinci used to hide information in his paintings and drawings. He sometimes used mirrors to write text, a naïve form of encryption. Now, try to hide information within DCT coefficients where majority values are very small; replace those near-zero values with your secret code.
4. Use a similar strategy as in Problem 3 to hide an image inside an image. Write a simple demo for encoding and decoding.
5. Assume you are a detective, and you want to check whether someone hid a message in an image. Design an algorithm to do so. Create a demo to show how it works and discuss the conditions and limitations.
6. Use chain code to convert the eye gaze path to letters. Discuss the compression ratio and limitations. Hint: Convert the eye gaze path in Figure 2.7 to Chain Code based on orientation and length of segments.
7. Make a Tangram from paper. Try to form a convex shape and concave shape.
8. The PSNR enables computers to measure image quality in the similar perceptual response to humans. Explain why.
9. Use both DCT and DWT to compress an image and evaluate the image quality with the PSNR. Compare the results with five images.
10. Select an image and compress it using DWT with energy retention of 10%, 5%, and 2%. Plot the curve of the PSNR and discuss the results.

3 Pattern Recognition

> The whole is different from the sum of its parts.
>
> —Wolfgang Köhler

3.1 INTRODUCTION

This chapter focuses on simple algorithms for automated pattern recognition. Intuitive models are often faster and more robust than overcomplicated ones in solving real-world problems. Here, we do not intend to cover all of the state-of-the-art methods of pattern recognition but only a few fundamental ones that benefit the applications of ambient diagnostics in the following chapters. We cover topics that include the following:

- How can we measure similarities between patterns?
- How can we cluster patterns?
- How can we classify patterns?
- How can we evaluate classification results?

3.2 SIMILARITIES AND DISTANCES

Similarity measurement is critical for pattern recognition. To match, cluster, or classify patterns, we need to know how similar they are. Dissimilarity and distances are the opposite of similarity. It is easy to convert them. For example, if a similarity value is between 0 and 1, then the distance would be (distance = 1 - similarity). This chapter only discusses essential measurements.

Euclidian Distance

Assume that we have two feature vectors $A = [a_1, a_2, \ldots, a_n]$ and $B = [b_1, b_2, \ldots, b_n]$, which are two points in n-dimensional feature space. If the number of attributes is fewer than or equal to three, we can just plot them with a spreadsheet. When the number of attributes exceeds three, we have to calculate the distance computationally by summarizing the segments of the distances between vectors at each dimension. The distance from A to B is given by

$$d(A,B) = \sqrt{(a_1 - b_1)^2 + (a_2 - b_2)^2 + \cdots + (a_n - b_n)^2} = \sqrt{\sum_{i=1}^{n} (a_i - b_i)^2} \qquad (3.1)$$

Cosine Angle Similarity

Given two feature vectors A and B, the cosine angle $cos(\theta)$ between the two is equal to their dot product divided by the product of their norms. The dot product is just the element-to-element multiply. The norm is the magnitude of a vector.

$$c(A,B) = \cos\theta = \frac{\sum\limits_{i=1}^{n} a_i \times b_i}{\sqrt{\sum\limits_{i=1}^{n} a_i^2} \times \sqrt{\sum\limits_{i=1}^{n} b_i^2}} = \frac{A^T \cdot B}{\|A\|\|B\|} \qquad (3.2)$$

Since the angle θ is in the range $[0, \pi]$, the resulting similarity will yield the value of

- +1 meaning exactly the same,
- −1 meaning exactly the opposite,
- 0 meaning independent, and
- in-between values indicating intermediate similarities or dissimilarities.

The cosine angle distance is

$$d_c(A,B) = 1 - \cos\theta \qquad (3.3)$$

For example, we have two vectors:

$$A = \begin{bmatrix} 1 \\ 2 \\ 3 \end{bmatrix} \quad B = \begin{bmatrix} 4 \\ 5 \\ 0 \end{bmatrix}$$

The vector dot product is

$$A^T B = \begin{bmatrix} 1 & 2 & 3 \end{bmatrix} \cdot \begin{bmatrix} 4 \\ 5 \\ 0 \end{bmatrix} = 1\times4 + 2\times5 + 3\times0 = 14$$

Their norms are

$$\|A\| = \sqrt{1^2 + 2^2 + 3^2} = 3.7417$$

and

$$\|B\| = \sqrt{4^2 + 5^2 + 0^2} = 6.403$$

$$\cos\theta = \frac{A^T \cdot B}{\|A\|\|B\|} = \frac{14}{3.7417 \times 6.403} \approx 0.5844$$

Let us look at a facial biometric similarity measurement case. Assume we have five male adults, A, B, C, D, and E, and we have biometric features 1 through 15 (Figure 3.1).[47] We can calculate the cosine similarities between them in the form of a similarity matrix (Table 3.1).

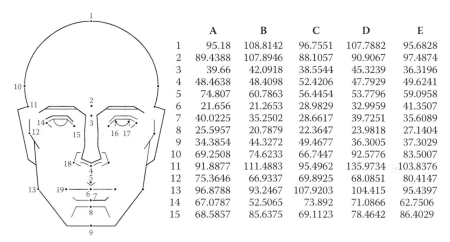

	A	B	C	D	E
1	95.18	108.8142	96.7551	107.7882	95.6828
2	89.4388	107.8946	88.1057	90.9067	97.4874
3	39.66	42.0918	38.5544	45.3239	36.3196
4	48.4638	48.4098	52.4206	47.7929	49.6241
5	74.807	60.7863	56.4454	53.7796	59.0958
6	21.656	21.2653	28.9829	32.9959	41.3507
7	40.0225	35.2502	28.6617	39.7251	35.6089
8	25.5957	20.7879	22.3647	23.9818	27.1404
9	34.3854	44.3272	49.4677	36.3005	37.3029
10	69.2508	74.6233	66.7447	92.5776	83.5007
11	91.8877	111.4883	95.4962	135.9734	103.8376
12	75.3646	66.9337	69.8925	68.0851	80.4147
13	96.8788	93.2467	107.9203	104.415	95.4397
14	67.0787	52.5065	73.892	71.0866	62.7506
15	68.5857	85.6375	69.1123	78.4642	86.4029

FIGURE 3.1   Fifteen facial biometric measurements (in columns) for five faces (A–E).

TABLE 3.1 Cosine Angle Similarity Matrix for the Five Subjects

	A	B	C	D	E
A	1	0.97892	0.98228	0.98904	0.97944
B	0.97892	1	0.97984	0.99147	0.98277
C	0.98228	0.97984	1	0.98621	0.99154
D	0.98904	0.99147	0.98621	1	0.99381
E	0.97944	0.9277	0.99154	0.99381	1

Jaccard Similarity Coefficient

If our feature vectors have binary values, we may use the Jaccard similarity coefficient. Given two feature vectors A and B, each with n binary attributes, the Jaccard coefficient is a useful measurement of the overlap that A and B share with their

---

[47] For more information about the definition of the facial biometric definitions, please refer to the book *Facial Geometry—Graphic Facial Analysis for Forensic Artists* by Robert M. George (Thomas, Springfield, IL, 2007).

attributes. Each attribute of A and B can be either 0 or 1. The total number of each combination of attributes for both A and B is specified as follows:

- M_{11} is the number of attributes when A and B both have a value of 1.
- M_{01} is when the number of attributes of A is 0 and the attribute of B is 1.
- M_{10} is when the number of attributes of A is 1 and the attribute of B is 0.

The Jaccard similarity coefficient is given as

$$J(A,B) = \frac{M_{11}}{M_{01} + M_{10} + M_{11}} \tag{3.4}$$

The Jaccard distance is

$$d_J(A,B) = 1 - J(A,B) \tag{3.5}$$

For example, assume we have three attributes for grouping patients: high cholesterol (HC), high blood pressure (HBP), and male (M). We have three patients, A, B, and C (Table 3.2).

TABLE 3.2 Jaccard Similarity Sample Data

	A	B	C
HC	1	1	0
HBP	1	0	1
M	1	1	0

$$J(A,B) = \frac{2}{2+1} = \frac{2}{3}, \quad J(B,C) = \frac{0}{2+1} = 0, \quad J(A,C) = \frac{1}{2+1} = \frac{1}{3}$$

Here, we find that patient A is more similar to patient B than to patient C.

Levenshtein Distance

In 2012, the Boston bomber Tamerlan Tsarnaev traveled to the volatile Dagestan region in Russia. The Federal Bureau of Investigation (FBI) was not able to track him because his name was misspelled on travel documents. When he got on the airplane, the agency misspelled his name, so it never went into the system that he actually went abroad. If the FBI had a Google-like search capability, which allows text matching with certain errors, the FBI would have not "dropped the ball."[48]

---

[48] http://www.dailymail.co.uk/news/article-2313061/Boston-bombings-FBI-didnt-know-Tamerlan-Tsarnaev-trip-Russia-misspelled.html

Imagine that we have some keywords or shapes that are transformed from image to text. We want to search the database with *partial matching*. We need to measure the errors during the matching process. Taking license plate matching, for example, does "A B C 1 5" match "A B D 4 5"? We notice that there are two errors. The number of errors in the letter matching is called the *Levenshtein distance*. The type errors include substitution, deletion, and insertion. For example,

dog $\rightarrow$ dag (substitution)
dog $\rightarrow$ dg (deletion)
dog $\rightarrow$ dogs (insertion)

The Levenshtein distance can be used for measuring the errors in text matching, for example, the shape matching encoded in the chain code. Assume we have three curves, A, B, and C (Figure 3.2). They can be converted to letters using chain code:

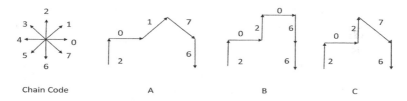

FIGURE 3.2   Three curves encoded with chain code.

A:	2	0	1	7	6	
B:	2	0	2	0	6	6
C:	2	0	2	7	6	

The Levenshtein distance between A and B is 3 (two replacements and one insertion). The Levenshtein distance between A and C is 1. Therefore, A and C are more similar compared to A and B.

3.3   CLUSTERING METHODS

k-Means

Assume we have n samples. How do we group them into k clusters so that the intracluster similarity is high but the intercluster similarity is low? The k-means[49] is one of the simplest clustering algorithms (Figure 3.3). The main idea is to define k centroids in k clusters and find the best centroid arrangement so that the square error is minimum:

---

[49] J. B. MacQueen. Some methods for classification and analysis of multivariate observations. In *Proceedings of 5th Berkeley Symposium on Mathematical Statistics and Probability*. University of California Press, Berkeley, 1:281–297, 1967.

$$J = \sum_{j=1}^{k}\sum_{i=1}^{n}\left\|x_i - c_j\right\|^2 \tag{3.6}$$

where $\left\|x_i - c_j\right\|^2$ is a chosen distance measured between a data point x_i and the cluster centroid c_j, and J is an indicator of the distance of the n data points from their respective cluster centroids.

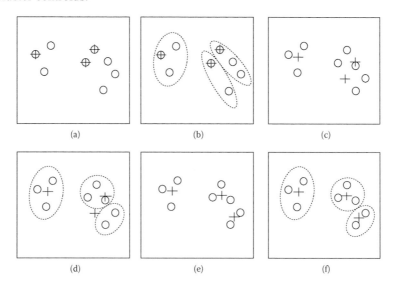

FIGURE 3.3 Clustering of eight samples based on the k-means method, given $k = 3$. The centroid (mean) of each cluster is marked by a plus sign. (a) First, three centroids are randomly assigned to three points. (b) Then, three clusters are formed and points are associated to the clusters based on the nearest neighbors. (c) The centroid for each cluster is recalculated. (d) Based on the new centroids, clusters are regrouped. (e) The centroid for each cluster is recalculated. (f) The clusters are regrouped based on the updated centroids. The process is repeated until the changes of centroids are less than a threshold.

The algorithm starts by randomly assigning k samples to be centroids. For each remaining sample, a sample is assigned to the cluster to which it is the most similar based on the distance between the object and the cluster mean. It then computes the new mean for each cluster. This process iterates until the criterion function converges.

The following is the pseudocode for k-means, assuming k is the number of clusters from n samples.

1. Randomly choose k samples as the initial cluster centers;
2. Do following recursively:
   Assign each sample to the cluster to which the sample is similar based on the mean value of the samples in the cluster.
   Update the cluster means of the samples for each cluster until no change.

The *k*-means is a simple algorithm that has been adapted to many problem domains. For more details, please read the tutorial slides written by Andrew Moore.[50] Also, there are many open sources available for the calculation.[51]

Like many other rudimentary algorithms in this book, simplicity does not always guarantee efficiency. The *k*-means is significantly sensitive to the initial randomly selected cluster centroids. Therefore, one should run the *k*-means algorithm multiple times to reduce this effect.

Dendrogram

It is desirable to organize clusters in a hierarchical structure. A dendrogram is one of the popular hierarchical clustering methods in bioinformatics. *Dendro* means "tree" in Greek. *Gram* means "graph." A dendrogram consists of many U-shaped lines that connect data points in a hierarchical tree. The height of each U represents the distance between the two data points being connected. It is a pairwise clustering method based on the distance matrix of attributes. In its simplest form, we can just use Euclidian distances.

There are two ways to make hierarchical clustering; one is to start from the bottom, with all the data points as clusters and then, at each step, merge two of them and put their centroid as the new point for further clustering with others. This is also known as "agglomerative nesting." The other one is called divisive and starts from the top, with everything in a big cluster, and at each step, a split toward the bottom is performed.

Figures 3.4A through 3.4E are examples of clustering five points situated in a two-dimensional (2D) plane. At the right in each is a dendrogram in progress.

There are packages for plotting dendrograms in MATLAB, for example. The function "dendrogram" generates a plot of the hierarchical binary cluster tree.

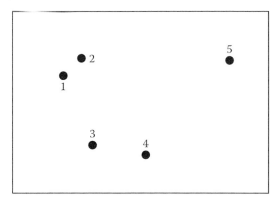

FIGURE 3.4A   An example of clustering five points on a two-dimensional plane where the distance between points 1 and 2 is the shortest.

[50] http://www.autonlab.org/tutorials/kmeans11.pdf

[51] http://www.mathworks.com/help/stats/kmeans.html

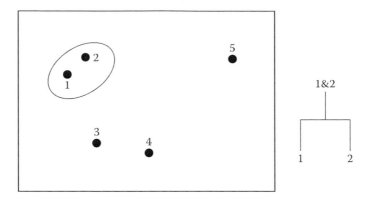

FIGURE 3.4B Merge points 1 and 2 and calculate their mean location as the centroid. The dendrogram is on the right.

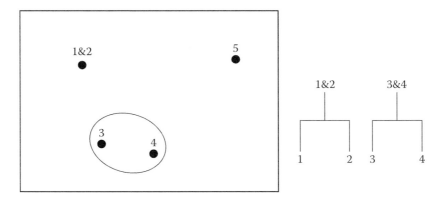

FIGURE 3.4C The next shortest distance is between points 3 and 4. Merge points 3 and 4 and calculate their mean location as the centroid. The dendrogram is on the right.

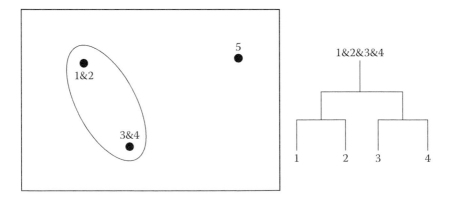

FIGURE 3.4D The next shortest distance is between merged points 1&2 and 3&4. Merge them and calculate their mean location as the centroid. The dendrogram is on the right.

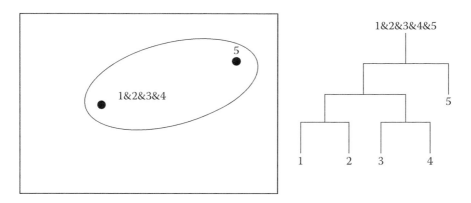

FIGURE 3.4E   Finally, let us group the merged point 1&2&3&4 and 5. The final dendrogram is on the right.

3.4   CLASSIFICATION METHODS

k Nearest Neighbor: Learn from Neighbors

The k nearest neighbor (k-NN) is the simplest classification method: the so-called lazy man's classifier. The main idea is to measure Euclidean distances between the test samples and training samples and make a majority vote decision based on k nearest neighbors. If $k = 1$, then just pick up the closest training sample as a classification result.

The k-NN method is a nonparameterized classification method, which means it does not build a model from the data. All it needs are training samples. However, k-NN needs a large amount of storage for training samples.

The pseudocode for k-NN is as follows:

1. Store training data in a matrix.
2. Input a test data in a feature vector and value of k.
3. Compute the Euclidean distances between the test data and training data.
4. Get k shortest distances.
5. Take a majority vote for which class is the nearest neighbor.

Let us look at a simple example. Assume we have two test variables x and y. The cases are plotted using their x, y coordinates as shown in Figure 3.5. Also, assume that the target variable has two categories, positive and negative. If we have a sample

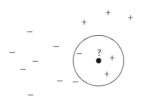

FIGURE 3.5   The k-nearest neighbor example, where k = 3. We have two "+" and one "-".

(plotted as the question mark), assume $k = 3$. We take the three nearest candidates and find two positives and one negative. Therefore, the result is positive.

Thanks to its simplicity, k-NN is faster and needs fewer training samples compared to other classifiers. When the number of samples is low, say, less than ten, k-NN works better than more supplicated models such as the Gaussian mixture model (GMM), which might simply quit working.

A disadvantage of the k-NN method is the time complexity of making predictions. Suppose that there are n training examples in m-dimension space. Then, applying the method to one test example requires $O(nm)$ time.

Radial Basis Function Network

The idea of the radial basis function (RBF)[52] is to simulate the neural network in the human visual system.[53] For example, for color vision we have three sensors: red, green, and blue. Each has its peak centered in the light spectrum. The farther from the center the input is, then the less activation there is.[54] Fortunately, our visual sensors can overlap each other well so that we have full coverage of the visible light spectrum (Figure 3.6).

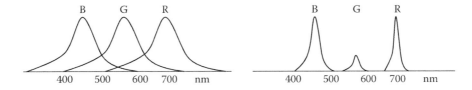

FIGURE 3.6 On-center, off-surround phenomenon in our vision system. The overlapped sensors cover the visible spectrum well in a smooth, solid, synthetic curve (left). The nonoverlapped sensors leave some blind spots on the spectrum (right).

This sombrero-like function is called the RBF. Assume c_i is the ith center, and $\|x - c_i\|$ is the distance between x and c_i. We have

$$\varphi(x) = G\left(\|x - c_i\|\right) \tag{3.7}$$

which is similar to the Gaussian function

$$G(y) = \exp\left(-y^2/\sigma^2\right) \tag{3.8}$$

where c is the center of the response peak. σ is a parameter called the spread, which indicates the selectivity of the neuron: Spread = 1/Selectivity. The larger the spread

[52] Christopher J. C. Burges. a tutorial on support vector machines for pattern recognition. *Data Mining and Knowledge Discovery* 2:121–167, 1998.

[53] http://www.cs.rit.edu/~lr/courses/nn/lecture/topic%204.pdf

[54] The LGN (lateral geniculate nucleus) description can be found at http://en.wikipedia.org/wiki/Lateral_geniculate_nucleus

is, the smoother the function approximation will be. Too large a spread means many neurons ignore fast changes. Too small a spread means many neurons may respond to trivial changes, and the network may not be generalized well.

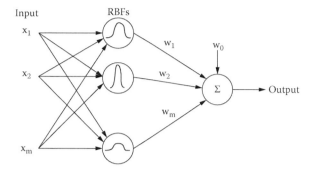

FIGURE 3.7   RBF network structure.

An RBF network has an input layer, a hidden layer, and an output layer (Figure 3.7). The neurons in the hidden layer contain Gaussian transfer functions whose outputs are inversely proportional to the distance from the center of the neuron.[55]

The output of the RBF network is a linear combination of the weighted RBFs.

$$F(X) = \sum_{i=1}^{N} w_i \cdot \varphi(X) \tag{3.9}$$

where X is the input vector.

How is the network trained? RBFs train in two stages, the first of which is unsupervised; the second is a linear supervised method. We can assume the spreads are fixed at the beginning. Choose the N data points themselves as centers. It remains to find the weights. We define

$$\varphi_{ji} = \varphi \left(\left\| x_i - x_j \right\| \right) \tag{3.10}$$

where φ is the RBF, and x_i and x_j are training samples. The matrix Φ of values φ_{ij} is called the interpolation matrix, which has the following property:

$$
\begin{bmatrix}
\varphi_{11} & \varphi_{12} & \cdots & \varphi_{1N} \\
\varphi_{21} & \varphi_{22} & \cdots & \varphi_{2N} \\
\vdots & \vdots & \vdots & \vdots \\
\varphi_{N1} & \varphi_{N2} & \cdots & \varphi_{N1}
\end{bmatrix}
\begin{bmatrix}
w_1 \\
w_2 \\
\vdots \\
w_N
\end{bmatrix}
=
\begin{bmatrix}
d_1 \\
d_2 \\
\vdots \\
d_N
\end{bmatrix}
\tag{3.11}
$$

---

[55] http://www.dtreg.com/rbf.htm

Let us abbreviate this as

$$\Phi W = D \tag{3.12}$$

where W is the weight vector, and D is the desired output vector over all training samples since the samples are both data points and centers. If Φ is nonsingular, then we can solve for weights as

$$W = \Phi^{-1} \cdot D \tag{3.13}$$

For exercises, we may use MATLAB's "newrb" function for RBF. The newrb function takes five arguments: input vectors, target class vectors, mean squared error goal, spread, and maximum number of neurons. The function returns a new radial basis network.

The RBF network is faster in training compared to other neural networks, such as backpropagation. It can recognize objects in real time. In a case study of voice recognition, the RBF algorithm outperformed the GMM and reached 94.8% accuracy.[56]

A few RBF-based neural network chips have been implemented with field programmable gate array (FPGA) technology; for example, Cognimem's CM1K chip has 1,024 neurons in parallel (Figure 3.8).[57] More details about the object detection and tracking can be found in the chapter on video analytics.

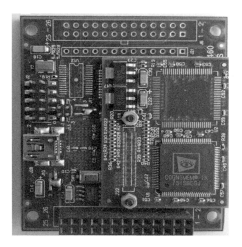

FIGURE 3.8 The neural network chip CM1K has 1,024 neurons (lower right corner) using the RBF neural network algorithm. The board is 5 × 5 cm with a 640 × 480 pixel black-and-white camera and can be used for simple pattern recognition tasks such as sign language recognition, face recognition, gender classification, and object tracking.

---

[56] http://arxiv.org/pdf/1211.2556.pdf
[57] http://www.cognimem.com/products/chips-and-modules/CM1K-Chip/index.html

Support Vector Machine

The main idea of a support vector machine (SVM) is to map data into a richer feature space and then construct a boundary plane to separate the data. The plane is called a hyperplane. It is a learning algorithm typically used for classification problems. A classifier boundary hyperplane can be written as

$$W^T \cdot X + b = 0 \qquad (3.14)$$

where X is the support vector on the hyperplane; W is a weight vector, namely, $W = \{w_1, w_2, \dots, w_n\}$; n is the number of attributes; and b is the scaler, often referred to as a bias. To optimize the classification, we want to make sure the data in each class has enough margins toward the hyperplane (Figure 3.9).

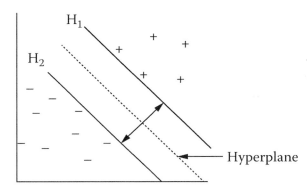

FIGURE 3.9   Hyperplane with plus plane (H_1) and minus plane (H_2) for margins.

To maximize the separation margin, the distance from the separating hyperplane to any point on H_1 is $1/\|W\|$, where $\|W\|$ is the Euclidean distance norm of W, that is $\sqrt{W \cdot W}$. By definition, this is equal to the distance from any point on H_2 to the separating hyperplane. Therefore, the maximal margin is $2/\|W\|$, which is equivalent to

Minimize $$\frac{1}{2} W^T W \qquad (3.15)$$

Subject to

$$W^T X_i + b \geq 1$$

and

$$W^T X_i + b \leq -1$$

Let us look at a toy problem. Assume we have two training data (Figure 3.10).[58] What is the separate hyperplane? $x_1 = 0$, and $x_2 = 2$.

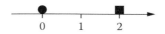

FIGURE 3.10   The two training data example.

We want to optimize

$$\min_{w,b} \frac{1}{2} w^2$$

Subject to constraints:

$$w \cdot 2 + b \geq 1,$$

$$w \cdot 0 + b \leq -1$$

We have $-b \geq 1$ and $2w \geq 1 - b \geq 2$. To satisfy these two constraints, we have $w \geq 1$. To minimize $\frac{1}{2} w^2$, the smallest possibility is $w = 1$. Therefore, the separating hyperplane is $x - 1 = 0$. So, the $x = 1$ is in the middle of the two training data.

However, in many real-world cases, it is not so easy to separate the datasets linearly. Taking a one-dimensional simple problem in Figure 3.11, for example, we have two types of data that are nested within one another. It is hard to separate them by Euclidean distances alone. Now, let us map the data to a two-dimensional feature space with the mapping function $\Phi(x)$ where the two types of data can be easily separated by a hyperplane. The mapping function can be linear, polynomial, an RBF, and so on. Let us try an RBF, as we discussed previously. The right part of Figure 3.11 shows the mapping result; the hyperplane can separate the two datasets with enough margins.

There are many open sources for SVM software: Spider (MATLAB), Weka (Java), SVMLight (C), and LibSVM (C++). All related tools are available through http://www.kernel-machines.org.

SVM is fast and robust in many applications. However, the weakness is that SVMs can only handle two-class outputs. For multiclass SVM, we may convert the multiclass problem into multiple binary classification problems.[59] Common methods include building binary classifiers that distinguish between one of the labels and the rest (one versus all). The one-versus-all case is done by a winner-takes-all strategy, in which the classifier with the highest output function assigns the class.

[58] S. H. Wu, CYUT. http://www.csie.cyut.edu.tw/~shwu/PR_slide/SVM.pdf
[59] Kai-Bo Duan and S. Sathiya Keerthi. Which is the best multiclass SVM method? An empirical study. In *Proceedings of the Sixth International Workshop on Multiple Classifier Systems. Lecture Notes in Computer Science* 3541:278, 2005.

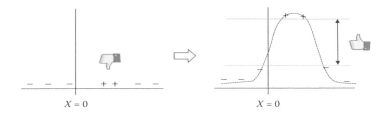

FIGURE 3.11   Map the one-dimensional data with a radial basis function to the two-dimensional feature space so that we can separate the two classes of data by planes with enough margins toward the border.

Eigenspace

The eigenspace method originated from the eigenface method that was initially developed in 1991 by Michael Turk and Alex Pentland. The idea is intuitive: Assume we have a database of known faces. We might be able to describe someone using a combination of those known faces.

The eigenface method is based on principle component analysis (PCA). The goal is to find the "feature-rich" faces, or so-called eigenfaces, as a basis for face-space. All of the training images are projected into this face-space, and the projection weights are stored as training data.

The eigenface method can be used to recognize objects other than faces. Here, let us take eye representation and recognition as an example. Eye detection is useful in the following chapter for fatigue detection.

For recognizing or classifying eyes, we need some features to represent a single eye image efficiently instead of just its pixels (Figure 3.12). A good solution is using the image's eigenvectors.

 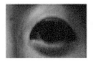

FIGURE 3.12   Samples from a training set.

First, let us find an "average eye." Assume we have a set of data that contains M sample images and N^2 features (pixels). This makes an $M \times N$ matrix F. Each column is an image.

$$F = \begin{bmatrix} F_{1,1} & \cdots & F_{1,m} \\ \vdots & & \\ F_{n,1} & \cdots & F_{n,m} \end{bmatrix} \tag{3.16}$$

The average of all sample images $\bar{F}$:

$$\bar{F}_i = \frac{1}{M} \sum_{j=1}^{M} F_{i,j} \tag{3.17}$$

So, $\bar{F}$ now contains the pixel values for an average eye. It is the average pixel values across all sample images. Here, we get an average eye from forty samples (Figure 3.13).

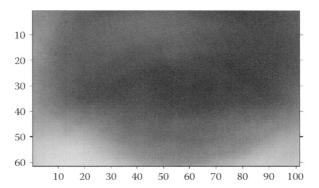

FIGURE 3.13   Average eye from forty samples.

We can see how each eye sample varies from the "mean" eye by constructing B. We call B the *mean-adjusted* matrix.

$$B = \begin{bmatrix} F_{1,1} - \bar{F}_1 & \cdots & F_{1,m} - \bar{F}_1 \\ \vdots & & \\ F_{n,1} - \bar{F}_n & \cdots & F_{n,m} - \bar{F}_n \end{bmatrix} \tag{3.18}$$

The differences have sign issues. Let us obtain the statistical covariance matrix C. To highlight the magic that is going to happen next, let us make a note about dimensions under each matrix.

$$\underset{n \times n}{C} = \underset{n \times m}{B} \cdot \underset{n \times m}{B^T} \tag{3.19}$$

Let us calculate the eigenvectors[60]:

---

[60] In MATLAB, calculating eigenvectors and eigenvalues only needs one line of code: [v, λ] = eig(a), where a is the input matrix, v is the eigenvectors, and λ is the eigenvalues.

$$\left(\underset{n\times m}{B}\cdot\underset{n\times m}{B^T}\right)\cdot\underset{n\times 1}{V_i}=\lambda_i\cdot\underset{n\times 1}{V_i}\tag{3.20}$$

The $\underset{n\times m}{B}\cdot\underset{n\times m}{B^T}$ is a large matrix ($n\times n$). Assume $\underset{m\times 1}{U}$ is m eigenvectors of $\underset{n\times m}{B^T}\cdot\underset{n\times m}{B}$, we have:

$$\left(\underset{n\times m}{B^T}\cdot\underset{n\times m}{B}\right)\cdot\underset{m\times 1}{U_i}=\lambda_i\cdot\underset{m\times 1}{U_i}\tag{3.21}$$

Multiple: $\underset{n\times m}{B}$

$$\left(\underset{n\times m}{B}\cdot\underset{n\times m}{B^T}\right)\cdot\underset{n\times m}{B}\underset{m\times 1}{U_i}=\lambda_i\cdot\underset{n\times m}{B}\underset{m\times 1}{U_i}\tag{3.22}$$

Therefore,

$$\underset{n\times 1}{V_i}=\underset{n\times m}{B}\cdot\underset{m\times l}{U_i}\tag{3.23}$$

where U are m eigenvectors of B^TB, and V are n eigenvectors of BB^T.

The advantage of this method is that one has to evaluate only a matrix of size M numbers and not N^2. Usually, $M \ll N^2$ as only a few principal components will be relevant. The amount of calculations to be performed is reduced from the number of pixels ($N^2 \times N^2$) to the number of images in the training set (M). Instead of computing at the pixel level ($n \times n$ features), we now can just use eigeneyes (m features), where each eye is a linear combination of all eigeneyes (Figure 3.14).

FIGURE 3.14   Sample eigeneyes.

Now, let's select the principal components. From M eigenvectors V_i, only M' ($M' \le M$) should be chosen, which have the highest eigenvalues. The higher the eigenvalue, the more characteristic features of an eye particular eigenvector describes. Eigenvectors with low eigenvalues can be omitted as they describe only a small part of features of the eyes. After M' eigenvectors V_i are determined, we construct eigeneyes, and the "training" phase of the algorithm is finished.

Now, let us reconstruct eyes (Figures 3.15 and 3.16). It was mentioned that each real image is a linear combination of all eigeneyes. Each real image is represented by a single vector of values in the eye space. To reconstruct an eye, we have to know its eye space coordinate vector $\left[\omega_1, \omega_2, ..., \omega_{M'}\right]$. Then, the real eye is the weighted sum of the eigeneyes.

$$I = \sum_{i=1}^{M'} V_i \cdot \omega_i + \overline{F} \tag{3.24}$$

where M', as before, is the total number of eigeneyes. For $M' = M$, the reconstruction is lossless; for $M' < M$, it is lossy and it degrades image quality.

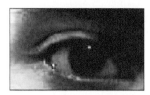 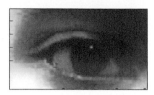

FIGURE 3.15 Original eye (left) versus reconstructed eye (right).

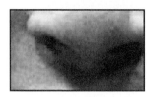 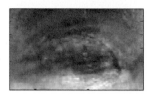

FIGURE 3.16 Input of a nose image sample (left) and the reconstruction result (right).

Detecting an eye from images is easy. We just need to compare the distances between stored eye samples and the reconstructed eye. If the test image is not an eye, then the distance between the stored eye image and the reconstructed image would be larger.

To recognize an input image, we can transform it into the eigenface components. The resulting weights form the weight vector $\{\omega_1,\ldots,\omega_{M'}\}$.

$$\omega_i = V_i^T \left(I - \overline{F}\right), \qquad i = 1,\ldots,M' \tag{3.25}$$

We can determine which eye class provides the best description for the input image by minimizing the Euclidean distance:

$$\Omega^T = \left[\omega_1, \omega_2, \ldots, \omega_{m'}\right] \tag{3.26}$$

$$\frac{\left\|\Omega - \Omega_k\right\|}{\left\|\Omega\right\|} \leq \varepsilon_k \tag{3.27}$$

where Ω_k is a vector describing the kth eye. ε_k is a threshold.

The Euclidean distance between two weighted vectors provides a measure of similarity between the corresponding images. If the Euclidean distance between the input image and other eyes exceeds some average threshold value, one can assume that the input image is not an eye at all. The Euclidean distance also allows one to construct "clusters" of eyes such that similar eyes are assigned to one cluster.

3.5   CLASSIFIER ACCURACY MEASURES

Confusion Matrix

The confusion matrix is a useful tool for analyzing how well a classifier performs against ground truth data. A confusion matrix for two classes is shown in Figure 3.17, where the rows are experimental results, and the columns are ground truths. For example, we have two classes: diseased (class 1) and nondiseased (class 2). The following terms are fundamental to understanding the utility of tests of a classifier:

- True positive (TP) or hit: the sample is positive, and the test is positive.
- False positive (FP) or false alarm: the sample is negative, but the test is positive.
- True negative (TN) or correct rejection: the sample is negative, and the test is negative.
- False negative (FN) or missed: the sample is positive, but the test is negative.

	Ground Truth +	Ground Truth −
Test +	TP	FP
Test −	FN	TN

FIGURE 3.17   The confusion matrix of 2 × 2 clinic diagnostic tests.

Sensitivity

The sensitivity is the proportion of the true positive samples over the total number of positive samples. The sensitivity of a test refers to the ability of the test to correctly identify those patients with the disease.

$$sensitivity = \frac{TP}{TP + FN} = \frac{TP}{P} \tag{3.28}$$

A test with 100% sensitivity means that the system correctly identifies all patients with the disease. A test with 70% sensitivity detects 70% of patients with the disease (true positives), but 30% with the disease go undetected (false negatives).

A high sensitivity is clearly important if the test is used to identify a serious but treatable disease (e.g., detecting colon cancer from a stool blood test). Screening the elderly population by stool blood test is a sensitive test. However, it is not very specific, and patients who have blood in their stool may not have colon cancer.

Specificity

The specificity is the proportion of the true negative samples over the total number of negative samples. The specificity of a test refers to the ability of the test to correctly identify those patients without the disease.

$$specificity = \frac{TN}{FP+TN} = \frac{TN}{N} \tag{3.29}$$

A test with 100% specificity means that the system correctly identifies all patients without the disease. A test with 90% specificity correctly reports 90% of patients without the disease as test negative (true negatives) but incorrectly identifies 10% of patients without the disease as test positive (false positives).

A test with a high sensitivity but low specificity results in many patients who are disease free being told of the possibility that they have the disease and are then subject to further investigation.

POSITIVE PREDICTIVE VALUE

The positive predictive value (PPV) shows the proportion of the test positives that are real positives.

$$Positive\ Predictive\ Value = \frac{TP}{TP+FP} \tag{3.30}$$

NEGATIVE PREDICTIVE VALUE

The negative predictive value (NPV) shows the proportion of the test negatives that are indeed negative.

$$Negative\ Predictive\ Value = \frac{TN}{TN+FN} \tag{3.31}$$

A Simple Example

Here, let us study a simplified problem. Assume we have the ground truth of five positive samples (+) and five negative samples (−). Then, P = 5, and N = 5.

Case I. The classifier shows all tests positive (Figure 3.18). TP = 5, and FP = 5.

$$\text{Sensitivity} = 5/5 = 100\%$$

$$\text{Specificity} = 0/5 = 0$$

The classifier appears to have a high hit rate but too many false alarms.

Case II. The classifier shows all tests negative (Figure 3.19). TN = 5, and FN = 5.

$$\text{Sensitivity} = 0/5 = 0$$

$$\text{Specificity} = 5/5 = 100\%$$

The classifier has a good rejection rate but too high a missing rate.

Case III. In the realistic scenario (Figure 3.20), we have TP = 4, FP = 2, TN = 3, and FN = 1. We have,

$$\text{Sensitivity} = 4/5 = 80\%$$

$$\text{Specificity} = 3/5 = 60\%$$

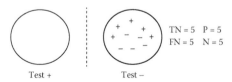

FIGURE 3.18   Case I: all tests positive.

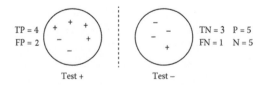

FIGURE 3.19   Case II: all tests negative.

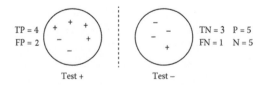

FIGURE 3.20   Case III: a more realistic dataset with some tests positive and some negative.

The classifier appears to have reasonable performance. Assume values of sensitivity and specificity are between 0 and 1. Let us plot the results on the sensitivity-specificity chart, called the receiver operator characteristic (ROC) curve (Figure 3.21). Using the curve, we can fine-tune the classifier's parameters to balance the two factors for an optimal solution.

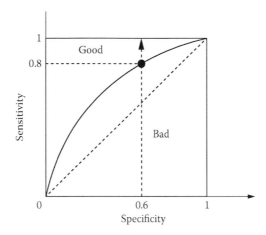

FIGURE 3.21   Receiver operator curve (ROC): The test results are above the AUC (area under the curve).

Receiver Operator Characteristic

The ROC curves were originally devised by radio receiver operators for tuning the system for optimal detection of enemy's aircraft during WWII. They are plots of 1-specificity or 100-specificity of a test on the x-axis against its sensitivity on the y-axis for all possible cutoff points. The area under the curve (AUC) represents the overall accuracy of a test. The larger the AUC, the better. The dotted line on the graph in Figure 3.21 represents the line of zero discrimination no better than 50/50 chances. In Chapter 10, we will study the application of the ROC in the wearable sensor design case.

3.6   SUMMARY

Pattern recognition algorithms are important to automatic diagnostic systems in which we want to take human factors out of the loop. In this chapter, we reviewed essential concepts for the recognition process. Similarities and distances are quality measurements for pattern matching or alignment. Here, we only covered measures that are related to ambient diagnostics, such as the cosine angle coefficient, which can be applied to biometric pattern recognition, alignment, and correlation analysis in social media.

For clustering, we reviewed two simple methods: k-means and dendrograms. The k-means method is widely used in machine learning, while the dendrogram is popular in bioinformatics. Putting the two in one place enables us to cluster the data in either planetary or hierarchic structures.

For classification problems, we have covered k-NN, RBF and SVM. Since k-NN and RBF have been implemented on a chip, perhaps it is time to develop an SVM chip. Besides, eigenspace was introduced as a classification method. This is based on the PCA method discussed in Chapter 2 for feature space reduction. The eigeneye case study shows that PCA can be used for both data transformation and pattern recognition. Finally, sensitivity and specificity are two essential measurements for evaluating classification quality.

PROBLEMS

1. Both Euclidean distance and cosine angle coefficient can measure the distance between feature vectors. However, there are some subtle differences in the two methods. Discuss the differences with numerical examples.
2. Given a set of human subjects A, B, and C, we have binary biometric features 1 through 5. Calculate the Jaccard index matrix among A, B, and C.

Feature	A	B	C
1	1	1	1
2	1	1	
3			1
4			1
5	1	1	

3. Use Chain Code to convert the outlines of 10 cars, 10 trucks, and 10 vans to numbers manually. Then, classify the feature vectors with Levenshtein distances. Analyze the classification results with a confusion matrix.
4. Based on Problem 3, improve the algorithm so that it can handle objects in different sizes.
5. Given five test samples and the Euclidean distance matrix that follows, plot a dendrogram.

	1	2	3	4	5
1	0				
2	2	0			
3	6	5	0		
4	10	9	4	0	
5	9	8	5	3	0

6. Given a one-dimensional classification problem illustrated in Figure 3.11, define an RBF so that the projected + and − points can be as far as possible.

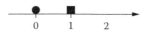

FIGURE 3.22 Support vector machine exercise problem.

7. Given two training samples at $X = 0$ and $X = 1$, find the hyperplane to separate the two using the SVM method (Figure 3.22).
8. Given a set of faces of both males and females, develop a gender recognition algorithm so that it can tell "male" or "female" whenever a new face is entered. Use the eigenspace approach to implement the algorithm. Hint: you may modify from a face recognition system because gender recognition is a subproblem of face recognition. Check out the MATLAB open source sample for face recognition.[61]
9. Assume you have a classification system that can tell the positive or negative results by tossing a coin. Consider two scenarios: tossing one coin and tossing two coins. Plot the ROC curves based on the sensitivity and specificity. Analyze the results in the report. Hint: for the one-coin case: the classifier would be the human's guess and the truth values would be coin sides. For example, if you guess "Head" (positive) and the coin lands on "Tail" (negative), then you will count that as a False Positive. After N tosses, you are able to calculate one data point for sensitivity and specificity. Repeat the process until you have enough data points to plot the ROC curve. For the two-coin case: same as the one-coin case, except one of the coins plays the role of the classifier and the other yields the truth value.
10. Given k-NN and SVM models, study the classification accuracy of the two models as the number of features (attributes) increases. Plot and discuss the trend.

---

[61] http://www.mathworks.com/matlabcentral/fileexchange/38268-eigen-face-recognition/content/New%20 folder/Mio.m

Section 2

Multimedia Intelligence

4 Sound Recognition

I recalled a well-known acoustic phenomenon: if you place your ear against one end of a wood beam the scratch of a pin at the other end is distinctly audible. It occurred to me that this physical property might serve a useful purpose in the case I was dealing with. I then tightly rolled a sheet of paper, one end of which I placed over the chest and my ear to the other. I was surprised and elated to be able to hear the beating of her heart with far greater clearness than I ever had with direct application of my ear. I immediately saw that this might become an indispensable method for studying, not only the beating of the heart, but all movements able of producing sound in the chest cavity.

—René-Théophile-Hyacinthe Laënnec, 1816

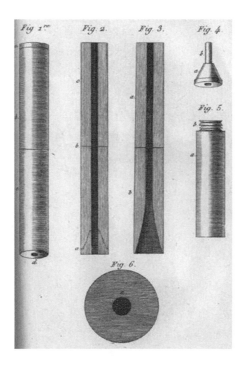

FIGURE 4.1 Early stethoscope invented by Rene-Theophile-Hyacinthe Laënnec in 1819. (From R. T. H. Launnec, *De l'Auscultation Médiate ou Traité du Diagnostic des Maladies des Poumons et du Cœur* - On mediate auscultation or treatise on the diagnosis of the diseases of the lungs and heart, published in Paris in 1819)

4.1 INTRODUCTION

Although stethoscopes have not changed much since 1819 (Figure 4.1),[62] digital technologies have evolved exponentially. In addition to sensing audio signals, we are
able to record, filter, and transmit audio data. All of these functions are available
in mobile phones today. Therefore, sound recognition is a "low-hanging fruit" for
ambient diagnostics. This chapter covers the following:

• Modern microphones
• Digital audio data formats
• Sound feature representation
• Sound pattern recognition

To show practical applications of the algorithms, we also study the cases of white
noise measurement at the workspace and asthma sound recognition.

4.2 MICROPHONE APPS

Mobile phones are revolutionizing healthcare in three ways: accessibility, quality,
and training. Mobile phones are affordable, and people can use them around the
clock to monitor and diagnose symptoms (Figure 4.2). Take asthma diagnosis,
for example: The sound of an asthma patient's breathing is widely accepted as a
symptom of disease.[62,63] A mobile phone can monitor airway diseases in real time
by recording and transmitting tracheal breath sounds.[64] Medical professionals can
replay, digitally share, and compare the data to improve the sensitivity and specificity of their medical diagnoses. Such a use of digital technologies would be especially
valuable for training medical students and junior doctors.

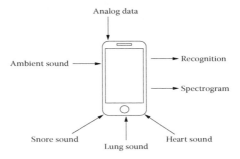

FIGURE 4.2 Sound recognition applications.

[62] M. A. Spiteri, D. G. Cook, and S. W. Clark. Reliability of eliciting physical signs in examination of the
chest. *Lancet* 2:873–875, 1988.

[63] H. Pasterkamp, S. S. Kraman, and G. R. Wodicka. Respiratory sounds: advances beyond the stethoscope.
American Journal of Respiratory Critical Care Medicine 156:974–987, 1997.

[64] K. Anderson, Y. Qiu, A. R. Whittaker, and Margaret Lucas. Breath sounds, asthma, and the mobile
phone. *Lancet* 358:1343–1344, 2001.

Today's smartphones are equipped with multiple microphones as well as advanced recording, signal-processing, and wireless transmission capacities. We can connect audio sensors to smartphones and laptops using the microphone analogical interface, Bluetooth, or Wi-Fi. This interface creates a "phone-centric peripheral" design arena.

It is worth noting that we can simplify sensory circuits by replacing analogical filters with digital filters in the processor. This is called "soft filter" approach.

Furthermore, automated sound recognition algorithms eliminate human factors, enabling real-time, persistent, quantitative diagnosis. Such technologies are especially useful for elderly people living independently, at intensive care units, and other personal care applications, such as monitoring blood pressure and blood sugar.

4.3 MODERN ACOUSTIC TRANSDUCERS (MICROPHONES)

Acoustic transducers convert vibrations into signals and vice versa. Early microphones were tubular or funnel-shaped devices that guided and amplified sound waves, such as ear trumpets made of animal horns, snail shells, wood, or metal. No matter what materials are used, all microphones have a diaphragm, a thin membrane skin, which is key for collecting the vibration.

Microelectromechanical System Microphones

The microelectromechanical system (MEMS) microphone is a tiny microphone on a chip. The pressure-sensitive diaphragm is etched directly into a silicon chip, comprising two capacitor plates. When a sound wave comes, the capacitor plates vibrate. This movement results in variation of the capacitance, producing either an analog or a digital output signal.

MEMS microphones are often accompanied with analog-to-digital converter (ADC) circuits and an integrated preamplifier (Figure 4.3). Therefore, MEMS microphones are more readily integrated with modern digital products, such as iPhones or Android phones, because of size and processing power. For most mobile phones today, there are at least two MEMS microphones inside: one on the front for acquiring voices and another on the back for canceling noises.

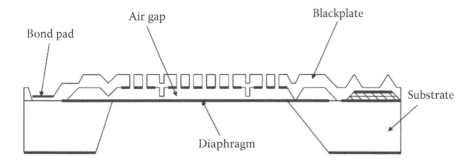

FIGURE 4.3 MEMS microphone structure.

Microphone Arrays

Microphone arrays consist of multiple microphones that function together as a stereo input device, similar to human ears. If we put microphones in different places, the sound will arrive at them at different times. So, we can calculate the location of the sound source based on the arrival difference. For more information about the processing algorithm, refer to Chapter 6 on Kinect sensors and a tutorial by McCowan.[65]

Microphone arrays can focus on speakers, freeing one from the need to wear a microphone near the face. However, arrays would be more expensive than a single microphone, and acoustic losses due to the distance from the sensor may occur.

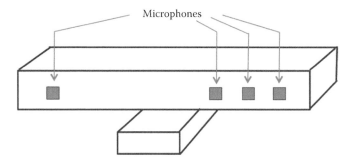

FIGURE 4.4   Kinect microphone array.

The good news is that the massive consumer market enables affordable microphone array products. For example, Kinect[66] was originally designed for an Xbox 360 peripheral and has four microphones in a line, three of them on the left side and one on the right. Kinect has several digital signal processors (DSPs) that process the complex algorithms for positioning, filtering, and merging data at the sensor side rather than at the computer side, freeing up more processing time to run applications such as games. Figure 4.4 shows the microphone array in a Kinect.

Fiber-Optical Microphones

A fiber-optic microphone converts acoustic waves into electrical signals by sensing changes in light intensity. Sound vibrations of the diaphragm change the intensity of light reflecting off the diaphragm in a specific direction. The moving light is then transmitted to a photodetector.

Fiber-optic microphones do not react to or influence any electrical, magnetic, electrostatic, or radioactive fields (Figure 4.5). Therefore, they are ideal for use where conventional microphones are ineffective or dangerous, such as inside magnetic resonance imaging (MRI) equipment environments. In addition, the distance

---

[65] Iain McCowan. Microphone arrays: a tutorial. http://www.idiap.ch/~mccowan/arrays/tutorial.pdf
http://www.idiap.ch/~mccowan/arrays/arrays.html
[66] http://www.wired.com/magazine/2011/06/mf_kinect/all/

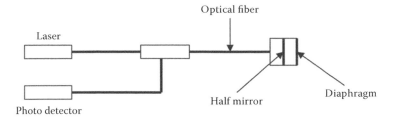

FIGURE 4.5   Fiber-optical microphone.

between the microphone's light source and its photodetector may be as large as several kilometers without need for any preamplifier or other electrical device. This makes fiber-optic microphones suitable for ambient or remote acoustic monitoring.

Laser Microphones

Laser microphones (Figure 4.6) often show up in James Bond movies because they pick up sound in a room from a window at a distance. The vibrations of the window change the angle of the reflected laser beam, so the motion can be reconstructed back to an audio signal.

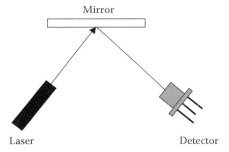

FIGURE 4.6   Laser microphone structure.

4.4   FREQUENCY RESPONSE CHARACTERISTICS

Sound travels through time. The number of times a molecule compresses over time determines its frequency or pitch. The human audible range is between 20 Hz and 20 kHz. Note that there is a slight peak at around 2–5 kHz, which luckily is the frequency zone of intelligibility for speech.[67]

Modern microphones often provide broader frequency response ranges and larger volume gains. However, microphones in mobile phones are often designed

[67] http://phonoscopy.com/SonicGeologic/SonicGeologic.html

to filter out lower frequencies that are distant from the normal human voice range (e.g., 50 Hz). Figure 4.7 shows a comparison between the human frequency response curve versus the iPhone 4 microphone's frequency response.

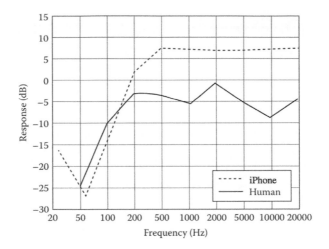

FIGURE 4.7 Human frequency response versus an iPhone 4 microphone's frequency response.

4.5   DIGITAL AUDIO FILE FORMATS

An audio file format is a file format for storing digital audio data on a computer system or digital media. This data can be stored uncompressed to preserve the fidelity or compressed to reduce the file size.

It is important to know the difference between a file format and an audio codec. A codec encodes and decodes the raw audio data, and the data itself is stored in a file with a specific audio file format. Most audio file formats support only one type of audio data. However, a multimedia container format may support multiple types of audio and video data.

Uncompressed Audio Formats (WAV and AIFF)

The most popular uncompressed audio formats include WAV (Windows and Linux) and AIFF (Max OS). The WAV, or Waveform Audio File Format, is a frequently used format in audio signal-processing tools such as MATLAB. The top-level definition of a WAV file is as follows:

- Format - the formated of the data file
- Cue points - a table of positions in the data
- Playlist - the play order for a series of cue points
- Associated data list - to attach labels to the data
- Wave data - the actual wave data

Uncompressed WAV files are large, so it is unwise to share WAV files over the Internet. The WAV format is suitable for high-quality recording, editing, or achieving professional applications.

The WAV format is limited to files that are less than 4 GB because of its use of a 32-bit unsigned integer to record the file size header, which is about 6.8 hours of CD-quality audio (44.1 kHz, 16-bit stereo). More often, the sound file we have to record exceeds this limit. The W64 format is therefore useful with the 64-bit header for much longer recording time.

Since the sampling rate of a WAV file can vary from 1 Hz to 4.3 GHz, and the number of channels can be as high as 65,536, people can use WAV files for nonaudio data. LTspice, for instance, can store multiple circuit trace waveforms in separate channels.[68] This is an attractive option for ambient diagnosis.

An AIFF file is grouped in several chunks; each chunk is identified by a chunk ID.[69] The typical chunks include: common chunk and sound data chunk.

Compressed Audio Formats (MP3 and Adaptive Multi-Rate)

MP3 is in fact a more frequently used compressed audio file format due to its smaller footprint, which allows faster Internet transmission, as well as lower consumption of space on memory media. MP3 is designed to preserve the overall character of the sound. However, it is a lossy compression. The greater the compression, the more sonic details are lost. MP3 usually discards extremely high and low frequencies. Further compression can diminish the differences between loud and soft sound patterns, weakening sound recognition capacities. If we had a deep compression, say, down to 64 kbps and lower, then it would flatten the sound wave and make the algorithms useless. Ideally, MP3 needs at least 192 kbps or greater to preserve most of the sound fidelity.

For mobile phones, the most frequently used mobile file format and audio codec is the Adaptive Multi-Rate (AMR), which is optimized for speech coding. AMR encodes narrowband (200- to 3,400-Hz) signals at variable bit rates ranging from 4.75 to 12.2 kbps. Many modern mobile phones can store short audio recordings in the AMR format.

Compressed audio files are not desirable formats for ambient diagnoses because they lose subtle auditory features that are important to recognition and classification models. For example, AMR cuts off the sound outside its 200 Hz, which is problematic for heartbeat or lung sound analyses. In addition, converting AMR or MP3 to WAV format introduces additional noise and further reduces the acoustic resolution. There are apps for recording WAV format data directly on mobile phones. Therefore, for ambient diagnoses, we should record the uncompressed WAV files instead of compressed AMR or MP3 files. With the increasing multicore processing power on today's mobile phones, it is possible to process the audio data locally on the phone instead of transferring a large amount of uncompressed data to the server.

---

[68] http://en.wikipedia.org/wiki/WAV
[69] http://en.wikipedia.org/wiki/Audio_Interchange_File_Format

Audio-Editing Tools

Audacity[70] is the most popular tool for recording and editing sounds. It is available for Windows, Mac, Linux, and other operating systems. Audacity is open source, and it can be used for recording live audio from microphones, line inputs, USBs, or Fireware devices; editing MP3, WAV, or AIFF sound files; and recording multiple channels at once. The most important feature of Audacity to ambient diagnostics is its sound analysis capacities, such as spectrogram view modes for visualizing frequencies and plot spectrum command for detailed frequency analysis (Figure 4.8).

FFmpeg is a cross-platform open source tool to record, convert, and stream audio and video.[71] The most notable part of FFmpeg is libavcodec, an audio and video codec library. FFmpeg is by far the most complete library for extracting audio tracks from video files and for transcoding multimedia files. However, FFmpeg is a big library written in C++/C, which requires a significant effort to recompile, maintain, and optimize.

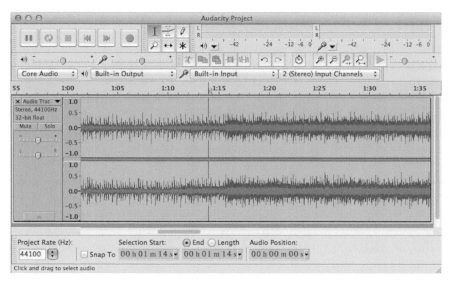

FIGURE 4.8   Audacity software screenshot.

4.6   HEART SOUND SENSING

The sound of the human heart is in the range of 20–100 Hz, a range that many microphones in mobile phones can pick up. However, mobile phones will need special digital amplifiers to boost the volume of the sound because normally they do not amplify well in this range. There are already apps that can amplify heartbeat sound, such as Blue FiRe for the iPhone, which is free to download. This app can boost gain up to 40 dB and record, replay, and transmit the sound data with the File Transfer

---

[70] http://audacity.sourceforge.net/
[71] http://www.ffmpeg.org/

Protocol (FTP). Figure 4.9 shows a screenshot of the heart sound wave, using Blue FiRe for iPhone.

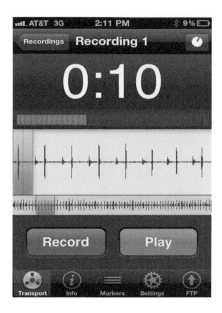

FIGURE 4.9 Heart sound recorded from iPhone 4 using Blue FiRe.

Another iPhone app, called iStethoscope, uses the iPhone's two microphones to record the sound of a heartbeat and e-mails the sound files to a user. To date, over one million copies have been downloaded.

4.7 LUNG SOUND SENSING

When a person breathes, lung sounds propagate through the lung tissue and can be heard over the chest wall. The tissue acts as a frequency filter with special characteristics based on pathological changes such as wheezing, crackling, and coughing. Therefore, medical professionals can diagnose respiratory diseases by acoustically analyzing lung sounds.

Lung sounds[72] can be classified into three categories: breath sounds, voice sounds, and adventitious sounds.[73]

Breath Sounds

Breath sounds include normal breathing sounds (vesicular sounds), bronchial breathing sounds, and soft breathing sounds (Figure 4.10).[74]

---

[72] http://www.stethographics.com/publications/1985_StateOfTheArt.pdf
[73] http://www.physio-pedia.com/Lung_Sounds
[74] http://www.drearleweiss.com/pdf/article_recording%20of%20breath.pdf

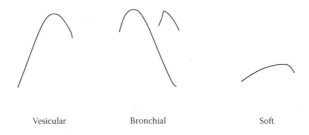

FIGURE 4.10   Breath sound patterns: normal or vesicular, bronchial, and soft.

Normal or vesicular sound is a long inhale and a short exhale (<500 Hz). Bronchial sound is a short inhale and a long exhale with a short, additional breath that follows (<200–4,000 Hz). Soft sound is a short inhale and a shorter exhale.

Voice Sounds

Voice sounds are filtered through the lung tissue, so they are normally incomprehensible to hear over the chest wall with a stethoscope.

Adventitious Sounds

Adventitious sounds include crackles, wheezes, mediastinal crunches, pleural rubs, and unclassified noises. *Crackles* are discontinuous explosive sounds. *Wheezes* are high-pitched or low-pitched continuous sounds caused by narrow airways. *Crunch* sounds are hoarse crackling sounds that are synchronous with heart contractions. *Pleural rubs* are discontinuous grating sounds that occur while breathing. Finally, *unclassified noises* are adventitious sounds that are not easily characterized by the other categories (e.g., rattles, squeaks, and gurgling).

Time-Amplitude Plot

Time-Amplitude plots of lung sounds are commonly used for diagnosis (Figure 4.11). The plot provides an overall view of acoustic characteristics in real time. In a time-expanded analysis, we stretch out the *x*-axis (time) to examine details of the acoustic phenomena more carefully. The zoomed display allows us to most easily see pattern distinctions between different types of lung sounds.[75]

Interference of Heartbeat Sounds with Lung Sounds

It is worth noting that heartbeats produce interference to lung sounds over the low-frequency components. The main components of heart sounds are in the range

---

[75] R. Murphy, S. Holford, and W. Knowler. Visual lung-sound characterization by time-expanded wave-form analysis. *New England Journal of Medicine* 296:968–971, 1977.

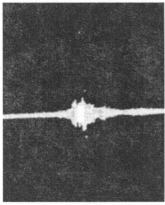 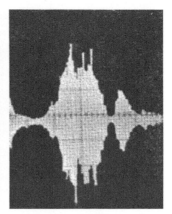

Normal (vesicular)   Acute asthmatic attack

FIGURE 4.11   Time-Amplitude plots of typical lung sounds showing the vesicular sounds with louder inspiration, of greater duration, and high pitched (left); and the acute asthmatic attack with bronchial sounds with prolonged loud, expiratory wheezing.

of 20–100 Hz, a range in which the lung sound has major components. High-pass filtering (HPF) with an arbitrary cutoff frequency between 70 and 100 Hz is not efficient in this case because lung sounds have major components in that range, particularly at low-flow rates. A study published in the *Journal of Medical and Biological Engineering and Computing* suggests that heart sound segments can be localized using multiresolution decomposition to reconstruct the lung sound.[76]

4.8   SNORE METER

Studies show that snoring is correlated with heart diseases because narrowed air ways do not allow enough oxygen to reach the heart. For scientists and physicians to examine sleep conditions, patients participate in sleep studies, in which they sleep in a lab where they are wired and monitored. Would it not make sense, however, that scientists and physicians would collect more natural data if patients could participate in the study while sleeping at home in their own beds? Thanks to consumer electronics, many lab experiments can now be conducted at home. For example, the snore meter smartphone app records sound samples and the number of snores and creates a histogram of the snore intensity (dB) (Figure 4.12).

4.9   SPECTROGRAM

A spectrogram is a three-dimensional visualization of sound patterns plotted in terms of *frequency, amplitude,* and *time.* A spectrogram is a powerful method for

---

[76] M. T. Pourazad, Z. Moussavi, and G. Thomas. Heart sound cancellation from lung sound recordings using time-frequency filtering, *Medical and Biological Engineering and Computing* 44(3):216–225, 2006.

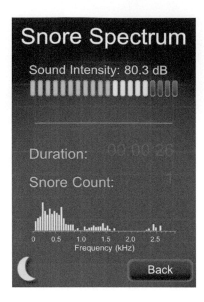

FIGURE 4.12   Histogram of the snore sound from the SnoreMeter app on the iPhone 4.

transforming invisible auditory signals into visible images. In contrast to the ampli-
tude-time plot, a spectrogram shows more frequency characteristics.

When representing an auditory signal, one might instinctively think of using
the Fourier transform. However, this mathematical transform assumes that a signal has infinite length, which is not true for the signal that we are studying, which
has limited length. The transform processes finite signals by infinitely repeating
the same signal, which creates discontinuities in the signal as interpreted by the
transform. This discontinuity leads to unwanted effects, called the Gibbs phenomenon, which manifests as overshoot and ripples surrounding the discontinuity during
reconstruction. Ultimately, the problem lies in trying to represent a non-band-limited
signal using a finite number of infinite-length basis functions. Therefore, *tapering*
or *windowing* is necessary to sample the signal. A smooth windowing function will
make the signal's ends connect smoothly by band limiting the signal and minimizing
unwanted artifacts of the transform.[77]

Richard W. Hamming, the mathematician who created the Hamming code, pro-
posed the Hamming window to sample an auditory signal (Figure 4.13). To compensate for the information loss caused by the Hamming Window, there is an overlap of
samples between each time slice.

We can construct the Hamming window as defined[78] by Equation 4.1. The next
step is to transform each of these slices of audio, where $w(n)$ is window function and
N represents the width of the window.

[77] Steven W. Smith. *The scientist and engineer's guide to digital signal processing.* California Technical,
Poway, 1997.
[78] Window function. http://en.wikipedia.org/wiki/Window_function, retrieved July 30, 2010.

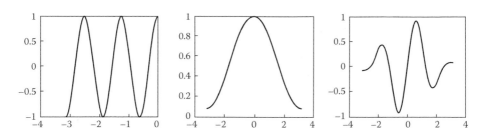

FIGURE 4.13 The signal wave (left) multiplied by the Hamming window (middle) generates the tapered signal (right). Note that the ends connect more smoothly.

$$w(n) = 0.54 + 0.46\cos\left(\frac{2\pi n}{N-1}\right) \tag{4.1}$$

The short-term Fourier transform (STFT) takes the Fourier transformation of windowed data in short periods. The discrete STFT is defined as $STFT(m,\omega)$, with signal $x(n)$, window $w(n)$, and frequency ω.

$$STFT(m,\omega) = \sum_{n=0}^{N-1} w[n-m] \cdot x[n] \cdot e^{-j\omega n} \tag{4.2}$$

In this case, m is the discrete time index, and ω is continuous, but in most typical applications, the STFT is performed on a computer using the fast Fourier transform, so both variables are discrete and quantized. The magnitude squared of the STFT yields the spectrogram, where the strength V is a function of time and frequency:

$$V = |STFT(\tau,\omega)|^2 \tag{4.3}$$

Spectrograms are often visualized using a three-dimensional plot, with the horizontal axis indicating time and the vertical axis indicating frequency and the intensity indicates the volume (magnitude). The magnitude of a frequency at a specific time is represented by the intensity or color of that point. Figures 4.14–4.16 show spectrograms of the first three seconds of each breath sound class in our training database. Brighter colors signify frequency components of higher magnitudes.

4.10 AMBIENT SOUND ANALYSIS

We do not live in a vacuum, so there are ambient sounds where we live and work. Sound pollution has become a new health concern. Regular exposure to loud noises can cause hearing loss, hypertension, and other diseases. There are a number of public health regulations about noise level in the workspace. However, persistent sound monitoring, and measuring noise frequency distribution, in particular, is expensive.

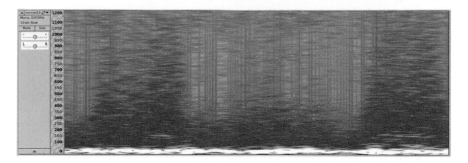

FIGURE 4.14   Spectrogram of a breathing sound.

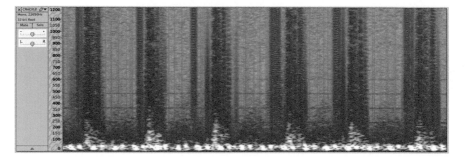

FIGURE 4.15   Spectrogram of a cracking sound.

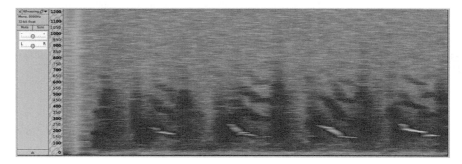

FIGURE 4.16   Spectrogram of a wheezing sound.

Thanks to sound spectrogram mobile phone apps, anyone can now measure sound noise anywhere and anytime. Figure 4.17 shows spectrograms of ambient sounds in daily life measured by the Spectrogram Pro app on the iPhone 4. From the spectrograms, we learn that the refrigerator generated a 200 Hz single-frequency sound from its compressor. In contrast, the microwave generated multiple-frequency sounds from its rotating table and fan, ranging from 100 to 210 Hz. Noises in a Starbucks café are mainly from human voices, ranging from 100 to 900 Hz in 60 dB. The loudest noisemaker is the vacuum cleaner, ranging from 100 to 850 Hz over 80 dB at a distance of 10 feet. Compared to the noises in Starbucks, which are random

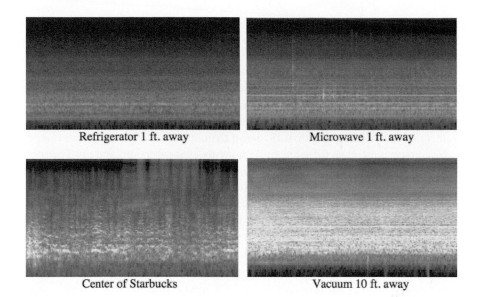

Refrigerator 1 ft. away   Microwave 1 ft. away

Center of Starbucks   Vacuum 10 ft. away

FIGURE 4.17 Spectrograms of ambient sounds using Spectrogram Pro on the iPhone: refrigerator, microwave, Starbucks, and vacuum.

and sparse, the vacuum cleaner bursts nonstop high-volume sounds across a broad audible spectrum.

Modern sound engineering can produce customized soundscape environments on demand. A *white noise* machine is a device that generates sound across all frequencies. White noise is used mainly to ensure privacy or promote concentration because it covers the largest spectrum range. Imagine turning on thousands of televisions simultaneously so that people in another room will not overhear a private conversation. Devices often produce colors of noise, rather than actual white noise, which has a harsh sound. For example, *pink noise* is a blend of high and low frequencies. *Brown noise* utilizes lower sound frequencies to generate a deep ambient rumble.

Recent studies show that white noise machines have negative effects on hearing loss, such as tinnitus symptoms and reduced spatial sensitivity.[79] Furthermore, continuous exposure to white noise sabotages the development of the auditory region of the brain, which may ultimately impair hearing and children's language acquisition. In one study,[80] young rats were exposed to constant white noise comparable to the random noise encountered by humans. The study's results suggest an explanation for the increase in language impairment development disorders over the last few decades.

Ergonomic injuries are the fastest-growing category of injuries in the United States today. They are now the leading cause of workers' compensation claims and can cause serious pain and temporary or permanent disability. The affordable mobile

---

[79] http://www.livestrong.com/article/184883-negative-effects-of-white-noise-machines/
[80] http://www.sciencedaily.com/releases/2003/04/030418081607.htm

phone spectrogram apps allow individuals to measure their own workplace noise levels, thereby empowering them to engage in conversations about and advocate for public and personal health standards.

Let us consider a real-world case study: a contemporary office building installed a white noise machine to help with privacy in the office. Employees in the building began to experience unexplained headaches, nausea, and hearing problems. Finally, one curious employee used the iPhone Spectrogram Pro app to take a sound measurement of the building. Figure 4.18 shows the comparative spectrograms that the employee measured when the white noise machine was turned off and on. The spectrograms show that the frequency of the constantly bursting white noise ranged from 161 to 280 Hz, which is not the correct range for white noise. Further tests showed that the noise was in a range similar to that of refrigerators and microwaves running simultaneously (Figure 4.17). After analyzing the data, environmental health and safety personnel and office managers permanently removed the white noise machine—a victory for ambient diagnostics.

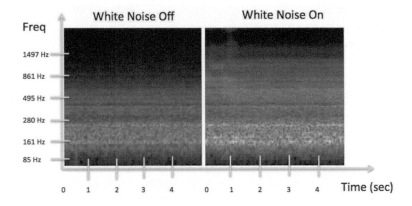

FIGURE 4.18   Spectrograms of the office environment with the white noise machine off (left) and on (right).

4.11   SOUND RECOGNITION

Traditional sound-based diagnostics depend on a doctor's sensitive hearing and acute vision to spot audio or spectrogram patterns. In contrast, automated sound recognition would enable continuous monitoring for early and mobile diagnoses without delay in data transmission.

An automated sound recognition algorithm often contains two stages: feature extraction and feature classification. The feature extraction process includes sampling raw audio signals, transforming the auditory data into frequency domain feature vectors, and compressing the feature vectors into lower feature dimensions. The feature classification process is normally a machine learning model. Just like humans, computers must learn to recognize certain sounds. To be able to classify sounds in supervised learning, we must carefully select and prepare a training dataset, then

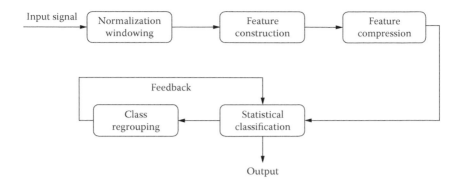

FIGURE 4.19 Overview of the training and testing algorithm for sound recognition.

train the computer with the feature vectors that were extracted. Finally, the computer will learn the feedback from the results and refine the class categories when necessary. Figure 4.19 shows an overview diagram of our approach.

Feature Extraction

To begin the feature extraction process, we can extract audio data from video or audio files and convert it into a WAV format. Audio data is preprocessed and normalized with filters to remove silent periods and noises. Then, we use STFT to convert the audio data into a spectrogram with Hamming windows and store the data in a three-dimensional matrix: frequency, magnitude, and time, where frequencies are normally in logarithmic scale. The matrix would create a feature space that might be too large to process quickly. We often need to use feature compression to reduce the features from high to low dimensions. Section 4.14 addresses the details of feature compression.

Feature Classification

There are many kinds of classifiers for sound feature recognition. The simplest is the nonparametric machine learning method, called k-nearest neighbor (k-NN), which finds the training sample whose distance to the test sample is shortest.

The support vector machine (SVM) is also a common choice. The SVM maps feature vectors to hyperplanes to maximize the distances between classes. Both k-NN and SVM have fewer training samples.

The Gaussian mixture model (GMM) is widely used in signal processing. The GMM calculates a probability value as a confidence indicator. The GMM is also similar to neural network architecture, such as radial basis function (RBF), which recognizes sophisticated patterns. However, the GMM needs more training samples than the k-NN and SVM.

We can achieve feature classification by evaluating the similarity between testing samples and clustered training samples. Because of computer limitations, we use the natural logarithm of sound features in calculations instead of the true values themselves. Multiplying many small values together would quickly result in underflows, or zeros. The property of the logarithm that reduces multiplication to addition helps resolve this problem.

We can detect patterns by letting the computer classify the test samples and output the log likelihood of the data that belongs to the determined class. If the similarity value is too low, the application will reject the data. However, one should be careful when determining the threshold for the probability value because there is no common global value suited for every case. The optimal threshold should be determined by hand, and the training database and the exact algorithms used will depend heavily on the clusters.

4.12   RECOGNIZING ASTHMA SOUNDS

Since the invention of the stethoscope, recognizing lung sounds has been an effective method for noninvasively diagnosing respiratory symptoms. However, such diagnoses have been a manual process for centuries. In this section, we explore computerized sound pattern visualization and recognition that aim to achieve repeatable and reliable automatic screening and monitoring, specifically for asthma.

Asthma, a common disease caused by narrowed airways, generates a significant acoustic feature: a wheezing sound ranging between 40 and 1,200 Hz. In this case study, we focus on how to recognize the wheezing sound pattern using a spectrogram.

A decibel-scaled spectrogram plot is essential to analyze recorded sample data because low frequencies of wheezing and normal breathing sounds make it difficult to see the details of the sound patterns. We can display spectrographs using the open source utility Audacity. Figure 4.20 shows the spectrogram of a normal breathing sound. Figure 4.21 shows the spectrogram of a wheezing sound with distinguished horizontal texture patterns.

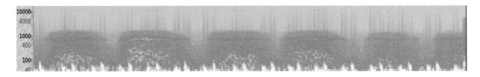

FIGURE 4.20   Spectrogram of a normal breathing sound.

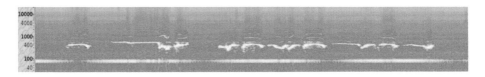

FIGURE 4.21   Spectrogram of a wheezing sound.

Given thirty normal breathing sounds and thirty wheezing sounds for training samples; and we also have fifteen normal breathing sounds and ten wheezing sounds for testing. We can convert the sound files to WAV format and used STFT to generate feature vectors in frequency, magnitude, and time dimensions. We then use k-NN to classify the input sample based on Euclidian distances between the training feature vectors and testing feature vectors. Table 4.1 shows the result of the simple example.

TABLE 4.1 Asthma Sound Recognition Results

	Breathing	Wheezing	Detection Rate
Breathing	13	2	87%
Wheezing	1	9	90%

4.13 PEAK SHIFT

To capture the essence of something, an artist often amplifies the differences and unique features of an object, which highlights the essential features and reduces redundant information.[81] This artistic process mimics what the visual areas of the brain have evolved to do by more powerfully activating the same neural mechanisms that were activated by the original object.[82] This psychological phenomenon is called the *peak shift* effect. Peak shift has been most widely understood concerning its applications in animal discrimination learning. In the peak shift effect, animals sometimes respond more strongly to exaggerated versions of training stimuli. For instance, a rat is trained to differentiate a square from a rectangle by being rewarded for recognizing the rectangle. The rat will respond more frequently to the object for which it is being rewarded, so much so that it will respond more frequently to a longer, narrower rectangle than to the original with which it was trained.

Here, we can also apply the peak shift principle to our sound recognition problem. For example, we can crop out the insignificant sound patterns and only store the representative patterns in the training data. In our case, we know the wheezing sound is a unique, sharp, high-pitched musical tone. By highlighting the 300- to 500-Hz range with horizontal, bright patterns, we can identify threshold ranges of frequency and magnitude, thereby removing nonsignificant patterns. Figure 4.22 shows the peak shift sampling windows that crop out the nonsignificant patterns for maximal discrimination in learning.

Our experiments showed that cropping the feature-rich patterns from raw data improves recognition accuracy. Based on forty training samples for wheezing sounds and normal sounds, after applying the peak shift preprocessing, the positive detection rate of the k-NN classifier rises from 33% to 89%.

Furthermore, if samples have distinguishable patterns and low noise, we can use simpler classifiers such as k-NN for recognition instead of more sophisticated ones such as the GMM, which needs more minimal training data than k-NN to run.

[81] Semir Zeki. *Inner vision: an exploration of art and the brain.* Oxford University Press, New York, 1999.
[82] V. S. Ramachandran and William Hirstein. The science of art: A neurological theory of aesthetic experience. *Journal of Consciousness Studies* 6(6–7):15–51, 1999.

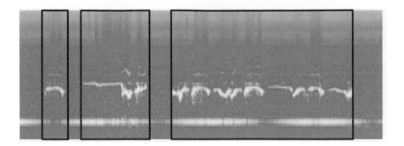

FIGURE 4.22   Peak shift processing.

4.14   FEATURE COMPRESSION

The STFT can generate a large feature space. To reduce the dimensionality across time segments, we can use principal component analysis (PCA) as discussed in Chapter 2. PCA transforms a dataset into a coordinate system in which the first component of the dataset corresponds to most of the variance in the data.[83] Each succeeding component accounts for the remaining variability in a decreasing manner. PCA decomposes the data and can be used to reduce dimensionality by keeping only the first few components. This implies information loss, but in such a way that the statistically most important features are preserved. After the PCA feature space compression, we can use the resulting feature vector to train a classifier in the training phase. Alternatively, after training, we can use the feature vector to classify new audio samples.

4.15   REGROUPING

In many cases, we do not know the acoustic correlations of sound classes. Classification results from machine learning may provide valuable feedback about acoustic correlation. When possible, we can *regroup* the highly correlated classes to a new class with a common name.

Audio classification results are often presented in the form of a confusion matrix, a table in which each row header is the actual audio class, and each column header is the detected audio class, as shown in Chapter 3. Given a reasonable classification procedure, one can use a confusion matrix as a guide for collapsing two classes if they are too close together in the chosen feature space. A confusion matrix is useful for recognizing falsely assumed dissimilarity between two classes.

In a confusion matrix, the number of correctly classified samples is shown in the matrix diagonal. Falsely classified ones will be found outside the diagonal. Misclassification for any of those two against any other third class will be comparatively low. Using this method, we can specify a margin we call a collapsing threshold. When we reach the collapsing threshold, two classes will collapse into one.

---

[83] Jon Shlens. A tutorial on principal component analysis: derivation, discussion and singular value decomposition, http://www.snl.salk.edu/~shlens/pca.pdf (accessed Nov. 12, 2013).

Let i and j be the indices of two arbitrary classes after a complete classification procedure. Furthermore, let R be the confusion matrix of $n \times n$ dimensions for n number of audio classes. The sum of row l of R can be defined as

$$S_l = \sum_{k=1}^{n} R_{l,k} \tag{4.4}$$

Then, we can define a Boolean expression B that, when it evaluates to true, causes classes i and j to be collapsed.

$$B_{i,j} = \begin{cases} \dfrac{R_{i,j}}{\left(S_i - R_{i,i}\right)} \geq t \; and \; \dfrac{R_{j,i}}{\left(S_j - R_{j,j}\right)} \geq t & True \\[2ex] Else & False \end{cases} \tag{4.5}$$

With t being the collapsing threshold, this expression is to be evaluated for each class pair i and j, where $i \neq j$.

4.16   NOISE ISSUES

Noise is undesirable because it negatively affects the processing of our target auditory data. In general, automated processing equipment like a computer cannot tell noise from useful data unless it has some knowledge about the nature of the noise itself. For classifications, noise within data can cause several problems. If the noise component of the data is too strong, then the feature extraction process will construct features of the noise, and the classifier will be trained to the nature of the unwanted data instead of the intended audio component.

Samples collected from audio sources are generally not noise free. Noise comes from many different sources, and it is possible to classify noise sources based on different criteria. One classification scheme, and maybe the most intuitive one, is noise origin, such as environmental noise from a crowd and the wind, transmission channel or processing noise (lossy compression), data corruption, or recording equipment (imperfections of the hardware). These are not all relevant in every case. For example, quantization noise is rarely an issue anymore because of modern technology. If the noise is statistically of a different nature than the audio that we originally targeted, it is also possible to filter out relatively strong noise. A random background noise can be easily filtered out from periodic waveforms, for example. On the other hand, filtering out strong crowd noise from a single person's speech can be challenging.

For sound classifier applications, if you expect that future data will not be noise free and that the noise cannot be or is not practical to remove, you should also use noisy audio samples for the training procedure. This allows the noise to be trained into the classification framework, making the model more immune and tolerant to the noise. In general, it is good practice to train the system on a relatively large number of sound samples even if they will only differentiate between a few classes. This is because of the huge variability of the audio samples, whose two largest contributors are variability in the source itself and noise.

The amount of noise that can be tolerated will be highly dependent on cases and implementations. For example, the nonspeech human sound classification is tolerant of noise if the signal-to-noise ratio (SNR) reaches approximately 50 dB.[84]

4.17   FUTURE APPLICATIONS

Mobile phones enable people to recognize and analyze sound in their home and work environments. Mobile phone microphones have rapidly improved, but there is room for further innovation. For example, Stethographics has developed a contactless stethoscope. The contactless stethoscope can detect heart and lungs sounds without touching a patient by shining a low-power optical laser onto the chest and detecting reflection. Using a fiber-optic interferometer, the device compares the source signal with the reflected signal and calculates the chest's vibrations. The contactless stethoscope will possibly be useful in the future for monitoring premature newborns and burn victims.

The growing presence of online medical case-sharing communities creates "crowd sources," which help to increase overall diagnostic quality through data mining and machine learning. Perhaps a more challenging task is understanding, annotating, and searching ever-growing online multimedia content. In many cases, we only need to know a broad range of clips before getting to further details, such as wheezing sounds. How can we search for similar sound data that does not have textual descriptions of the sound?

Finally, sound recognition can go beyond auditory vigilance of anomalous sounds and has potential uses in video triage, healthcare, robotics, and security. Using a passive sensing mode, sound recognition is an affordable watchdog.

4.18   SUMMARY

Sound recognition is an essential method for ambient diagnosis. In this chapter, we reviewed contemporary microphones, including MEMS, fiber-optical, and laser sensors. We covered audio data file formats, including WAV, AIFF, MP3, and AMR, as well as the audio editing tools Audacity and FFmpeg. We introduced the Hamming window, which tapers sound signals, and the STFT, which extracts acoustic features and uses PCA to compress the feature vector. Finally, we discussed problems with noisy data and future applications for sound recognition technologies.

---

[84] Wen-Hung Liao and Yu-Kai Lin. Classification of non-speech human sounds: feature selection and snoring sound analysis. In *Proceedings of the 2009 IEEE International Conference on Systems, Man and Cybernetics.* San Antonio, TX, Oct. 11-14, 2009.

PROBLEMS

1. In 1816, Dr. René-Théophile-Hyacinthe Laënnec discovered that he could hear heart sounds more clearly and loudly using mediate auscultation (a stethoscope) rather than immediate auscultation (putting an ear on the chest). This seems counterintuitive. Similar to a garden hose, an increase in the length of a tube will decrease the pressure at the end of the hose as a result of friction and other internal forces. The same effect occurs when the tubing length of a stethoscope is increased. However, in the case of stethoscope tubing, change in length is relatively small, resulting in a decrease in acoustic pressure that is not detectable by the human ear. In addition, as tubing length increases, resonant frequency decreases, meaning that an increase in tubing length provides a better response to lower-frequency sounds. Many heart sounds fall below 150 Hz, which is considered low frequency. Because the human ear is least sensitive to low-frequency sounds, improved low-frequency response is advantageous. Design an experiment to demonstrate this phenomenon.

2. Record ambient sounds such as those from a microwave oven, vacuum, refrigerator, fan, or television in WAV format. Plot spectrograms for ambient sounds.

3. Develop an algorithm to classify the recorded sound files in Problem 2. Report the positive detection rate, missing rate, and false-positive rate in a confusion matrix.

4. After completing Question 3, test whether the *frequency* in a logarithm scale yields better results than a linear scale.

5. After completing Question 3, test whether the *magnitude* in a logarithm scale yields better results than a linear scale.

6. Record sound samples of a bus approaching at a bus station. Plot the spectrograms. Use the Hamming window to obtain the signal frames. Develop an algorithm to detect a bus in sound files using the k-NN. Analyze the sensitivity and specificity of the bus detector.

7. Based on Problem 6, crop the bus samples to keep only the bus signal in the sampling window (see Figure 4.22) and run the algorithm again. Compare the results.

8. Based on Problem 6, crop the bus sample within a particular frequency range and run the algorithm again. Compare the results.

9. Record the approaching and departure sounds of buses and cars. Visualize the data in spectrograms. Study the so-called Doppler effect (the frequency of the sound decreases as the object leaves the sensor and the frequency increases as the object approaches). Develop a simple algorithm to estimate the speed of the buses and cars.

10. If you have an iPhone, download the apps iStethoscope and Blue FiRe. Record the heart sound. Compare the results from the two apps. Summarize findings in a report.

5 Color Vision

5.1 INTRODUCTION

Color is a perception of a light, which can be described as a frequency or a wavelength. Color is a key medium for ambient diagnostics, ranging from skin inspection to colorimetric sensors for smell and chemical compounds. This chapter discusses

- Human color vision
- Color sensors
- Color spaces
- Color segmentation
- Color calibration

In this Chapter, cases of tongue imaging and colorimetric sensors for blood and urine tests and smells of bacteria are also studied.

5.2 COLOR SENSING

Color sensing consists of three elements: light, reflection, and a sensor (Figure 5.1). To see colors, we need a light. To recognize objects, we need to know their reflection and absorption properties. To capture color images, we need a color sensor.

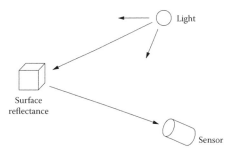

FIGURE 5.1 Color perception from light and reflection sources.

Rapidly growing colorimetric sensors, mobile imaging, computing, and telecommunication technologies enable us to develop affordable personal diagnostic devices.

There are three main applications of human color vision in ambient diagnosis: direct color sensing, indirect color sensing, and remote color sensing.

Direct color sensing is to see the color with the bare eyes (e.g., skin inspection and blood-in-urine detection). *Indirect color sensing* normally involves a physical or chemical reaction that converts a surface of the material to a color. An example is the pH test paper, which converts chemical content into a visible color. *Remote color sensing* involves electronic media to sense, compress, transfer, and display the color from a remote site. For example, a doctor visually examines a patient via a telemedicine system. In this case, the apparent color of a surface varies with illusion, viewpoints, and material properties. A color calibration is needed.

5.3   HUMAN COLOR VISION

Human color vision originates from a basic instinct for survival. For prehistoric humans, the shift in diet from tiny nocturnal insects to red, yellow, and blue fruits, as well as leaves whose nutritional value was color coded in various shades of green, brown, and yellow, propelled the emergence of a sophisticated system for color vision.[85]

The eye structure is complicated (Figure 5.2). It is made up of many layers: On the outside, there is a tough protective layer; then, there is a pigmented vascular layer that stops light from going through; and the innermost layer is the retina, which is composed of many layers itself. The outermost layer contains two types of light-sensitive cells: rods and cones. The cones are scattered among the rods except for in a spot called the fovea near the center, where there are only cones.[86]

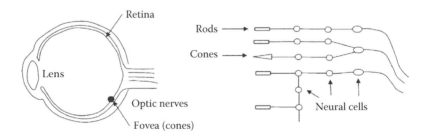

FIGURE 5.2   Human eye structure: retina with light-sensitive rods and cones.

There are three types of cones, which are responsible for color vision; each class is sensitive to one of three overlapping ranges of wavelengths of light, which cover the spectral wavelengths of visible lights from 400 to 800 nm, with maxima at 436, 546, and 580 nm (Figure 5.3). Both rods and cones have an outer segment, loaded with light-sensitive pigment in a stack of flattened membrane bags.

Human color vision is diverse. First, not everyone's color vision is equal. Some people are even color-blind. The color-sensing function can change during the aging

---

[85] V. S. Ramachandran. *The tell-tale brain.* Norton, 2011, p. 42.
[86] David H. Hubel. *Eye, brain and vision.* Scientific American Library, Freeman, New York, 1987.

process. For example, the impressionist painter Claude Monet is believed to have developed cataracts later in life, and the effect may be seen in his paintings. Tones in his later paintings became muddy; whites and green colors became yellow.

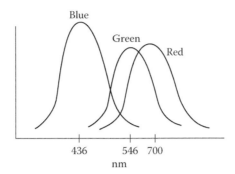

FIGURE 5.3 Color spectrum sensitivity of humans when the peaks are 436, 546, and 700 nm.

Human vision has color consistency. The visual system is constantly adapting to changes in the environment and compares the various colors in a scene to reduce the effects of the illumination. If a scene is illuminated with one light and then with another, as long as the difference between the light sources stays within a reasonable range, the colors in the scene appear relatively constant to us. This was studied by Edwin Land in the 1970's and led to his theory of color constancy.

5.4 COLOR SENSORS

Digital cameras are affordable color sensors; this is especially true for the cameras on mobile phones. Despite their tiny size, the structures of digital cameras are more sophisticated than we can imagine. The quality has been improving dramatically. For example, within merely 5 mm in depth, a phone camera normally contains over six lens components. Behind the lens, there are sensor circuits and a light-sensitive surface on the CMOS (complementary metal oxide semiconductor) image sensor chip.

In a CMOS sensor, each pixel has its own light-to-voltage conversion, and the sensor also includes amplifiers, noise correction, and digitization circuits, so that the chip outputs digital bits. These overhead functions increase the design complexity and reduce the area available for light capture. With each pixel doing its own conversion, uniformity is lower, but it is also massively parallel, allowing for high-speed processing. CMOSs are suitable for high-volume, space-constrained applications where image quality requirements are low. This is a perfect fit for phone cameras and webcams (Figure 5.4).

In a CCD (charge-coupled device), on the other hand, every pixel's signal is transferred through each output node to be converted to voltage and sent out as an analog signal. Because the pixel can be devoted to light capture, the output's uniformity is high, but at the expense of system size. CCD cameras are suitable for high-end applications such as medical imaging.[87]

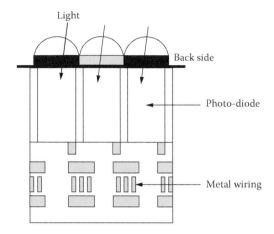

FIGURE 5.4   Back-side illumination of a digital camera in a mobile phone.

Due to the small imaging sensor size, a point-and-shoot camera in dim environments often results in noisy pictures. A larger light-sensitive chip would produce better low-light shots, but it is very expensive. The solution is the back-side illumination (BSI) structure where the light-sensitive silicon surface is placed on top of metal wires, meaning that light will strike the silicon directly, delivering better low-light shots, compared to front-side illumination (FSI) image sensors. Also, the angle at which light can reach the sensor is increased; this enables the use of lenses that are shorter in height. This can slim down camera phones even more.

Similar to human vision, CMOS color sensors have three types of color receptors: red, green, and blue (RGB). Each color receptor has a spectral sensitivity. Figure 5.5 shows the typical spectral sensitivity characteristics of a digital camera.

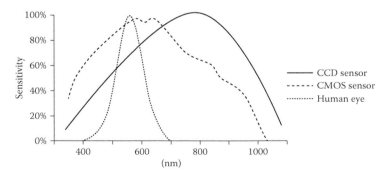

FIGURE 5.5   Spectral sensitivity characteristics for CMOS and human eye.

---

[87] Dave Litwiller. CCD vs. CMOS: facts and fiction. *Photonics Spectra* January 2001.
   https://www.teledynedalsa.com/public/corp/Photonics_Spectra_CCDvsCMOS_Litwiller.pdf

Amazingly enough, many CMOS color sensors can sense near-infrared light (750–1,050 nm), which is both good news and bad news. The good news is that the camera can be used for near-infrared imaging (e.g., detecting infrared light); the bad news is that it causes noises in visible light imaging. Therefore, most digital cameras use an infrared filter to remove the near-infrared light.

5.5 COLOR-MATCHING EXPERIMENTS

In 1853, German scientist Hermann Grassmann conducted the first color-matching experiment. He used three lamps with spectral distributions R (λ = 700 nm), G (λ = 546 nm), and B (λ = 436 nm) and weight factors $r(\lambda)$, $g(\lambda)$, $b(\lambda)$ to match the color impression of the fourth lamp the color impression $F(\lambda)$. Figure 5.6 shows the experimental layout.

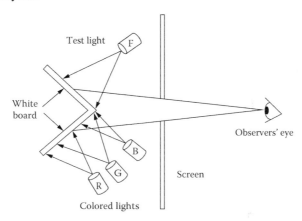

FIGURE 5.6 Layout of Hermann Grassmann's color-matching experiment.

The color impression for the test light $F(\lambda)$ is:

$$F(\lambda) = r(\lambda) \cdot R + g(\lambda) \cdot G + b(\lambda) \cdot B \tag{5.1}$$

In many cases, the match is possible. For example, when the weight factors are in photometric units, we have

$$White\ Light = 1.0000 \cdot R + 4.5907 \cdot G + 0.0601 \cdot B \tag{5.2}$$

However, in other cases, the test color $F(\lambda)$ is saturated. So, we have to mix a certain amount of R to match the color.

$$F(\lambda) + r(\lambda) \cdot R = g(\lambda) \cdot G + b(\lambda) \cdot B \tag{5.3}$$

$$F(\lambda) = -r(\lambda) \cdot R + g(\lambda) \cdot G + b(\lambda) \cdot B \qquad (5.4)$$

This is the introduction of "negative" colors. The equal sign means "matched by." It is generally possible to match a color by three weight factors, but one or even two can be negative. Figure 5.7 shows the resulting *tristimulus values*, which are three values that are used together to describe a color and are the amounts of three reference colors that can be mixed to give the same visual sensation as the color considered.[88]

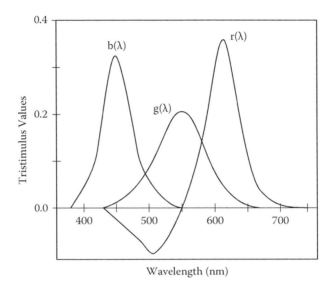

FIGURE 5.7   The original XYZ color-matching function that has negative values.

To avoid negative RGB numbers, the International Commission on Illumination (CIE) introduced a coordinate system CIE XYZ in 1931. For a spectral pure color F with a fixed wavelength λ in the diagram the three values, the color can be mixed by the three standard primaries X, Y, and Z:

$$F(\lambda) = x(\lambda) \cdot X + y(\lambda) \cdot Y + z(\lambda) \cdot Z \qquad (5.5)$$

This linearizes the perceptibility of color differences. Figure 5.8 shows the experimental results after using the XYZ coordination system.

Equation (5.6) is the linear mapping between CIE XYZ and RGB at the luminance D65, where D means daylight. Why do we need the luminance? We need lighting to see the color. Imagine you are walking outside on a night with a full moon. What color can you see? Monitors are assumed D65, but for printed paper, the standard illuminant is D50.

---

[88] N. Ohta and A. Robertson. *Colorimetry: fundamentals and application.* Wiley, New York, 2006.

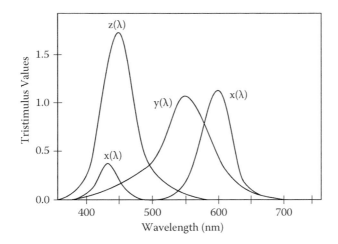

FIGURE 5.8   The XYZ color-matching function that avoids negative RGB values.

$$\begin{bmatrix} X \\ Y \\ Z \end{bmatrix}_{D65} = \begin{bmatrix} 0.4124 & 0.3576 & 0.1805 \\ 0.2126 & 0.7152 & 0.0722 \\ 0.0193 & 0.1192 & 0.9505 \end{bmatrix} \begin{bmatrix} R \\ G \\ B \end{bmatrix}_{D65} \quad (5.6)$$

Therefore, this transformation is recommended if the data are used for printing:

$$\begin{bmatrix} X \\ Y \\ Z \end{bmatrix}_{D50} = \begin{bmatrix} 0.4361 & 0.3851 & 0.1431 \\ 0.2225 & 0.7169 & 0.0606 \\ 0.0139 & 0.0971 & 0.7141 \end{bmatrix} \begin{bmatrix} R \\ G \\ B \end{bmatrix}_{D65} \quad (5.7)$$

CIE XYZ is an absolute color space (is not device dependent). Each visible color has nonnegative coordinates X, Y, Z.

5.6   COLOR SPACES

Color spaces are normally represented by a three-dimensional (3D) system. Here, we introduce RGB, L*a*b*, and HSV (hue, saturation, and value) spaces.[89],[90]

RGB Space

The RGB color space is an intuitive color model because the human visual system also works in RGB color channels. From the three colorants, one can make all possible colors. The RGB system is normally represented in three bytes $(2^8)^3 = 16$ million distinct color codes, but human eyes can only distinguish thousands. In computer

---

[89] Color conversion algorithms. http://www.cs.rit.edu/~ncs/color/t_convert.html
[90] Gernot Hoffmann. CIE color space. November 2, 2010. http://www.fho-emden.de/~hoffmann/

programming, we often use the RGB values in a 3D array, ranging from [0, 0, 0] to [255, 255, 255].

The most commonly used RGB color space is sRGB. The sRGB is a standard RGB color space created by HP and Microsoft in 1996 for measurements on monitors, printers, and the Internet. The sRGB color space is designed to match typical home and office viewing conditions, instead of the typical dark lab environment used for commercial color matching.

Converting a color image to a grayscale image is simply taking an average of the three colors. Assume I is the intensity of the pixel:

$$I = (R + G + B)/3 \tag{5.8}$$

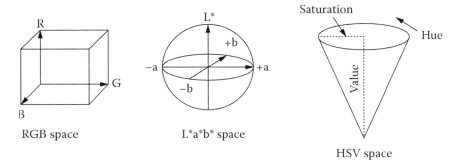

FIGURE 5.9   RGB, L*a*b*, and HSV color spaces.

CIE L*a*b* Space

CIE L*a*b* is mainly used to measure color lighting. It is a nonlinear transformation of XYZ into coordinates L*, a*, b*. CIE 1976 L*a*b* was intended to mimic the logarithmic response of the eye (Figure 5.9).

The three coordinates of CIE L*a*b* represent the lightness of the color ($L^* = 0$ yields black, and $L^* = 100$ indicates diffuse white; specular white may be higher); its position between red/magenta and green (a^*, negative values indicate green while positive values indicate magenta), and its position between yellow and blue (b^*, negative values indicate blue and positive values indicate yellow). The asterisks (*) after L, a, and b are pronounced *star* and are part of the full name since they represent L^*, a^*, and b^*. L*a*b* decomposes a trichromatic space to the luminance illumination and two-dimensional chrominance space.

If we ignore the illumination factor, then we can compress the pixel data to two dimensions. Coloring information is referred to the color of the white point of the system, subscript n.

$$L* = \begin{cases} 116 \cdot \left(Y/Y_n\right)^{1/3} - 16 & \text{for } Y/Y_n > 0.008856 \\ 903.3 \cdot Y/Y_n & \text{otherwise} \end{cases}$$

$$a* = 500 \cdot \left(f\left(X/X_n\right) - f\left(Y/Y_n\right)\right)$$

$$b* = 200 \cdot \left(f\left(Y/Y_n\right) - f\left(Z/Z_n\right)\right)$$

where

$$f(t) = \begin{cases} t^{1/3} & \text{for } t > 0.008856 \\ 7.787 \cdot t + 16/116 & \text{otherwise} \end{cases} \tag{5.9}$$

HSV Space

HSV (hue, saturation, and value) commonly measures paint colors. The HSV model was created by A. R. Smith in 1978. It is based on such intuitive color characteristics as tint, shade, and tone (or family, purity, and intensity).

$$H = \arccos \frac{\frac{1}{2}\left((R-G)+(R-B)\right)}{\sqrt{\left((R-G)^2 + (R-B)(G-B)\right)}} \tag{5.10}$$

$$S = 1 - 3\frac{\min(R,G,B)}{R+G+B} \tag{5.11}$$

$$V = \frac{1}{3}(R+G+B) \tag{5.12}$$

Fortunately, MATLAB has functions for the conversions between color spaces. Assume M is the input matrix:

G = rgb2gray(M);

Lab = rgb2lab(M);

RGB = lab2rgb(M);

HSV = rgb2hsv(M);

RGB = hsv2rgb(M);

Color Gamut

A color gamut is a subset of colors that can be accurately reproduced in a given circumstance, such as a given output device or a given color space. In color theory, the gamut of a device or process is that portion of the color space that can be represented, or reproduced. When certain colors cannot be expressed within a particular color model, these colors are said to be out of gamut. For example, the CIE L*a*b* color space cannot be expressed in the RGB color space on a monitor; the color is out of gamut in the RGB color space (Figure 5.10).

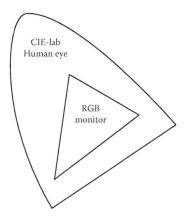

FIGURE 5.10 Color gamut Venn diagram for the CIE L*a*b* space and RGB monitor color space.

Color Compression

In digital image processing, we can use L*a*b* to decompose a trichromatic space to the luminance illumination and two-dimensional chrominance space. If we ignore the illumination factor, then we can compress the pixel data to two dimensions.

In digital video products and compression algorithms, the luminance and chrominance are encoded in different lengths since our eyes are more sensitive to the change of luminance than colors.

The YCrCb color compression format is commonly used by European television studios and for image compression work. Y is luminance (perceptual brightness), Cr is chrominance red channel, and Cb is chrominance blue channel (Figure 5.11).

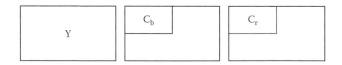

FIGURE 5.11 Decomposition of a color image into Y, Cb, and Cr channels at a 4:2:0 compression (4:4:4 is all channels in full resolution, 4:2:2 is Cr and Cb in half the horizontal resolution of Y, and 4:2:0 is Cr and Cb in one-fourth the resolution of Y).

The conversion from RGB to YCrCb is as follows:

$$Y = 0.299R + 0.587G + 0.114B$$

$$C_b = 0.564(B - Y) \qquad (5.13)$$

$$C_r = 0.713(R - Y)$$

YIQ color compression is commonly used by the National Television System Committee (NTSC) television systems in North America. Assume Y is the luminance value; I (red-cyan) and Q (magenta-green) are chromaticity values. The relationship between YIQ and RGB spaces is as follows:

$$Y = 0.30R + 0.59G + 0.11B$$

$$I = 0.60R - 0.28G - 0.32B \qquad (5.14)$$

$$Q = 0.21R - 0.52G + 0.31B$$

The multimedia formats JPEG and MPEG use YUV encoding. Similarly, assume Y is luminance and U and V are chromaticity. The conversion of RGB to YUV is as follows:

$$Y = 0.30R + 0.59G + 0.11B$$

$$U = 0.493(B - Y) \qquad (5.15)$$

$$V = 0.877(R - Y)$$

YCrCb, YIQ, and YUV allow us to encode luminance and chromaticity values in different resolutions in which our eyes can hardly perceive the difference.

5.7 COLOR SEGMENTATION

Color segmentation is a simple approach for object detection and classification. Color-based methods, however, are not robust because they are sensitive to the imaging environments and variation of the object's color. For example, color-based methods normally work well in a well-controlled lighting environment such as microscopic imaging. However, they perform poorly in many uncontrollable environments, such as outdoors, or with incoherent color features, such as skin colors of different races. If the face recognition system was trained with Caucasian faces, then it may not be able to detect an African American face. There is a video that provides an example of the problem.[91]

By all means, skin detection is important for human detection, face detection and tracking, hand tracking, tongue inspection, gesture recognition, and other video and image applications, such as a filter for pornographic content on the Internet. Skin features allow fast processing, and it is robust to geometric variations of the skin patterns. It is robust under partial occlusion and resolution changes. It can eliminate the

---

[91] http://www.youtube.com/watch?v=R-vGGBBPyIc

need for cumbersome tracking devices or artificially placed color cues. Studies suggest that human skin has a characteristic color that is easily recognized by humans. However, skin color depends on race, lighting conditions, and emotion. Here we discuss two approaches: pixel-based and region-based methods.

Pixel-Based Method

This section discusses the pixel-based method.[92,93,94,95,96] For color segmentation, we convert the color space to L*a*b* so that we can ignore the lighting factor and only consider the two-dimensional chromatic space $a*$ and $b*$ (Figure 5.12). Studies showed that removing the illumination component not only generalizes the training dataset but also increases the overlap between the object and background pixels.[97]

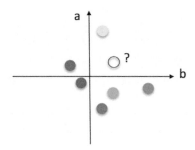

FIGURE 5.12   The k-nearest neighbor for color segmentation in L*a*b* space. The circular points are skin color markers (training samples).

Assume we want to detect a color in an image (e.g., a human skin tone). We would first to create a color marker by taking n samples and calculate the mean of the sample colors $S_{a,i}$ and $S_{b,i}$, where a and b are color values in L*a*b* and i is the index.

For skin detection, we need to see whether the Euclidean distance between the color marker (training samples) and the input pixel color (a and b) is less than a threshold T. If we want to detect or classify m colors based on n color markers, we can use the k-nearest neighbor method. Assume k is the number of Euclidean distances to be considered for the nearest neighbors.

[92] V. Vezhnevets. A survey on pixel-based skin color detection techniques. In *Proceedings of Graphicon* pp. 85–92, 2003.

[93] Michael J. Jones and James R. Rehg. Statistical color models with application to skin detection. *International Journal of Computer Vision* 46:81–96, 2002.

[94] D. Zarit. Comparison of five color models in skin pixel classification. Proceedings of RATFG-RTS'99, page 58, ACM Digital Library, 1999.

[95] A. Albiol, L. Torres, and E.J. Delp. Optimum color spaces for skin detection. In *Proceedings of the 2001 International Conference on Image Processing*, 1:122–124.

[96] Min C. Shin. Does color space transformation make any difference on skin detection? Sixth IEEE Workshop on Applications of Computer Vision, 2002 (WACV 2002).

[97] N. Rasiwasia. Color space for skin detection—a review, online. http://www.svcl.ucsd.edu/~nikux/skin/ Color%20Space%20for%20skin%20segmentation.ppt

$$D = \sum_{i=1}^{K} \sqrt{\left(S_{a,i} - a\right)^2 + \left(S_{b,i} - b\right)^2} \leq T \qquad (5.16)$$

If the summary of distances to the skin color is shorter than the background, then the color is classified as a skin tone. To improve the accuracy, we can use statistical methods found in the references or the regional-based method discussed next.

Region-Based Methods

The idea of region-based methods is to take the shape information into account during the detection stage. To do so, we need additional models, such as those for shape, size, texture, and so on.

For example, we can define an edge template for a facial area, using the edge filter on a black-and-white image for extraction.[98] Compose an average face using edges, scaled to mean zero. The peak of edge response is the centroid of the face.

We can count the region-based edge outlines that have clearly identifiable connected regions. To avoid too many small regions, scaling down the image can generate larger segmented regions.

In addition, we can use proportion of height and width for filtering. For face shapes, we know that the height is larger than the width. Figure 5.13 shows an example of face detection based on color and edge information.

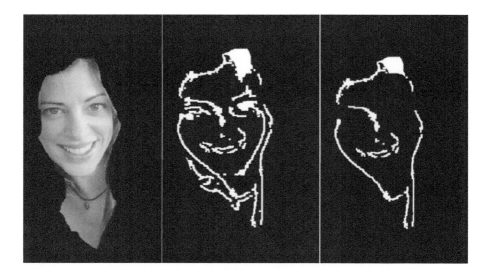

FIGURE 5.13 Region-based color segmentation: segmented skin area (left), regions from edge detection (middle), and reduced region by using lower-resolution image (right).

---

[98] In MATLAB, the edge detection function is edge('matrix','canny').

5.8   COLOR CONSISTENCY CALIBRATION

In diagnoses, we have to take images from different lighting conditions using different cameras. How can we get the same perception of a color from different lighting conditions or cameras? Here, we study how to use the embedded color calibration checkboard to preserve color consistency.[99] Figure 5.14 shows a typical miniature board with 24 color patches, numbered from top left to bottom right row by row. Each color patch has ground-truth values (sRGB and L*a*b*).

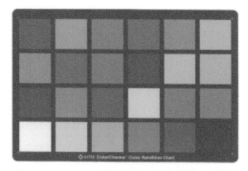

FIGURE 5.14   Color calibration board. More details can be found at http://en.wikipedia.org/wiki/ColorChecker.

Given n patches from an input image, we have a color matrix X_{ij}, where i is the index of the patch, and j is the color channel index. Let us consider a three-dimensional color space. Assume we have the ground truths for the color values on each patch Y_{ij}, where i is the index of the patch and j is the color channel index. We then can find a linear 3×3 color calibration matrix $\underset{3\times3}{A}$. Note that we have the underscore notation to illustrate the dimensions of the matrix. For example, 3×3 means a matrix with 3 by 3 elements.

$$
\underset{n\times3}{Y} = \underset{n\times3}{X} \cdot \underset{3\times3}{A} =
\begin{bmatrix}
y_{11} & y_{12} & y_{13} \\
y_{21} & y_{22} & y_{23} \\
y_{31} & y_{32} & y_{33} \\
\vdots & & \\
y_{n1} & y_{n2} & y_{n3}
\end{bmatrix}
=
\begin{bmatrix}
x_{11} & x_{12} & x_{13} \\
x_{21} & x_{22} & x_{23} \\
x_{31} & x_{32} & x_{33} \\
\vdots & & \\
x_{n1} & x_{n2} & x_{n3}
\end{bmatrix}
\cdot
$$

$$
\begin{bmatrix}
a_{11} & a_{12} & a_{13} \\
a_{21} & a_{22} & a_{23} \\
a_{31} & a_{32} & a_{33}
\end{bmatrix}
\tag{5.17}
$$

---

[99] http://www.babelcolor.com/main_level/ColorChecker.htm

The squared error between the input color and the ground truth is

$$\varepsilon^2 = \left\| \underset{n \times 3}{X} \cdot \underset{3 \times 3}{A} - \underset{n \times 3}{Y} \right\|^2 \tag{5.18}$$

Let us minimize the squared errors:

$$\min \left\| \underset{n \times 3}{X} \cdot \underset{3 \times 3}{A} - \underset{n \times 3}{Y} \right\|^2 \tag{5.19}$$

We have:

$$= \left(\underset{n \times 3}{X} \cdot \underset{3 \times 3}{A} - \underset{n \times 3}{Y} \right)^T \left(\underset{n \times 3}{X} \cdot \underset{3 \times 3}{A} - \underset{n \times 3}{Y} \right)$$

$$= \left(\underset{3 \times 3}{A^T} \cdot \underset{3 \times n}{X^T} - \underset{3 \times n}{Y^T} \right) \left(\underset{n \times 3}{X} \cdot \underset{3 \times 3}{A} - \underset{n \times 3}{Y} \right)$$

$$= \underset{3 \times 3}{A^T} \cdot \underset{3 \times n}{X^T} \cdot \underset{n \times 3}{X} \cdot \underset{3 \times 3}{A} - \underset{3 \times 3}{A^T} \cdot \underset{3 \times n}{X^T} \cdot \underset{n \times 3}{Y} - \underset{3 \times n}{Y^T} \underset{n \times 3}{X} \cdot \underset{3 \times 3}{A} - \underset{3 \times n}{Y^T} \cdot \underset{n \times 3}{Y} \tag{5.20}$$

Now, take a gradient of this expression[100] and set it to zero:

$$2 \underset{3 \times n}{X^T} \cdot \underset{n \times 3}{X} \cdot \underset{3 \times 3}{A} - \underset{3 \times n}{X^T} \cdot \underset{n \times 3}{Y} - \underset{3 \times n}{X^T} \cdot \underset{n \times 3}{Y} = 0$$

$$\underset{3 \times n}{X^T} \cdot \underset{n \times 3}{X} \cdot \underset{3 \times 3}{A} = \underset{3 \times n}{X^T} \cdot \underset{n \times 3}{Y}$$

$$\underset{3 \times 3}{A} = \left(\underset{3 \times n}{X^T} \cdot \underset{n \times 3}{X} \right)^{-1} \cdot \underset{3 \times n}{X^T} \cdot \underset{n \times 3}{Y} \tag{5.21}$$

Finally, we obtain the 3×3 color calibration matrix A for n pixels. Assume we have an image with $(r \times c)$ pixels. At row r, each column j of the input image X, we can calculate the output column j in the calibrated image Y'.

$$\underset{r \times 3}{Y'_j} = \underset{r \times 3}{X_j} \cdot \underset{3 \times 3}{A} \qquad j = 1, 2, \ldots, c \tag{5.22}$$

An example of the calibration process is shown in Figure 5.15, including the original image and the calibrated results. The color version of this figure is available for download from the publisher's web site.

---

[100] For a list of properties, see http://en.wikipedia.org/wiki/Matrix_calculus

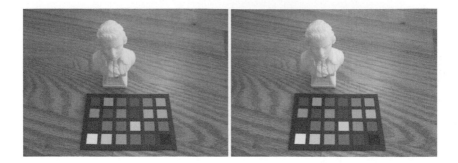

FIGURE 5.15   Color calibration result: original (left) and reconstructed image (right).

5.9   SURFACE COLOR DIAGNOSIS

Color vision is a primitive diagnostic method. For over two thousand years, physical inspection has been a unique and important diagnostic method of traditional Chinese medicine (TCM). For instance, observing abnormal changes in the tongue can aid in diagnosing diseases. Clinical statistics show that there are significant changes of surface color, coating, shape, and dorsum shape of the tongues of the patients with digestive diseases versus the tongues of healthy patients.

Modern Western medicine also uses tongue color for health diagnoses (e.g., in diagnosing vitamin B_{12} deficiency).[101] Vitamin B_{12} is required for proper red blood cell formation, neurological function, and DNA synthesis. It is naturally found in the animals we eat, such as seafood. Although the animals themselves do not synthesize the vitamin, bacteria that live symbiotically within the animals form B_{12} as a by-product. Vegetarians normally can obtain B_{12} from breakfast cereals. Dietary supplements also provide an animal-free source, and while it acts fundamentally the same as natural sources, it is not readily absorbed. Studies show that only a very small fraction of the B_{12} provided in pill form actually is used; the rest is converted into incredibly bright yellow urine (which is discussed in Chapter 12). Deficiencies in B_{12} result in symptoms of fatigue, headaches, depression, and weight loss, among others. This is easily seen on the tongue, which can turn pale, swell, and bleed. Figure 5.16 shows an example of B_{12} deficiency symptom.

Unfortunately, TCM requires an experienced doctor to inspect the tongue with his or her bare eyes. The human factors in the inspection have a significant impact on the accuracy and repeatability of the diagnostic method.

A computerized tongue inspection system is necessary for quantitatively measuring the physical appearances of the tongue so that the inspection results can be repeatable and comparable. Ultimately, it is desirable to build affordable devices for ambient diagnosis.

To achieve this, first we need to calibrate color tongue images under different lighting conditions and with different cameras. In 2002, Cai introduced a linear

---

[101] http://ods.od.nih.gov/factsheets/VitaminB12-HealthProfessional/

color calibration method with CIE L*a*b* color, which was one of the early attempts to build an affordable tongue diagnostic system.[102]

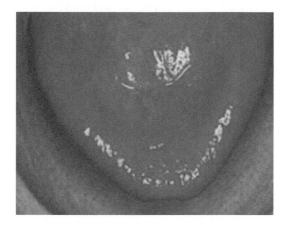

FIGURE 5.16 Vitamin B_{12} deficiency can make the tongue swell, bleed, and turn a strawberry color. (Adapted from C. Scully and D.H. Felix, *British Dental Journal* 199:639–645, 2005. Courtesy of *British Dental Journal* with license number 3195840452758).

To ensure color consistency under different lighting conditions, we must calibrate the color, in particular, the white balance and the interpretation of sensor input from the digital camera. The interpretation of the sensor's color signals will depend on the sensor itself and the software of the camera and in general will be different across camera vendors and models. With a digital camera, the input images are represented in an sRGB absolute color space.

By having some areas in an image with known physical colors, it is possible to estimate the real color of other areas. Here, we can embed a color calibration board in each of the tongue images. Then, using the known physical color patches of such a board and the observed colors of the same board in the image, we can calculate a color calibration matrix. In this case, a Munsell ColorChecker Mini[103] can be used in experiments. We can embed the board in each image by placing the board near the tongue during imaging acquisition. The image should be taken under sufficient lighting conditions, and no shadows should be cast on the board or on the tongue proper. The board should be slightly facing the light source instead of directly perpendicular to the plane of the camera lens to ensure that the board receives enough light. Before imaging, the exposure should be set so that no under- or overexposure occurs. The white balance should be set to the closest that corresponds to the current lighting conditions (e.g., set to fluorescent or incandescent light in an office environment). Then, the image should be captured with good focus.

---

[102] Yang Cai. A novel imaging system for tongue inspection. In *Proceedings of IEEE IMTC*, Anchorage, Alaska, 2005.

[103] At the end of 2010, the ColorChecker Mini had been replaced by the X-Rite ColorChecker Passport product.

Using the color consistency calibration model discussed, we can recover the realistic color under normal lighting. Figure 5.17 shows the result after the calibration. Table 5.1 and Table 5.2 summarize the color errors before and after calibration, respectively.

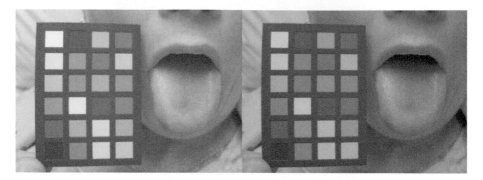

FIGURE 5.17   Recovering the tongue color: original (left) and result (right).

TABLE 5.1 Error before Calibration

	Red	Green	Blue
Mean error	135.71	63.90	62.70
Max error	242.00	201.00	224.00
Min error	7.00	0.00	0.00
Error STD	63.71	53.41	59.93

TABLE 5.2 Error after Calibration

	Red	Green	Blue
Mean error	14.73	7.38	9.94
Max error	48.00	41.00	52.00
Min error	0.00	0.00	0.00
Error STD	9.50	7.90	8.33

There are further developments for improving the color calibration methods. For example, Cao et al. developed a device specifically for acquiring tongue images to solve the problem of lighting variations and color calibration.[104] Other efforts aim to map physical features of the tongue to the semantic features in terms of TCM, such as purple color, grimy coating, and papillae.[105,106] This approach enables TCM doctors to understand the computational results. However, the approach has two problems: The verbal descriptions of the TCM tongue types vary from person to person, and the mapping alone does not warrant an accurate disease diagnosis model. To go beyond the heuristic mapping between semantic TCM features and diseases, a computational classifier is needed.

---

[104] Meiling Cao, Yiheng Cai, Changjiang Liu, and Lansun Shen. Recent progress in new portable device for tongue image analysis. In *2008 International Conference on Neural Networks and Signal Processing*, Nanjing, 2008, pp. 488–492.

[105] Chuang-Chien Chiu. A novel approach based on computerized image analysis for traditional Chinese medical diagnosis of the tongue. *Computer Methods and Programs in Biomedicine* 61(2):77–89, 2000.

[106] Bo Pang, David Zhang, Naimin Li, and Kuanquan Wang. Computerized tongue diagnosis based on Bayesian networks. *IEEE Transactions on Biomedical Engineering* 10:1803–1810 (2004).

Several classifiers based on machine learning have been developed to represent the correlation between tongue features and diseases. For examples, Cai et al. used radial basis function neural networks for diagnosing precancerous colon polyps.[107] Li et al.[108] used kernel principal component analysis (PCA) and Gabor wavelets to construct global and local features. Wang et al.[109] used color segmentation and a nearest neighbor classifier to classify the tongue surface and color. Pang and Wang, et al.[110,111] used a Bayesian network model to classify common diseases based on the tongue image. The model is also used for diagnosing appendicitis.[112]

The support vector machine (SVM) method has also been used for tongue diagnoses. Gao and Hui, et al.[113,114] conducted a comparative study between the SVM classifier and the Bayesian network for tongue diagnosis. The study concluded that the SVM produced better results. Building a classifier is trivial these days because most of the models are widely available online. Typical machine learning models do not describe which features are really significant to the diagnosis. How to validate the results of a classifier is critical.

Recently, researchers also explored new features through image processing and multispectrum imaging. For examples, Li et al. used a hyperspectral imaging technique to improve classification of tongues based on color.[115,116] Spectrum imaging provides more accurate tongue feature measurements. However, it normally requires special hardware and special lab environments that are less accessible to home users.[117]

---

[107] Y. Cai, G. Li, T. Mick, Sai Ho Chung, and B. Pham. Ambient diagnostics. In *Ambient intelligence for scientific discovery, LNAI*. Springer-Verlag, New York, 2005, pp. 224–247.

[108] W. Li, J. Xu, C. Zhou, and Z. Zhang. A novel method of tongue image recognition. In *Fifth International Conference on Computer and Information Technology (CIT'05)*, Shanghai, 2005, pp. 586–590.

[109] Ibid.

[110] Pang et al., Computerized tongue diagnosis.

[111] H. Wang and X. Zong. A new computerized method for tongue classification. In *IEEE Proceedings of the Sixth International Conference on Intelligent Systems Design and Applications, 2*. Washington, DC, 2006, pp. 508–511.

[112] Bo Pang, David Zhang, and Kuanquan Wang. Tongue image analysis for appendicitis diagnosis. *Information Sciences* 175(3):160–176, 2005.

[113] Z. Gao, Lai-Man Po, W. Jiang, X. Zhao, and H. Dong. A novel computerized method based on support vector machine for tongue diagnosis. In *Third International IEEE Conference on Signal-Image Technologies and Internet-Based System,* Shanghai, 2007, pp. 849–854.

[114] Siu Cheung Hui, Yulan He, and Doan Thi Cam Thach. Machine learning for tongue diagnosis. In *6th International Conference on Information, Communications and Signal Processing*, Singapore, 2007, pp. 1–5.

[115] Qingli Li and Z. Liu. Tongue color analysis and discrimination based on hyperspectral images. *Computerized Medical Imaging and Graphics* 33(3):217–221, 2009.

[116] Qingli Li, Yiting Wang, Hongying Liu, and Zhen Sun. AOTF based hyperspectral tongue imaging system and its applications in computer-aided tongue disease diagnosis. In *3rd International Conference on Biomedical Engineering and Informatics*, Yantai, 2010, pp. 1424–1427.

[117] Xu Jiatuo, Liping Tu, Hongfu Ren, and Zhifeng Zhang. Diagnostic method based on tongue imaging morphology. In *The 2nd International Conference on Bioinformatics and Biomedical Engineering,* 2008, pp. 2613–2616.

5.10   COLORIMETRIC PAPER SENSOR: LAB ON PAPER

Using paper in diagnostic tests is not entirely new.[118,119,120] Pregnancy test kits soak up urine and diabetes test kits soak up blood in the home and are administered by untrained eyes. The colorimetric paper sensor is a chemistry laboratory that fits on a postage stamp and costs less than a penny. The new approach is to miniaturize diagnostic tests so they can move into the field with tiny pumps and thread-thin tubes so a drop of blood or urine could soak its way through a square of filter paper etched with tiny channels (Figure 5.18). Along the pathway, the fluid is diffused with dried proteins and chemically triggered dyes, and the thumbnail-size square could be a minilaboratory, which can be run by the millions on an ink-jet printer or a 3D printer.

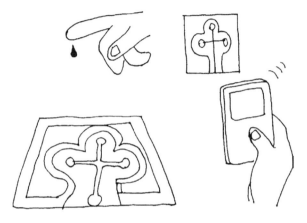

FIGURE 5.18   Colorimetric paper sensor: a drop of blood as the input, a cell phone as the image analyzer and the telemedicine media.

The key component of this technology invented by George Whitesides' lab is the microfluid channels in the multiple-layer paper where a patient's blood is soaked into the forked channels with embedded reactive chemicals to produce the diagnostic colors—similar to the home pregnancy test kit, except that the chips are smaller and cheaper and test for multiple diseases simultaneously. Instead of a simple positive or negative reading, the results also illustrate the severity of the disease. The chips can quickly identify those people living in remote parts of the world who warrant more serious medical attention.

[118] C. J. Musto, S. H. Lim, and K. Suslick. Colorimetric detection and identification of natural and artificial sweeteners. *Analytical Chemistry* 81:6526–6533, 2009. http://www.scs.illinois.edu/suslick/documents/us6495102b1.p1.pdf

[119] C. Zhang and K. S. Suslick. Colorimetric sensor arrays for soft drink analysis. *Journal of Agricultural Food Chemistry* 55:237–242, 2007.

[120] C. Zhang, D. P. Bailey, and K. S. Suslick. Colorimetric sensor arrays for the analysis of beers: a feasibility study. *Journal of Agricultural Food Chemistry* 54:4925–4931, 2006.

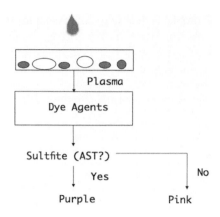

FIGURE 5.19   Liver test process.

Taking liver tests for example, the paper diagnostic sensor assesses the level of the enzyme aspartate transaminase (AST) in the blood. The AST level is elevated when liver cells break down. When a drop of blood reaches the back of the square of paper, it seeps through a membrane with pores that only allow the clear plasma to pass. Then, the next layer contains two dried chemicals. If AST is present, then it binds to the two chemicals, causing a reaction to release sulfite. The next layer contains a methyl dye that is normally blue but becomes colorless when sulfites attach to it. It is printed over a pink background, so the spot looks purple. If the layer changes to light purple, the blood contains dangerous levels of AST (Figure 5.19).[121]

The pseudocode of the liver test is as follows:

1.   Drop a blood sample on the test paper.
2.   Filter out red blood cells and white blood cells.
3.   If AST exists, then bind the two dried chemicals and release sulfite.
4.   If sulfite exists, then the paper turns to purple.

The user can use a mobile phone to take a photo of the test paper with a color calibration board around it. The program processes the color calibration, locates the individual diagnostic sensors on the paper, and classifies the sensory data. The results can be wirelessly transmitted to medical professionals for further diagnosis.

5.11   COLORIMETRIC SMELL SENSORS

The olfactory system is a primitive sensor for mammals. Olfactory signals are directly connected to our nervous systems, triggering alertness, emotion, and memory. Smells are effective indications of diseases such as infection of the gum and

---

[121] G. Whitesides. Cool, or simple and cheap? Why not both? *Lab Chip* 13:11, 2013. http://gmwgroup. harvard.edu/pubs/pdf/1173.pdf

skin, as well as digestion problems. Bacteria emit a complex mixture of chemicals as by-products of their metabolism. Each species of bacteria produces its own unique blend of gases, and even differing strains of the same species will have an aromatic "fingerprint," with bacteria simply micron-size chemical factories that exhaust pollutants. The new colorimetric smell sensor technology[122,123,124] is for detecting and distinguishing among different odorants (Figure 5.20).

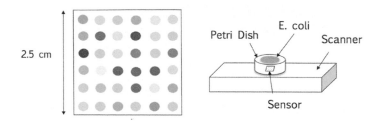

FIGURE 5.20 Colorimetric sensor array used for bacterial identification experiments (Modified from Professor K. S. Suslick's articles with permission. James R. Carey, et al. *Journal of the American Chemical Society* 133:7571–7576, 2011.)

The artificial nose is an array of 36 pigment dots that change color when they sense chemicals in the air. Researchers spread blood samples on sample dishes (Petri dishes) of a standard growth gel, attached an array to the inside of the lid of each dish, and then put the dishes upside down onto an ordinary flatbed scanner. Every thirty minutes, they scanned the arrays and recorded the color changes in each dot. The pattern of color change over time is unique to each bacterium. The progression of the pattern change is part of the diagnosis of which bacteria it is, similar to time-lapse photography, a motion of the frames over time (Figure 5.21).

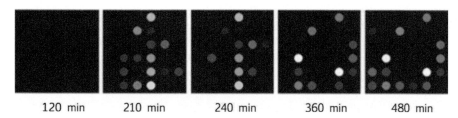

| 120 min | 210 min | 240 min | 360 min | 480 min |

FIGURE 5.21 The time-lapse images of the colorimetric sensor array with the cultured *Escherichia coli* bacteria in a petri dish, developed by Ken S. Suslick of the University of Illinois. The black background is a difference map of the color change after exposure minus before exposure. (Modified from Ken Suslick's articles with permission. James R. Carey, et al. *Journal of the American Chemical Society* 133:7571–7576, 2011)

---

122 B. Suslick, L. Feng, and K. S. Suslick. Discrimination of complex mixtures by colorimetric sensor array: coffee aromas. *Analytical Chemistry* 82(5):2067–2073, 2010.

123 N. A. Rakow and K. S. Suslick. A colorimetric sensor array for odour visualization. *Nature* 406:710–714, 2000.

124 James R. Carey, Kenneth S. Suslick, et al. Rapid identification of bacteria with a disposable colorimetric sensing array. *Journal of the American Chemical Society* 133:7571–7576, 2011. Online edition.

Given their broad sensitivity, the chemical-sensing arrays also could enable breath diagnosis for a number of conditions (e.g., using these arrays to diagnose sinus infections and screen for lung cancer).

The pseudocode for the smell sensor is as follows:

1. Spray sample on the colorimetric sensor paper.
2. Use grow gel to culture the sample.
3. Repeat every 30 minutes.
4.   Color imaging.
5.   Until terminate time.
6. Feature dimension reduction.
7. Clustering analysis.

Principal component analysis can be used to reduce the dimensions of features to the three most important principal components based on all trials of bacterial strains and controls. The resolution between bacterial classes is in fact much better than can be shown by any 3D PCA plot because the first three principal components account for only 79% of the total variance.

A case study of all of the ten strains of bacteria, including *Enterococcus faecalis* and *Staphylococcus aureus*, showed that bacteria were identified with 98.8% accuracy within ten hours, a clinically important time frame. For example, hospitals have used blood cultures as the standard for identifying blood-borne bacterial infections. The major problem with clinical blood culturing is that it takes too long. The process usually takes 24 to 48 hours. After a culture is positive, doctors still need to identify which species and strain of bacteria is present, a process that can take up to another day. Therefore, in 72 hours doctors may have diagnosed the problem, but the patient may already have died.

5.12   SUMMARY

Color vision has two major applications in ambient diagnosis: human color perception and automated computer color vision. Both human vision and computer vision are nonlinear to color stimuli. Color spaces were introduced to linearize the color expressions and mimic human color impression. Those equations are not just mathematical creations but are based on painstaking color-matching experiments and "data mining" in the 1930s. Color compression allows us to encode luminance and chromaticity values in different resolutions, in which our eyes can hardly perceive the difference because our retina is more sensitive to luminance changes rather than chromaticity changes.

Color sensors are simulations of human color vision (e.g., RGB channels). Color segmentation is a simple way to detect skin and other color-rich objects. However, color in an image is not a robust feature because of the impact of lighting, reflection, and distance. A color calibration is needed to reduce the color noises so that the color values can be measured correctly. The calibration model plays an essential role in color-based diagnostic methods, such as tongue imaging, based on TCM. Finally, two groundbreaking colorimetric methods are introduced here: chemical sensors on paper and smell sensors. Both are affordable to make based on existing technologies. The color values can either be inspected by the user or processed on a mobile phone automatically.

PROBLEMS

1. Some animals have better color vision than humans; for example, mantis shrimps have twelve color pigments versus the three that are in human eyes.[125] Write a survey about animal color vision and discuss potentials in diagnostics.
2. In digital video products and compression algorithms, luminance and chrominance are encoded in different lengths since our eyes are more sensitive to the change of luminance than colors. Design an experiment using a computer to test the assumption.
3. In 1996, the team of computer vision expert David Forsyth developed a remarkable algorithm for detecting a naked body in an image.[126] Read the related literatures on that web page. Summarize the algorithm in a pseudo-code. Write a description of the algorithm. Discuss its potential in ambient diagnosis.
4. For the color calibration algorithm, how many sample pixels are needed as a minimum?
5. The Muncell ColorCheck board takes away about half the space of the image. Design an alternative that can save more space for imaging the tongue.
6. Given an uncalibrated color image with Muncell ColorCheck board embedded, reproduce the color image that is close to its original color under an ideal lighting situation.
7. Design an algorithm that can automatically find the centers of color patches on the ColorCheck board.
8. Select ten of your own photos and reduce them to a size of 6 × 6 pixels each. Use the PCA method to reduce the feature dimensions.
9. Use a dendrogram and k-means to cluster the data from Problem 8. Compare the results.
10. Select ten color portraits. Segment the skin color in RGB and L*a*b* spaces. Compare the results.

---

[125] https://en.wikipedia.org/wiki/Mantis_shrimp
[126] http://luthuli.cs.uiuc.edu/~daf/tracking.html

6 Kinect Sensors

> The Kinect is more than a toy: it is a revolution in the making.
>
> —The New Scientist

6.1 INTRODUCTION

Kinect is derived from the words *kinetic* and *connect*. It is a revolutionary imaging sensor featuring a depth sensor that consists of an infrared projector and imaging sensor, a color camera, and a multiarray microphone enabling acoustic source localization and ambient noise suppression. Thanks to brave hackers that the open source application programming interfaces (APIs) are possible. Now, Kinect can be sold as a stand-alone sensor. It has been broadly used for many applications relevant to ambient diagnostics, including robotics, three-dimensional (3D) modeling, biometrics, training, clothes fitting, and motion capture (Figure 6.1).

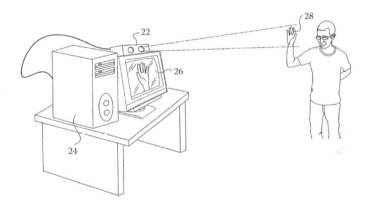

FIGURE 6.1 Pictorial schematic of a system for 3D mapping. (Illustrated in Alexander Shupunt and Zeev Zalevshy's U.S. patent US8390821 B2, assigned by Prime Sense Limited, filed May 8, 2007.)

This chapter addresses the following questions:

- Is Kinect a revolution?
- How does Kinect work?
- How does Kinect track objects?
- How does Kinect compare gestures?
- How does Kinect recognize gestures?

- How does Kinect make a high-resolution surface model?
- How can Kinect be used for measuring biometrics?
- How does Kinect locate the sound source?

6.2   THE KINECT REVOLUTION

The Kinect is integrated with many new concepts of the digital age, including vision on chip, disruptive price, overdrive design, fabless industry, and crowdsourcing.

Vision on Chip

For decades, developers have tried to make sensors that recognize and track human gestures in 3D space. Stereovision is designed to mimic human perception to create a 3D model, but it does not work well in low-lighting conditions; infrared sensors can track human motion in the dark, but they usually require infrared reflective markers on the body they are tracking. Besides, these sensors are so expensive that they are only used in highly technical environments such as research labs, robotics, and industry. Two decades ago, robotics scientists made a bold attempt to build a mobile robot for homes using a 3D navigation and tracking system. The project failed due to the complexity and, above all, cost of the system. Finally, PrimeSense, an Israel-based company, made a breakthrough by putting the 3D imaging system on a chip for consumer products.[127] Kinect has made many computer vision textbooks obsolete because it can replace those complex vision algorithms for object detection, tracking, and recognition with much simpler, faster, and more robust algorithms.

Disruptive Price

From November 2010, when it was first released, to February 2013, Kinect sales have reached 24 million units worldwide. The price dropped from the original US$249 to US$105. Developers are using the Kinect to replace high-end vision systems for mobile robots, surveillance, 3D imaging, and so on.

Overdrive Design

Kinect integrates multiple sensors, including a 3D imaging sensor, an RGB (red-green-blue) camera, an array of four microphones, and three accelerometers. The overdrive style design creates an abundance of applications that reach beyond the original product design, similar to trendy smartphone designs. Developers and users have more sensors and functions than one might expect.

Fabless Industry

PrimeSense is a fabless company in the digital age. *Fabless* is a movement in hardware industries that treats hardware development similar to software engineering: The

---

[127] http://www.primesense.com

companies research, design, test, and market the blueprint of chips; have the so-called intellectual property core (IP core) in house; but outsource manufacturing to other companies around the world. Partnering with Microsoft, PrimeSense developed Kinect for Xbox game systems; the company also developed its own product Asus.

Crowdsourcing

The first launch of Kinect triggered worldwide excitement among hackers. Unlike other game controllers, the Kinect has a USB port to connect it to a personal computer (PC) as well as an Xbox. Unfortunately, Microsoft did not release any PC drivers for the device, which was a barrier between the Kinect and a PC.

Adafruit Industries offered a bounty of US$2,000 to anyone who would provide an open source driver for this cool USB device. The winner was Héctor Matín, who produced Linux drivers that allow the use of both the RGB camera and the depth image from the Kinect. The open source drivers opened a door to many Kinect applications, which were spurred on by the Internet with YouTube videos and blogs about them. In 2010, PrimeSense released its own drivers and programming framework for the Kinect, called OpenNI. In 2011, Microsoft released the noncommercial Kinect SDK (software development kit) and then, in 2012, a commercial version for Windows.

Kinect indeed is a milestone of an ongoing technical revolution in which the mass market and hackers have made it a reality.

6.3   HOW DOES IT WORK?

Kinect is a 3D imaging sensor. It uses a structured lighting method to create a depth map. Let us explore more details.

Structured Lighting

To obtain a 3D image, Kinect uses an infrared light projector to cast invisible coded dots on the object (Figure 6.2). The advantage of the infrared light is that it works well in the dark, and it does not interfere with people's visible world.

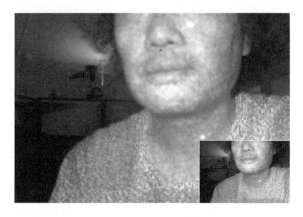

FIGURE 6.2   Coded infrared dots for structured lighting.

Assume we project a straight line that contains many dots to a flat wall. It will be a straight line from the view of a camera. But, if the surface is not flat, then the projected line will be bent. The greater the curvature, the farther away from the original straight line the object would be.

As we know the distance between the projector and the camera and the angles of the projector and the camera with respect to the horizontal line, we can calculate the depth of the surface based on triangulation. This gives the video console the depth of every pixel, creating a depth map in black-and-white pixels, with more white indicating something is closer and more black indicating something is farther away. Figure 6.3 illustrates the concept of the structured lighting imaging system.

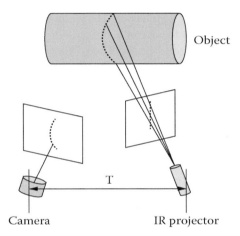

FIGURE 6.3   Depth information is processed using triangulation where T is the distance between the camera and the infrared projector.

Open Source SDKs

There are a few open source SDKs for the Kinect: OpenNI, NITE, OpenKinect, and Microsoft's Kinect for Windows SDK. Processing libraries such as Simple-OpenNI use the middleware architecture, which decouples sensors from applications. They also provide a broad spectrum of APIs, such as tracking, skeleton detection, and so on (Figure 6.4).

For example, NITE middleware includes both a computer vision and a framework that provides the application with gesture-based UI (User Interface) controls. This includes the following algorithms: (1) *Scene segmentation* is a process in which individual users and objects are separated from the background and tagged accordingly; (2) in *hand point detection and tracking*, users' hands are detected and followed; and (3) for *full-body tracking*, based on the scene segmentation output, users' bodies are tracked to output the current user's pose—a set of locations of body joints.

In addition, the 3D Point Cloud Library (PCL) and Python-based SimpleCV also have interfaces to acquire the Kinect data.

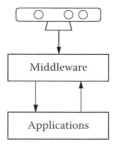

FIGURE 6.4   Kinect software architecture.

6.4   OBJECT TRACKING

Tracking hands or legs is useful for ambient diagnoses. Some examples include evaluating the level of tremor of patients with Alzheimer's disease, recovery progress of stroke patients, or effectiveness of physical therapies for sports injuries. Figure 6.5 shows a demonstration scene of the hand tracking with Kinect and the trajectory display, or "graffiti," as a result of the hand movement.

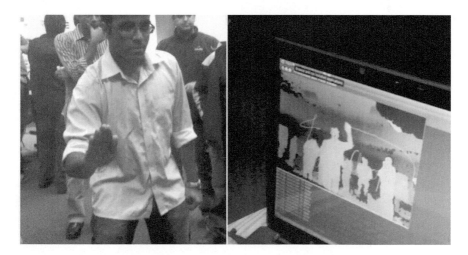

FIGURE 6.5   Hand tracking and the trajectory display, or so-called graffiti, as a result of the hand movement.

Object tracking is an essential function of Kinect. The infrared projector creates coded dots, and the infrared camera receives the structured lighting image and creates the depth map. Then, the open source API is able to segment the depth map into a foreground and background based on depths (Figure 6.6). Further cleanups include watershedding the connected areas and removing noises and the background. For hand tracking, assume the tracked hand is the closest object in front of the Kinect. A simple cutoff depth can easily extract the hand area, including the tip of the hand (Figures 6.7–6.9).

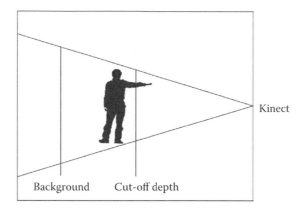

FIGURE 6.6   Point cloud filter based on thresholds of depth.

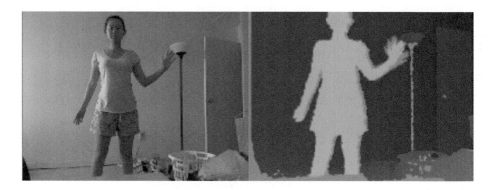

FIGURE 6.7   Colored image from the RGB camera (left) and the depth map from the infrared camera (right).

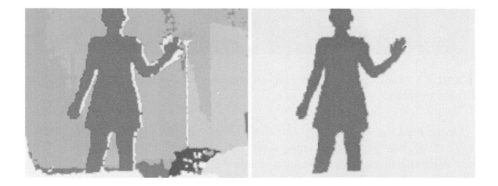

FIGURE 6.8   Segmented objects and background based on the depth map and thresholds (left) and the filtered figure (right).

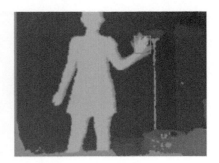

FIGURE 6.9   The detected hand area (left) and the segmented image (right).

Skeletal Tracking

The current open sources for Kinect also provide the tracking function for human figure joints, enabling skeleton animations. For example, OpenNI, NITE, and Microsoft can track up to twenty joints. The definitions of the joints are shown in Figures 6.10 and Figure 6.11.

Kinect SDK can track two people in detail at the skeleton level and up to four persons for the locations of their center of mass only.

Combining Tracking Joints of Hands and the Body

NITE provides tools that enable application writers to design the flow of the application according to hand movements. For an application that uses NITE controls, a session is a state in which the user is in control of the system using his or her

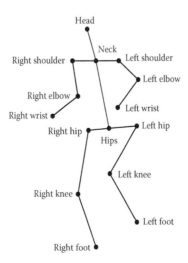

FIGURE 6.10   Skeleton definition for human figure joints.

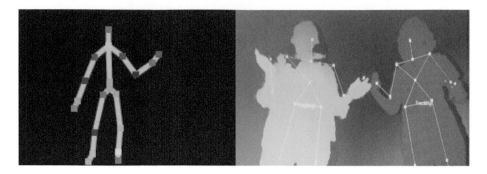

FIGURE 6.11   Skeletal tracking (left) and two-person tracking with segmentation (right).

hand. During the session, the hand point has persistent ID and tracked by the system. A session typically starts with the user requesting to gain control by performing a predefined hand gesture (e.g., waving). This hand gesture is referred to as the "focus gesture." This is the gesture that, once identified, is interpreted by the system as a request from the user to gain control. Then, the user's hand is tracked. The session ends when the user's hand disappears.

The Skeletal Viewer API is designed for tracking the skeleton of the human body. TipTep, on the other hand, is designed for tracking the skeleton of the hand. We can combine the two to track the body skeleton and hand skeleton simultaneously.

However, the two programs are not able to read frames from the same Kinect stream. This problem can be resolved by using the open source library NITE2, which contains both the skeleton-tracking method and hand-tracking method. The NITE2 library also provides the confidence measurement function "getPositionConfidence." If the 3D joint is confident, or stable, then the method will return 1; otherwise, it will return 0. NITE2 can detect whether the 3D joint is confident. If both connected joints are confident, then the skeleton will draw in colors defined by the developer.

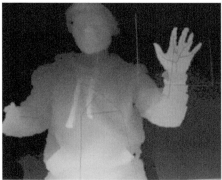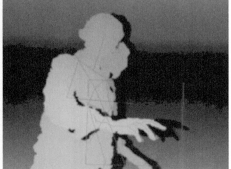

FIGURE 6.12   Tracking the hand and body skeleton by implementing the TipTep method. (Contributed by Bing Yang, with permission.)

TipTep Skeletonizer is a middleware, based on the OpenNI platform, which provides tools and APIs that can be used to extract the geometric skeleton of the hand from depth images.[128] Based on OpenNI, we can develop a program for tracking the body and hand skeleton at the same time. By using OpenNI.lib, we can access the Kinect Stream, and the NiTE2.lib provides a method to obtain skeleton depth frames, from which we can obtain the position of the center of the palm. Then, we can further apply the algorithm used by TipTep within this to detect the whole-hand skeleton (Figure 6.12).

6.5   GESTURE ALIGNMENT

Given two time sequences of gesture features (e.g., angles or positions of joints), we want to evaluate the feature distance between the two. For example, in physical therapy, we often need to evaluate the progress of gesture control by comparing the time-space sequences. Figure 6.13 shows two time-space sequences of gestures in Tai Ji exercise. How similar are the two and how do we measure their alignment?

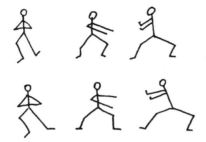

FIGURE 6.13   Two Tai Ji gesture sequences. Are they similar?

Traditional measurements such as Euclidean distance will produce a poor similarity score (Figure 6.14). A more elastic and intuitive alignment measurement is expected. This would allow similar shapes to match even if they are out of phase in the time axis.

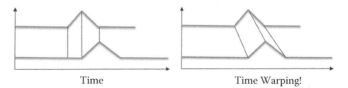

Time   Time Warping!

FIGURE 6.14   Evaluating two time sequences. The Euclidean distance produces poor similarity score (left). The elastic and intuitive alignment measurement allows similar shapes to match even if they are out of phase in the time axis (right).

---

[128] http://youtu.be/nkFgnlPteUQ

Dynamic Time Warping

Dynamic time warping (DTW)[129] can be used to find the best alignment between time sequences $A[1], \dots , A[m]$ and $B[1], \dots , B[n]$ (Figure 6.15). Here we arrange a two-dimensional (2D) matrix $(n \times m)$ for A and B. The goal is to find the minimal total distance between them.

$$P = \underset{P_s}{\arg\min}\left\{\sum_{s=1}^{k} d(P_s)\right\} \tag{6.1}$$

where $d(P_s)$ is the distance between i_s and j_s. P is called the warping function.

Intuitively, if A and B are perfectly aligned, P would be the shortest path along the diagonal line from the left bottom to the top right corner of the matrix.

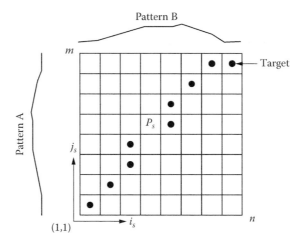

FIGURE 6.15   Dynamic time warping in this alignment evaluation matrix is used to find the shortest path between the bottom left corner (1,1) and the top right corner (m,n).

DTW Constraints

Dynamic time warping is an NP-complete problem. The number of possible warping paths against the size of the grid is exponentially explosive. To solve the problem, we have to reduce the search space by adding restrictions on the warping function, including the warping window, monotonicity, continuity, boundary conditions, and slope constraint.

Boundary conditions: $i_1 = 1$, $i_k = n$ and $j_1 = 1$, $j_k = m$. The alignment path starts at the bottom left and ends at the top right. This is an essential constraint for

---

[129] http://www.phon.ox.ac.uk/jcoleman/old_SLP/Lecture_5/DTW_explanation.html

every DTW algorithm (Figure 6.16). This guarantees that all features are considered, not just a portion of them.

Warping window: $|i_s - j_s| \leq r$, where $r > 0$ is the window length. A good alignment path is unlikely to wander too far from the diagonal. Also, this constraint significantly reduces the search space. Therefore, the warping window is a common constraint in many DTW implementations (Figure 6.17). This guarantees that the alignment does not try to skip different features and become stuck at similar features.

Monotonicity: $i_{s-1} \leq i_s$ and $j_{s-1} \leq j_s$. The alignment path does not go back in the time index (Figure 6.18). This guarantees that features are not repeated in the alignment.

Continuity constraint: $i_s - i_{s-1} \leq 1$ and $j_s - j_{s-1} \leq 1$. The alignment path does not jump in the time index. This guarantees that the alignment does not omit important features (Figure 6.19).

Slope constraint: $(j_{S1} - j_{S2})/(i_{S1} - i_{S2}) \leq p$ and $(i_{S1} - i_{S2})/(j_{S1} - j_{S2}) \leq q$, where q is the number of steps in the *x* direction, and *p* is the number of steps in the *y* direction. After *q* steps in *x*, one must step in *y* and vice versa. This ensures the path is not too steep or too shallow. (Figure 6.20).

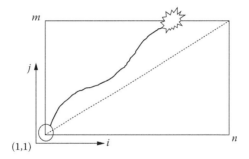

FIGURE 6.16   Boundary constraint. The alignment path always starts at the bottom left and ends at the top right.

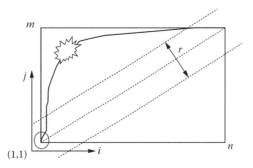

FIGURE 6.17   The warping window constraint reduces the search space to a narrow area along the diagonal.

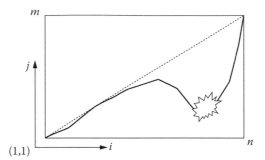

FIGURE 6.18 Monotonicity constraint forces the alignment path to move forward. This constraint helps to fix the misalignment when the path goes backward.

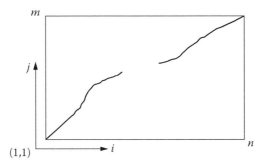

FIGURE 6.19 Continuity constraint is necessary to make sure the alignment path does not overlook some features.

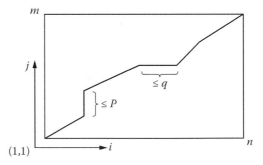

FIGURE 6.20 Slope constraint is used to ensure the alignment path is along the diagonal, not too steep or too shallow. This image on the right shows a poor slope path scenario where the feature matching is not evenly spread.

DTW Algorithm

The algorithm for DTW is an iterative process (Figure 6.21). Let the initial condition of the goal function $g(i, j)$ be set to $g(1,1) = d(1,1)$. We have

$$g(i,j) = \min \begin{cases} g(i,j-1)+d(i,j), \\ g(i-1,j-1)+d(i,j), \\ g(i-1,j)+d(i,j). \end{cases} \tag{6.2}$$

The time-normalized distance is

$$D(A,B) = g(n,m)/(n+m) \tag{6.3}$$

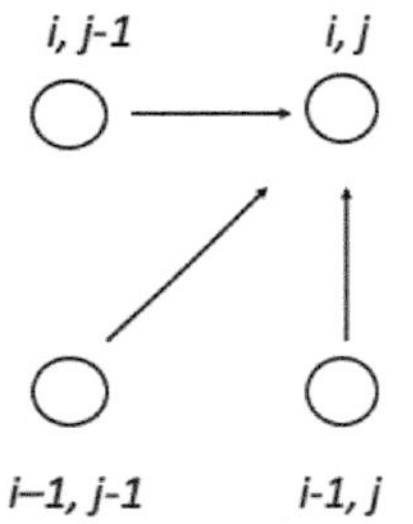

FIGURE 6.21   Illustration of dynamic time warp algorithm in the two-dimensional matrix.

Here is how the DTW algorithm works in pseudocode:

1. Start with the calculation from the bottom left corner and set g(1, 1) = d(1, 1).
2. Calculate the first column g(i, 1) = g(i − 1, 1) + d(i, 1).
3. Calculate the first row g(1, j) = g(1, j) + d(1, j).
4. From the second row and second column, calculate from left to right and from bottom to top with the rest of the grid:
    g(i, j) = min(g(i, j − 1), g(i − 1, j − 1), g(i − 1, j)) + d(i, j).
5. Trace back the best path through the grid starting from g(n,m) and moving toward g(1,1).

Here is a simple example. Assume we want to evaluate the difference between the two gestures shown in Figure 6.22.[130]
We have a one-dimensional input signal:

$$\begin{array}{ccccc} A[t] = & 0 & 1 & 1 & 2 \\ B[t] = & 1 & 1 & 2 & 3 \end{array}$$

---

[130] http://www.phon.ox.ac.uk/jcoleman/old_SLP/Lecture_5/DTW_explanation.html

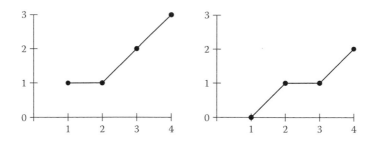

FIGURE 6.22   Test pattern $B[t]$ (left) and reference pattern $A[t]$ (right).

The two signals appear to have a similar trend. They both go upward with similar slopes. However, there are subtle differences.

To calculate the similarity between them, let us use a matrix of the squared distance between $B[t]$ and $A[t]$: $D = (B[t] - A[t])^2$ (Figure 6.23). There is a short path with small numbers close to the diagonal, indicating which samples of $B[t]$ are closest in value to those of $A[t]$. These are marked with underscores: $P = 1 + 0 + 0 + 0 + 1 = 2$.

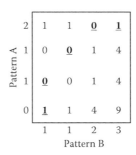

FIGURE 6.23   Example of the DTW algorithm.

The DTW algorithm has been implemented in MATLAB, providing an open source module for applying DTW to many applications,[131] including speech recognition, handwriting recognition, multimedia processing, and gesture recognition.

6.6   GESTURE RECOGNITION

DTW for Gesture Recognition

Here we apply DTW to gesture recognition, using the skeleton joint positions from Kinect (Figure 6.24). Compared to many existing gesture-tracking models that rely on features of color, texture, and background, the Kinect-based method is much more robust because it uses the infrared depth map to predict joint positions. It can even work in dark environments.

---

[131] http://www.ee.columbia.edu/~dpwe/resources/matlab/dtw/

Kinect SDK tracks 3D coordinates of R joints (typically up to twenty) given in Figure 6.10 in real time (thirty frames per second). A feature vector consists of 3D coordinates of these R joints and is of dimension $3 \times R$ (e.g., 60) as follows:

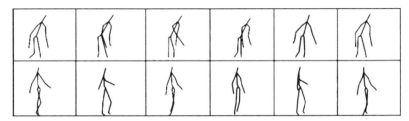

FIGURE 6.24 Skeletal data of walking sequences: crippled (top) and normal (bottom) gestures.

$$f_k = \left[x_1, y_1, z_1, ..., x_R, y_R, z_R \right] \qquad (6.4)$$

where k is the index of the skeleton frame at time $t = k$. A gesture sequence is the concatenation of N such feature vectors.

Assume we have another gesture sequence with feature vector $h_k = [x_1, y_1, z_1, ..., x_R, y_R, z_R]$. To compare the two gesture sequences, we want to find the minimal warping path cost in the DTW function:

$$DTW(f, h) = \min_{g_1 ..., g_R} \left\{ \sqrt{\sum_{k=1}^{R} g(i_k, j_k)^2} \right\} \qquad (6.5)$$

To eliminate variations in the feature vectors due to a person's size, orientation, or distance to the Kinect,[132] preprocessing for data normalizations for the feature vectors is necessary. For example, we can normalize the feature vector with the distance between the left and right shoulders to eliminate the size factor.

To make life easier, we normally set the two sequences to have the same length. In this case, the Euclidean distance between two sequences can be used for DWP.

In many practical cases, we only need to use a portion of joint positions. For example, if we want to track a sign language gesture, then we just need to use the upper body joints and ignore the rest of the joints. In some cases, we may assign weights to the joints. This can be implemented in the weighted warping cost function. For more details, please refer to a publication by Celebi et al.[133]

---

[132] P. Doliotis et al. Comparing gesture recognition accuracy using color and depth information. In *Proceedings of PETRA 2011*, Crete, Greece, 2011.

[133] S. Celebi et al. Gesture recognition using skeleton data with weighted dynamic time warping. In *Proceedings of VISAPP 2013*, 2013.

Performance Comparisons

From comparing the performance of DTW to other algorithms such as hidden Markov models (HMMs), studies show that DTW gives higher performance than HMMs and strongly support the use of DTW.[134]

Comparing the performance of Kinect versus color camera-based gesture recognition, results show that Kinect-based gesture recognition is far more robust than other methods.

Open Source

CodePlex is the open source for Kinect SDK DTW for gesture recognition.[135] It uses skeletal tracking in 2D vectors. The open source includes a gesture recorder, recognizer, and sample gestures. Users can save their own gestures for later use.

6.7   SURFACE MODELING

Imagine a patient shows up in the clinic office with a swollen face. The doctor may just make a visual or tactile exam. Can we measure the patient's surface in 3D? It would be helpful in plastic surgery, physical therapy, infection diagnoses, and telemedicine. Kinect is an affordable 3D imaging sensor. It can be conveniently set up on a desktop as shown in Figure 6.25.

However, Kinect was not originally optimized for surface modeling because the resolution of the infrared dots is too low to reconstruct a smooth surface. To improve

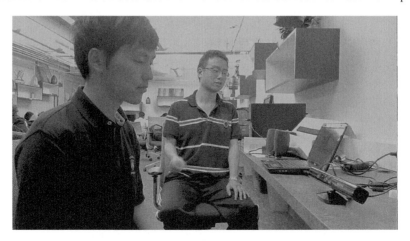

FIGURE 6.25   Kinect 3D imaging setup in an office environment. The system can build a 3D model within one second.

---

[134] Josep Maria Carmona and Joan Climent. A performance evaluation of HMM and DTW for gesture recognition. Progress in pattern recognition, image analysis, computer vision, and applications. *Lecture Notes in Computer Science* 7441:236–243, 2012. http://link.springer.com/chapter/10.1007%2F978-3-642-33275-3_29

[135] http://kinectdtw.codeplex.com/

the resolution, we can use the superresolution method by fusing multiple scans from different angles.

Multiscan Fusion

A simple approach for multiscan fusion is to take three scans while the person sits on a rotating chair: left, front, and right. This makes data-model registration easier because these three scans have the same rotational z-axis.

To reconstruct 3D surfaces from multiple scans, the iterative closest point (ICP)[136] algorithm is commonly used (Figure 6.26). The algorithm is a point-based registration method. It iteratively translates and rotates one of the two point clouds to minimize the distance between the points of two raw scans. The transformation process will stop when the criterion is satisfied.[137]

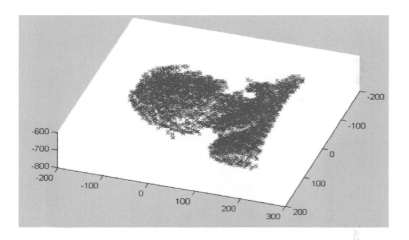

FIGURE 6.26   3D points plotted in MATLAB.

Fortunately, there are several open sources for the ICP algorithm. One example is MeshLab, an open source mesh-processing tool that includes a GNU general public license implementation of the ICP algorithm. CloudCompare, an open source point and processing tool that includes an implementation of the ICP algorithm, is another. PCL is an open source framework for n-dimensional point clouds and 3D geometry processing. It includes several variants of the ICP algorithm. Open source C++ implementations of the ICP algorithm are available in VTK and ITK libraries.

Combining the three scans indeed increases the number of 3D surface points. In fact, the number of points increases from 18,659 to 63,896—about three times as many points. However, fusion of multiple scans also brings noise to the 3D surface

---

[136] http://en.wikipedia.org/wiki/Iterative_closest_point
[137] Paul J. Besl and N. D. McKay. A method for registration of 3-D shapes. *IEEE Transactions on Pattern Analysis and Machine Intelligence* 14(2):239–256, 1992.

due to the noise in sensing and registration (Figure 6.27). A low-pass filter is needed to smooth the surface.

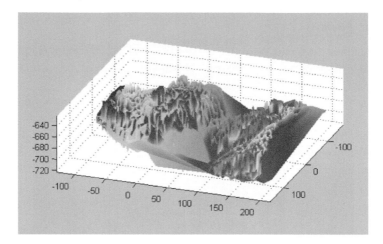

FIGURE 6.27   Fusion of multiple scans creates a highly noisy surface. Here is the sample of the result using MATLAB.

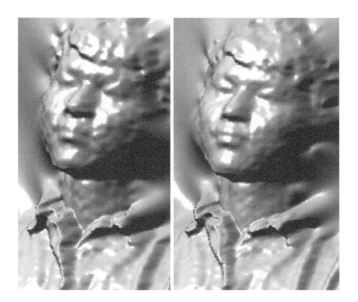

FIGURE 6.28   The reconstructed 3D surface with single scan (left) and the result of the fusion of multiple scans (right).

Rendering

After the fusion process, the 3D points become vertices of mesh triangles. The surface normal vectors are calculated to indicate whether the surface is pointed to the inside or outside. A ray-tracing algorithm is used to render the reconstructed 3D surface. Fortunately, many open source graphics libraries provide these functions, such as MATLAB, OpenGL, PCL, and MeshLab. Figure 6.28 shows the results of the reconstructed face using a single scan and fusion of three scans after low-pass filtering.

The reconstructed 3D models can be saved as Wavefront's OBJ format, which contains mapped color texture and mesh data, or stereolithography (STL) format for 3D printing. In the medical domain, DICOM format is commonly used, which is compatible with radiological images and videos such as magnetic resonance imaging (MRI), computed tomography (CT), positron emission tomography (PET), X-ray, and so on.

6.8 BIOMETRIC MEASUREMENT

Imagine a weight meter is embedded in the carpet of a living room. Can we ubiquitously measure each family member's body mass index (BMI = weight/height) without asking for the individuals' names during measurement? Here, we need to detect each individual's biometric measurements.

User Recognition

With the Kinect, users can be recognized by simply measuring the height of each person in the room. Whenever a user enters the field of view of the Kinect, the system starts to track the person, finds the highest and lowest points defining the person's body, and extracts the height of the person from those points. At the same time, the software skeletonizes the user and tracks the proportions of the user's limbs to use as a footprint to match the user with previously saved information. If the footprint is similar to an existing user, then the system recognizes the person and retrieves the data from previous readings.

The Kinect's skeleton-tracking data can help to characterize a user in the multi dimensional vector. Configuring the feature vector is rather tricky. If one uses the absolute joint coordinates, then the representation will be too sensitive to the poses and distances. To make a more robust feature vector, we should use the proportional measurement (e.g., the ratio of the upper arm length over the upper leg length or the length ratios of the triangular shape on the chest). So, these features are ratios instead of absolute values. To compare any two users' biometric data, we just calculate the n-dimensional distance between the two feature vectors $A = [a_1, a_2, \ldots, a_n]$ and $B = [b_1, b_2, \ldots, b_n]$. We first do a vector subtraction:

$$
\begin{bmatrix} a_1 \\ a_2 \\ \vdots \\ a_n \end{bmatrix} - \begin{bmatrix} b_1 \\ b_2 \\ \vdots \\ b_n \end{bmatrix} = \begin{bmatrix} c_1 \\ c_2 \\ \vdots \\ c_n \end{bmatrix} \tag{6.6}
$$

and then calculate the magnitude of the subtracted vector, the Euclidean distance:

$$\|C\| = \sqrt{c_1^2 + c_2^2 + c_3^2 + \ldots + c_n^2} \qquad (6.7)$$

By subtracting the input vector with all the stored user feature vectors, we can recognize the user by measuring the minimal distance.

Height Estimation

The detection of the user's height can be estimated by two methods: directly tracking the point cloud or calculating from the skeletal-tracking data.

To use the first method, we just need to find out the highest and the lowest points of the user point cloud so that we subtract their y coordinates and find the real height of the user in centimeters.

The second method is a bit tricky. We have to add the links between the joints vertically, from the bottom to the top. Kinect provides the x, y, and z coordinates of twenty skeleton joints. The height is the sum of the lengths of the following line segments: head, spine, hip, knee, and ankle. As Kinect only gives the center of the head joint, we need to add a few centimeters to the estimated height, say, thirty centimeters. The results of experiments showed that the errors are within two centimeters, which is reasonably accurate for calculating BMI.

6.9   SOUND SOURCE LOCATION

Kinect has a four-microphone array. By analyzing the audio differences between each of the four audio streams, Kinect can determine the location of the sound source (Figure 6.29). The Kinect SDK beta API does not provide the distance for the audio event though, only the angle, and only one angle is provided.

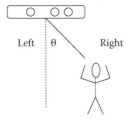

FIGURE 6.29   Sound source location by Kinect.

Assume a sound wave front arrives at the angle θ, perpendicular to a line joining the two microphones *M1* and *M2*. In Figure 6.30, the microphone on the left (*M1*) receives the sound a little later than the one on the right (*M2*) because the left edge of the wave has to travel an extra distance p.

This can be expressed as the equation

$$\sin \theta = p/d \qquad (6.8)$$

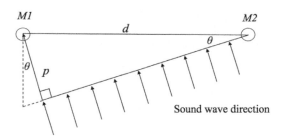

FIGURE 6.30 Sound wave front triangulation calculation.

The sound arrival delay can also be defined in terms of sound velocity and time:

$$p = c \cdot \Delta t \qquad (6.9)$$

where c is the speed of sound (in meters/second), and Δt is the time delay (in seconds) between the wave reaching $M1$ and $M2$. These two equations can be merged to be one equation for θ:

$$\theta = \sin^{-1}\left(c \cdot \Delta t / d\right) \qquad (6.10)$$

Unfortunately, this method can only sense the location of the sound source in angle but not in distance. To include the distance information, we have to measure the strength of the sound signals from a microphone array. Typically we need at least three microphones to be able to triangulate the position of the sound source.

Sensing the location of the sound source at home enables Kinect to estimate the user's position outside the camera range. It has potential in ambient diagnoses, such as activity analysis and telemedicin, when the location of the user is relevant.

For more information about the binaural localization library in Java, please refer to "Java Programming Techniques for Games. Kinect 15. Kinect Mike." Draft #1 on 14th of March 2012: http://fivedots.coe.psu.ac.th/~ad/kinect/ch15/kinectMike.pdf.

6.10 SUMMARY

In this chapter, we explored various applications of the Kinect device outside its original intended purpose. The Kinect device is useful in ambient diagnostics because it is packed with powerful sensors, it is affordable, it is rich in open source ecosystems, and it can be closely connected to many individual's lives, such as playing video games and watching television.

With structured lighting, 3D object tracking using Kinect is simpler than conventional methods such as stereoscopic imaging. Using depth thresholding, the moving objects can be segmented and tracked. In addition, skeletal tracking provides a more robust way to study a gesture's trajectories, so-called air graffiti, for the level of tremor of patients with Alzheimer's disease, recovery progress of stroke patients, or effectiveness of physical therapies for sports injuries.

With the DTW algorithm, we can evaluate gesture alignment or recognize gesture sequences.

The Kinect can also be used for 3D surface modeling. To improve the spatial resolution, the ICP algorithm can be used to fuse the multiple data scans.

Finally, the sound wave front triangulation model was introduced to explain Kinect's sound source location function.

PROBLEMS

1. Evaluate the difference between the following two gesture sequences in Euclidean distance:

$x(t)$:	1	1	2	3	2	0	
$y(t)$:	0	1	1	2	3	2	1

2. Based on the same input data in Problem 1, evaluate the two gesture sequences with the best alignment path.
3. Given two-dimensional joint position sequences $x(t)$ and $y(t)$, calculate the best alignment path with the DTW algorithm.

$x(t) =$

−0.87	−0.84	−0.85	−0.82	−0.23	1.95	1.36	0.60	0.0	−0.29
−0.88	−0.91	−0.84	−0.82	−0.24	1.92	1.41	0.51	0.03	−0.18

$y(t) =$

−0.60	−0.65	−0.71	−0.58	−0.17	0.77	1.94
−0.46	−0.62	−0.68	−0.63	−0.32	0.74	1.97

4. Discuss the potential applications of the Kinect for elderly care at home. Write a report with references and analysis.
5. Given two sequences of gesture data from the Kinect, how do you normalize the feature vectors so that the center of the shoulder would be the original coordinate system for all the datasets? Describe the method with drawings and text. Use the Kinect data to prove it. Write a report to summarize the experiments and discuss the results.
6. One of the limitations of the Kinect is its distance to the user. Test the actual visible range for the Kinect you have and plot the space in 3D. Find solutions for the Kinect to have a farther or closer range. Hint: try optical solutions or multiple Kinects. Compare the solutions with analytical reasoning and data when possible.
7. Use ICP or other methods to merge multiple scans of your foot. Use MeshLab or Blender to visualize the result. Study the filters and discuss the effects in the report. Discuss the relationship between number of scans and the improvement in the final appearance.

8. Export your 3D model from the Kinect to STL format and use a 3D printer to build the physical model. Discuss (A) digital filters needed to improve the surface quality and (B) potential applications in ambient diagnosis.

9. Set up the Kinect in a conference room. Have at least three people sit in front of the Kinect. Test the sensitivity of the sound source location in the following conditions: (A) one person speaks, (B) two people speak, and (C) three or more people speak. Analyze the results and write a report.

10. Use open sources or write your own code for a demonstration to recognize a sign language. Define at least twenty-six gestures, test with three subjects, and test multiple times. Use a confusion matrix to summarize the classification results. Discuss the robustness of the algorithm, including the answer to questions such as "Does the system work with the left hand after being trained with the right hand?"

11. Use the Kinect to create interactive art; for example, draw snow angels with the Kinect. Develop a demonstration for the project and discuss the potential for rehabilitation and ambient diagnosis.

12. The Kinect has an accelerometer. Discuss its applications with data, give examples, and provide analysis.

13. The Kinect is capable of tilting up and down. Add an Arduino-controlled step motor to the Kinect so that it can yaw from left to right. Show the demonstration to the class and discuss the potential for ambient diagnosis.

7 Video Analysis

> Our nature consists in motion; complete rest is death.
>
> —Blaise Pascal

7.1 INTRODUCTION

A video camera is a versatile sensor for monitoring and diagnosing. It is so affordable that many people have more than one on their phones, cars, or computers. In this chapter, we combine visualization and analytic algorithms to make video analytics an intuitive task. The goal is to extract dynamic features in videos for ambient diagnostic applications. We will study the following:

- Moving object detection
- Object tracking
- Shape description
- Video summarization
- Activity recognition
- Video magnification

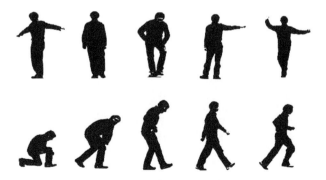

FIGURE 7.1 Human activity blobs extracted from webcam videos. Even though they are in very low resolution, we still can recognize the activity of the figure.

7.2 OBJECT DETECTION BY MOTION

Given a set of video frames and assuming the camera is stationary, how do we extract the moving foreground and remove the static background? Figure 7.1 shows a desirable scenario, where the moving objects are extracted as binary blobs. A binary blob is the simplest visual form of a shape description. It is so important that intelligence analysts often refer to video analytics as "blobology." Here, we introduce three basic background subtraction methods: frame subtraction, approximate median, and Gaussian mixture model (GMM).[138]

To obtain binary blobs, we need to do some preprocessing. First, we reduce the resolution of the frames to speed up computation since it is a time-consuming process, and it is not necessary to have high resolution for this. As a rule of thumb, a factor of five to ten reduction is reasonable. Then, we convert the original image to a grayscale image. We then use an appropriate grayscale threshold to produce a binary image and fill in any interior holes in the shape.

Read and Write Video Frames

A video consists of frames. Our first task is to read the frames of a video and write frames to a video file. MATLAB, OpenCV, and other video-processing toolboxes have the frame reading and writing functions. In Appendix A, there is a MATLAB sample code for reading frames from a video file and writing frames to a video file.

Frame Subtraction

Frame subtraction is the simplest way to extract the moving object from the video. Assume the camera is stationary; p_i is the pixel value of the current frame, and p_{i-1} is the pixel value of the previous frame. If their pixel difference is larger than a threshold T, then the pixel is the moving foreground. Otherwise, the pixel is the background.

$$|p_i - p_{i-1}| > T \qquad (7.1)$$

Pseudocode for frame subtraction is as follows:

```
1.    read first_frame
2.    prev_frame = first_frame
3.    while (frames remaining)
4.            current_frame = read next_frame
5.            for (each pixel)
6.                    delta = | current_frame – prev_frame |
7.                    if(delta > threshold)
8.                            foreground_pixel = current_frame
9.                    else
10.                           foreground_pixel = 0
11.                   end
12.           end
13.           prev_frame = current_frame
14.           filter foreground_pixel
15.   end
```

---

[138] Sample MATLAB code for frame subtraction and approximate median is available at http://www.eetimes.com/design/automotive-design/4017685/Background-subtraction-part-1-MATLAB-models

The results of background subtraction are binary, creating a binary image, where foreground figures are blobs.

However, frame subtraction is sensitive to noises in the video and is very sensitive to the threshold. In addition, it is sensitive to objects' speed and the camera's frame rate. If the object moved too fast or the frame rate were low, then results would be poor.

Approximate Median

The approximate median algorithm makes a more advanced assumption about the background of the video. Here, we assume the background is consistent over the short term but can still change over longer periods of time. This assumption helps prevent short-term noise while still being able to accommodate a dynamic scene.

The algorithm is called approximate median because it behaves like a low-pass filter to the background model. For example, if we take one pixel out of a sequence of frames, we initiate the pixel as the background. When a man passes the pixel, its intensity value will change. The Approximate Median algorithm waits for a short period of time to see if its intensity value returns to the original value. If so, then the Algorithm does not change its background model. Otherwise, the background will be updated with the current intensity value at the pixel (Figure 7.2).

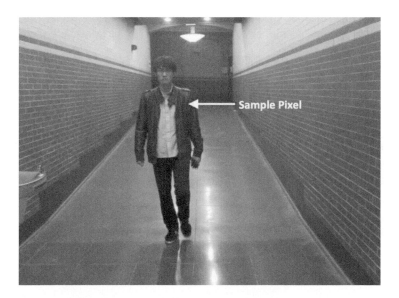

FIGURE 7.2 Examining one pixel out of a sequence of frames while a man passed through the pixel location. Note that the shadow on the floor may create noise.

Note that long-term changes, such as shadows changing as time passes, result in pixel value changes that are below the threshold. These changes are integrated into the median background value without ever entering the foreground scene.

The pseudocode for the approximate median is

```
1.    read first frame
2.       median_frame = first frame        % assume the first frame is the median
3.    while (frames remaining)
4.              current_frame = read next_frame
5.             for (every pixel)
6.                         delta = | current_frame – median_frame|
7.                         if (current_frame_pixel > median_pixel)
8.                                  median_pixe l + 1
9.                        else
10.                                 median_pixel - 1
11.                        end
12.                       if (delta > threshold)
13.                                  foreground_pixel = current_frame_pixel
14.                      else
15.                                 foreground_pixel = 0
16.                      end
17.              end
18.   end
```

Figure 7.3 shows the results of the approximate median algorithm, including (a) the original video frame, (b) the reconstructed background, (c) the extracted foreground, and (d) the filtered foreground figure. We can see that the extracted foreground figure has her shadow attached because the shadow is also a moving object. The filter fills the holes and smooths the edges and texture in the foreground.

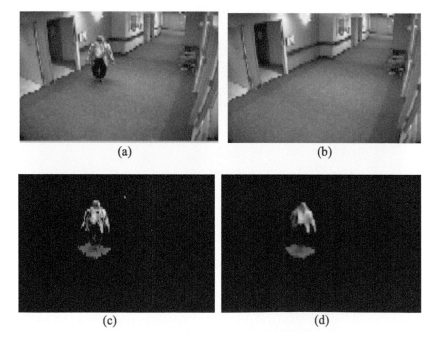

(a)   (b)

(c)   (d)

FIGURE 7.3 Approximate Median method: (a) original video, (b) background model, (c) foreground extracted, and (d) filtered foreground.

Gaussian Mixture Model

Gaussian Mixture Model (GMM) is to build a high-fidelity background model, which can be expressed as:

$$F(x) = \sum_{i=1}^{k} w_i \cdot e^{\frac{-(x-\mu_i)^2}{\sigma_i^2}} \tag{7.2}$$

where u_i is the mean of the background pixel values in each Gaussian function; w_i is the weight; and σ_i is the standard deviations of each component (where higher weight and lower σ_i mean higher confidence). There are typically three to five Gaussian components per pixel.

Unfortunately, the GMM needs more frames for training, and it is more computationally expensive than the other two methods. According to the author's test results, GMM does not generate better segmentation results than the approximate median method. Therefore, GMM is not recommended as the first choice.

The approximate median often generates decent foreground segmentation for outdoor and indoor videos. It outperforms Frame Subtraction and GMM methods in many cases.

Nonfixed Camera Segmentation

The last three segmentation methods are based on the assumption of the video from a stationary camera. What if the camera is moving? For example, we want to extract the moving humans from the videos from a wearable camera. So far, there are very few successful object extraction algorithms for mobile video data. Here, we introduce a simple but effective heuristic approach. Figure 7.4 shows a sample result. The pseudocode for segmentation from a moving camera is as follows:

1. For every frame:
2.   Determine global motion between the current and previous frames;
3.   Store this motion in a transformation matrix;
4.   Warp current frame based on the motion and
5.   Find the current temporal gradient (compared to actual frame)
6.   Label segments:
7.   Threshold the gradient based on running average of last 4 frames
8.   Label the nonzero segments
9.   Find blobs:
10.   Compute masses and bounds for every label
11.   Get the center of mass of every segment
12.   Extract blobs:
13.   Threshold the masses of the blobs
14. End loop for frames

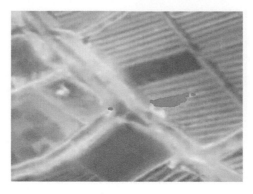

FIGURE 7.4   Result of the moving object extraction from the video from a moving camera.

7.3   OBJECT TRACKING

Object tracking is in fact object detection over time. Tracking needs to detect objects to initiate the position. Since object detection is always noisy, tracking algorithms often act like filters to obtain a smooth trace from imperfect lighting and obscured scenes, such as the popular Kalman filter. Many tracking algorithms also predict the trajectory of objects so that we do not have to detect objects in each frame.

However, predicting trajectory is a nontrivial task. So far, most common prediction models are linear transports of particles, such as the particle filter.

Perhaps the simplest approach is to use a threshold for detecting objects and marking their locations. For example, given a sequence of grayscale frames, find the object with intensity larger than one. In Figure 7.5, the pixels on the object are highlighted in bold. The same process can be repeated for the following frames.

	Frame 1	Frame 2	Frame 3
	0 0 0 0 1	0 0 0 0 1	0 0 0 0 1
Original	0 3 3 0 0	0 0 **3 3** 0	0 0 0 **3 3**
(intensity)	0 **5 4** 1 0	0 0 **5 4** 1	0 0 0 **5 4**
	0 0 0 0 0	0 0 0 0 0	0 0 0 0 0
	0 0 0 0 0	0 0 0 0 0	0 0 0 0 0
Tracking	0 **1 1** 0 0	0 0 **1 1** 0	0 0 0 **1 1**
(T > 2)	0 **1 1** 0 0	0 0 **1 1** 0	0 0 0 **1 1**
	0 0 0 0 0	0 0 0 0 0	0 0 0 0 0

FIGURE 7.5   Illustration of object tracking based on an intensity threshold $T > 2$.

Note that the simple problem in Figure 7.5 does not have a filter or a prediction model. In many cases, the tracking results are not always reliable. Given consecutive sample frames, we can model the intensity distribution of an object, assuming the distribution does not change during the tracking period (in fact, this is not true). Here, we would like to discuss two relatively simple and general methods: mean shift and radial basis function (RBF).

Mean Shift

Assume we have n data points x_i, and $K(x)$ is a kernel to model how much x distributes to the estimation of the mean. Then, the sample mean m at x with kernel K is given by

$$m(x) = \frac{\sum_{i=1}^{n} K(x - x_i) x_i}{\sum_{i=1}^{n} K(x - x_i)} \qquad (7.3)$$

The difference $m(x) - x$ is called the mean shift, where

$$K(x) = k \|x\|^2 \qquad (7.4)$$

k is called the profile of K, and $k > 0$, $k(x) \geq k(y)$ if $x > y$.

The pseudocode for the mean shift algorithm (Figure 7.6) is as follows:

1. Draw the tracking target on the first frame.
2. Iteratively move tracking point to its mean.
3. In each iteration, let x equal to $m(x)$.
4. Stop when $|m(x) - x| <$ threshold.

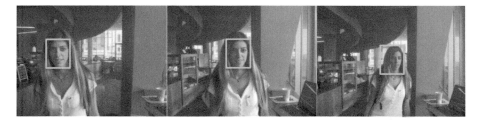

FIGURE 7.6   A sample result of Mean-Shift tracking algorithm.

Radial Basis Function

As we discussed in Chapter 3, the RBF is a versatile neural network that can be used for pattern recognition. Here, we use RBF for object tracking.[139] RBF is relatively fast because many RBF algorithms can be divided into two stages: clustering and weight computing. Each stage can be optimized for speed.[140]

The pseudocode for the RBF-based tracking is as follows:

1. Draw the tracking target on the first frame
2. Use the first n frames as a training data for the RBF model.

---

[139] MathWorks. *MATLAB neural network toolbox manual* (in MATLAB type: help nn). http://www.mathworks.com/help/pdf_doc/nnet/nnet_ug.pdf

[140] T. Yamaguchi, T. Takai, and T. Mita. Self-organizing control using fuzzy neural networks. *International Journal of Control* 56:2, 1992.

3. Do
4.   Use the current frame as the input for the RBF model
5.   Display the result in a bounding box
6.   Read next frame
7. Stop when done

Figure 7.7 shows a real-time object tracking result from the RBF neural network chip. It can start tracking the face after a fraction of a second, and it can tolerate size changes and limited rotation angles.

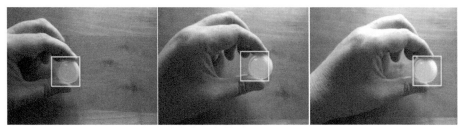

FIGURE 7.7   Radial basis function tracking results.

7.4   SHAPE DESCRIPTIONS

Shape description is critical for recognition and classification. Here, we introduce basic descriptors: bounding box, centroid, proportion, convex hull, contour, polar coordinate profile, and active contour. For more details, please read one of the best tutorials.[141]

Bounding Box, Centroid, and Proportion

Given binary foreground blobs, the simplest shape description is to put a rectangular bounding box around those blobs. The center of the bound box is approximately assigned as the centroid of the blob. The size of a bounding box itself does not tell us much information. However, if the box is compared to other boxes in the same image, the intrinsic proportions of sizes are helpful for recognition or classification. For example, an adult man is normally bigger than a dog (Figure 7.8). Similarly, the width-to-height ratio can describe the object's proportion features; for example, an adult human's height is longer than his or her width, while a dog's proportion is the opposite.

Human instincts use the knowledge about proportions of the world. It is common sense to us. Encoding those aspects of common sense would simplify our algorithms and speed the processing time.

[141] A. Ashbrook and N. A. Thacker. Tutorial: algorithms for 2-dimensional recognition. Tina Memo No. 1996-003. http://www.imageprocessingplace.com/downloads_V3/root_downloads/tutorials/Tutorial--Algorithms%20for%202-D%20Object%20Recognition.pdf

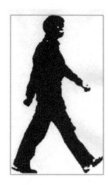

FIGURE 7.8 Bounding boxes of an adult man and a dog. The proportions of the width-to-height ratio and sizes reveal the differences between normal humans and dogs.

Convex Hull

Bounding boxes do not have a shape description. In many cases, we want to describe the outer perimeter of the shape but not too many small details (e.g., for a rough convex contour of a walking space). Given a set of points, how do we determine which support the "outer perimeter"? This is similar to putting a rubber band around a set of points. The minimal area of the convex region is called the *convex hull*, in which all the inner points are ignored (Figure 7.9).

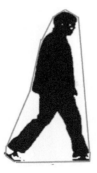

FIGURE 7.9 Shape description with Convex Hull. The envelope shows the motion energy over frames.

The simplest convex hull algorithm is explained in Figure 7.10. The pseudocode for the convex hull is as follows:

1.   Divide points in two subsets.
2.   Repeat:
3.   Find the maximal distance point from the line.
4.   Remove the points inside the triangle.
5.   Stop until no more point left.

There are many open source codes for calculating the convex hull. For example, a sample code is available.[142] For planar data sets, Eddy's QuickHull is a fast algorithm, and its complexity is $O(nh)$.[143]

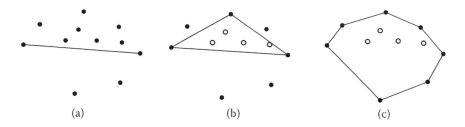

(a)   (b)   (c)

FIGURE 7.10   Convex Hull algorithm: (a) divide points in two subsets. (b) find farthest point from the line and remove the points inside the triangle. (c) repeat until no more points are left.

Contours

Contours are edges along the object that can be obtained from the binary blobs. Usually, blobs contain holes and noisy edges. To remove the noises, we can use binary image processes dilation and erosion operators (Figure 7.11).

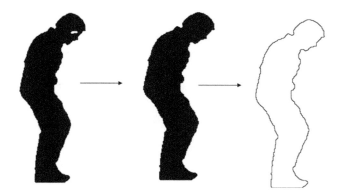

FIGURE 7.11   Original blob, dilation and then erosion, and contour extraction process.

Dilation bleeds one or more layers of pixels around the blob edges. Erosion, on the other hand, removes one or more layers of pixels around the blob edges. Dilating a couple of times and then eroding one or more times normally can remove small holes in the blob. Then, use an edge detection algorithm to extract the border contours.

---

[142] http://softsurfer.com/Archive/algorithm_0109/algorithm_0109.htm#chainHull_2D
[143] W. Eddy. A new convex hull algorithm for planar sets. *ACM Transactions on Mathematical Software* 3(4):398–403, 1977.

Note that dilation and erosion would change the shape a little bit. The more layers of dilation or erosion there are, the more distortion there will be.

Polar Coordinate Profile

In Chapter 2, we studied the polar coordinate profile representation method. The beauty of this method is that it can transform a two-dimensional (2D) feature space to a one-dimensional (1D) feature space—so it greatly simplifies problems. However, omitting shape details may create other problems. The polar coordinate profile is useful in video analysis because of (1) scale invariance (size does not matter); (2) rotation invariance (any rotated version of the contour should have no impact on the recognition); and (3) shift invariance (the shape doesn't change if it moves). The polar profile is also called the centroid contour distance curve (CCDC).[144]

How do we find the centroid? In many cases, we can draw a rectangular bounding box around the shape and put the centroid at the center of the bounding box. If we have prior knowledge about the shape, then we may use the knowledge to locate the centroid; for example, we put the centroid to the belly button of a human blob.

Then, we can plot the polar coordinate profile. Each point along the contour is defined by its distance from the centroid and its angle around the boundary from some arbitrary reference. By default, we normally begin at the zero degree in the counter-clockwise direction. We may also normalize the boundary to the [1, 0] range for scale invariance.

Human shape is complex. For some values of angle, there may exist a number of different values of radial distance. To avoid the problem, we may just use the smallest or the largest distance values at each angle, but this would reduce the accuracy of the shape representation.

How can we match polar coordinate profiles extracted from a scene with those from the training set? The matching process can be done by sliding the test profile along the candidate profiles and finding a significant fit.

Given a polar coordinate profile, we have at least three methods for matching it with known profile templates: Nearest Neighbor, Dynamic Time Warping (DTW), and Fourier Transform (FT).

Nearest neighbor is the simplest. For angles from 0 to 360, summarize the Euclidian distance between the template profile and the polar coordinate profile in terms of radius. The profile with the minimal distance is a match.

Dynamic Time Warping incorporates feature point alignment during the matching process (e.g., aligns peaks to peaks and valleys to valleys). As discussed in Chapter 6, DTW is computationally expensive. However, with some constraints, such as search window, slope, ending point, and monotony, approximate solutions can be obtained within a reasonable time frame.

Fourier Transform converts the 1D polar coordinate profile to a Fourier series (Figure 7.12). We can use the fast Fourier transform (FFT) to make the conversion. After the FFT, the contour is represented by the infinite series of Fourier coefficients.

---

[144] http://homepages.cae.wisc.edu/~ece533/project/f06/karrels_ppt.pdf

What is the physical meaning of these coefficients? The high-frequency terms describe microscopic details in the profile, while the low-frequency terms describe the metaphor, or macroscopic shape of the profile without details. In light of this, we can use a low-pass filter to remove the curvy details while keeping the high-level description of the profile (Figure 7.13). According to Zahn et al., the first ten Fourier coefficients should be enough to represent many 2D shapes for the problems, such as recognizing hand-written numbers.

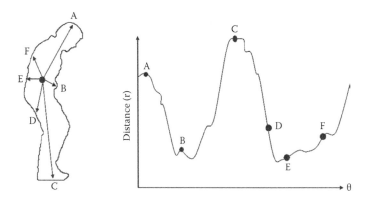

FIGURE 7.12 A two-dimensional shape and its polar coordinate profile (r, θ) plot.

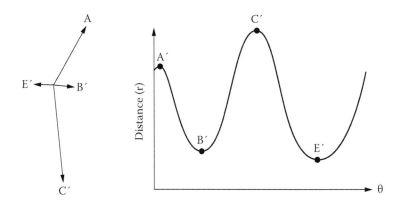

FIGURE 7.13 Use the low-pass filter to remove small details on the contour.

Active Contour

An active contour is an elastic 2D template based on a few landmark points. The term *active* represents the dynamics of the shape deformation. The active contour model is also called a "snake" because the points move sideways like a snake.[145] The model

---

[145] http://homepages.inf.ed.ac.uk/cgi/rbf/CVONLINE/entries.pl?TAG709

can be used to fit the template to a contour of an object, where the gradient along the contour along the object is maximal. The elastic snake has a number of control points (Figure 7.14). Normally, the snake contour is an open-ended curve. There are three parameters for controlling the points: *gradient attraction* in the image, *stiffness* of the snake curve, and *continuity* of the snake points.

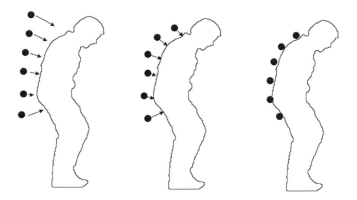

FIGURE 7.14   The point distribution model of a shape defined by six points.

An active contour can help to draw a smooth contour around the object. However, it has several limitations. For example, it is sensitive to the initial position of the control points, and it only works on grayscale images. There are several open source sample codes available online (e.g., the MATLAB version).[146]

7.5   VISUALIZATION OF VIDEO DATA

Video Summarization

Watching recorded footage in real time is very time consuming. Most video-editing software offers a "nonlinear" operation for manually moving the frame cursor backward and forward to find the interested point. However, our vision system can only catch up to the video images at thirty frames per second, and we will not see everything if we move the frame cursor too fast. Therefore, we need to find a way to reduce the information in the video. Video summarization[147] is playing an increasingly important role in the digital age. It aims to minimize visual data while retaining patterns of interest. The basic video summarization methods include time lapse, thumbnails, and superimposition.

A *time-lapse movie* is a video with reduced temporal resolution. In this digital age, a time-lapse movie can be easily produced from a full-speed video by skipping every *n* frames per second. This definitely reduces the footprint of the video.

Thumbnails can be organized in a timeline or calendar. This reduces spatial resolution and creates an overview of the video.

[146] http://www.mathworks.com/matlabcentral/fileexchange/28149-snake-active-contour
[147] http://www.cs.utexas.edu/~grauman/courses/spring2008/slides/Video_Summarization.pdf

Superimposition puts multiple frames onto one image. Figure 7.15 shows an example of the historical 1884 image *History of a Jump* by Thomas Eakins.

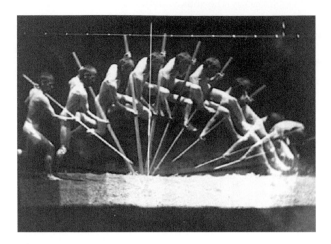

FIGURE 7.15   Superimposition using multiple exposures in this classic photograph, *History of a Jump* by Thomas Eakins in 1884. (From http://figuredrawings.com/Eakins-Photographs. html.)

Figure 7.16 is an example of superimposed frames for the traffic analysis in the hallway of a nursing home. For each pixel, we can sum up the values of n frames for each channel and then normalize the result to make sure that the values do not exceed the limit.

$$S_R = \frac{\sum_{i=1}^{n} R_i}{n} \tag{7.5}$$

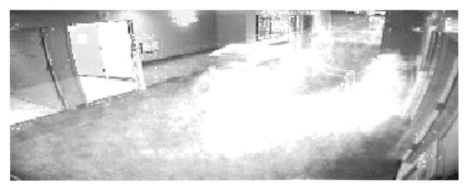

FIGURE 7.16   Superimposition of the traffic in a nursing home.

In the superimposed image, the white color area indicates the heavy traffic near the elevator. It shows that it is not a good idea to store things such as wheelchairs in that area.

More abstract methods include line tracing, histogram, heat map, convex hull, and scene map. Let's explore further.

Line History Image

For the line history image (LHI) method (Figure 7.17), assign the pixel values on the line to an array [x, t, v] and convert the array to an image, where x is the position of the line, t is the time length, and v is the value of the pixel at position x and time t.

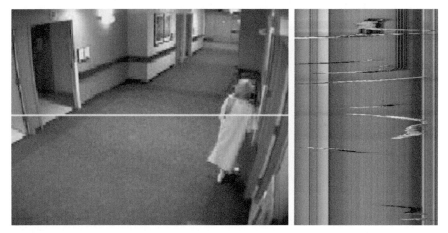

FIGURE 7.17 Sample result of line history image (LHI): original video (left) and the LHI (right).

Histogram

A histogram is a profile of colors or intensity of pixels (Figure 7.18). It is a simple and fast method to distinguish scene segments, detect scene changes, or detect an object based on its color or intensity signatures (e.g., daytime vs. nighttime or indoors vs. outdoors).

Heat Map

A heat map is a 2D histogram of repeated events (e.g., traffic patterns in the hallway of a nursing home). Similar to a histogram, a heat map is nonparameterized. The accumulation of the events on particular pixels can be converted to a pseudocolor map. Figure 7.19 shows an example of the traffic pattern in the hallway of a nursing home where we found that the area in front of the elevators was a hot spot. A heat map can summarize a very long CCTV (closed-circuit television) video as an intuitive pseudocolor image.

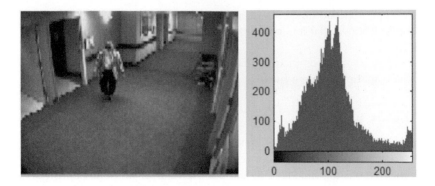

FIGURE 7.18   Original image (left) and histogram of the intensity (right).

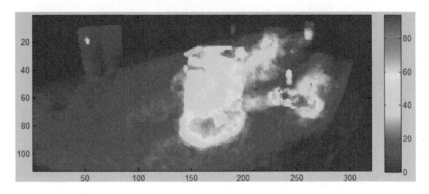

FIGURE 7.19   The heat map of the traffic in the hallway of a nursing home.

7.6   ACTIVITY RECOGNITION

A motion energy image (MEI) is an envelope of the moving pixels. Given a sequence of frames, MEI superimposes all the moving pixels onto one image, creating an outline of the motion energy area.

Given an image sequence $I(x, y, t)$, we have binary images indicating regions of motion $D(x, y, t)$. The binary MEI $E(x, y, t)$ is

$$E(x,y,t) = \bigcup_{i=0}^{t} D(x,y,t-i) \qquad (7.6)$$

Note that the values of $D(x, y, t)$ and $E(x, y, t)$ are binary: either one or zero. Now, let us look at a case study. Assume a hand moves from left to right. The MEI is shown in Figure 7.20. Note that the right corner of the MEI has some rough edges. This is because of the shadow of the hand.

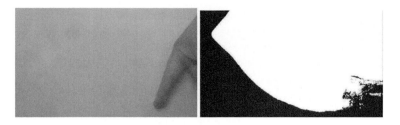

FIGURE 7.20 Motion energy image (MEI): The hand moves toward right in the original video sequence (left) and the MEI result (right)

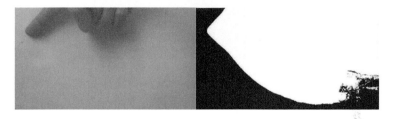

FIGURE 7.21 Motion energy image (MEI): The hand moves toward left in the original video sequence (left) and the MEI result (right)

Now, let us move the hand backward, from right to left. Figure 7.21 shows the same MEI simply because MEI only summarizes the moving pixels without considering the motion direction, speed, or history.

To analyze the gesture directions, we have to use the Motion History Image (MHI), which is about the changes of pixel intensity over time (Figure 7.22).

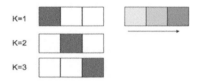

FIGURE 7.22 Motion history image of a moving pixel.

Normally, an MHI $H(u, v, k)$ at time k and location (u, v) is defined by the following equation:

$$H(u,v,k)= \begin{cases} d = 255, & \textit{if the pixel is recent} \\ 0, & \textit{if the pixel is never moved, or} \\ & H(u,v,k-1)=0 \\ H(u,v,k-1)-s & \textit{if } H(u,v,k-1) \neq 0 \end{cases} \quad (7.7)$$

where s is the reduction value for intensity level change, and d is the maximum duration a motion is stored. In general, d is chosen as the constant 255, allowing the MHI to be easily represented as a grayscale image with a depth of one byte. Thus, an MHI pixel can have a range of values, whereas an MEI is its binary version that can easily be computed by thresholding $H > 0$.

Now, let us compute the MHI with the same video sequence of the moving hand (Figures 7.23 and 7.24).

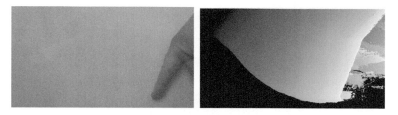

FIGURE 7.23   Motion history image (MHI) result of the hand moving from left to right

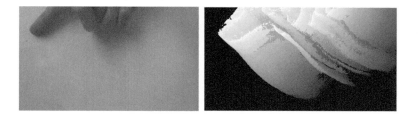

FIGURE 7.24   Motion history image (MHI) result of the hand moving from right to left..

7.7   COLOR AND MOTION AMPLIFICATION

The best is the last. Color and motion amplification is a breakthrough in video analytics. Researchers at the Massachusetts Institute of Technology (MIT) showed that it is feasible to measure people's body pulse patterns remotely using a webcam.[148] The amplification process contains three filters: the spatial filter, temporal filter, and infinite impulse response (IIR) filter. The spatial filter blurs the image to remove the spatial noises. The temporal filter removes the unwanted wave frequencies. The IIR filter is a digital filter for optimal transformation.

Spatial Filtering

The Gaussian blur is a spatial filter that uses a Gaussian function for calculating the transformation on each pixel in the image. For a 2D Gaussian function, we have

---

[148]   http://people.csail.mit.edu/mrub/vidmag/

$$G(x, y) = \frac{1}{2\pi\sigma^2} e^{-\frac{x^2+y^2}{2\sigma^2}} \tag{7.8}$$

where x is the distance from the origin in the horizontal axis, y is the distance from the origin in the vertical axis, and σ is the standard deviation of the Gaussian distribution. A Gaussian blur filter is similar to the low-pass filter in the frequency domain (see Figure 2.22).

Temporal Filtering

The ideal band-pass filter (Figure 7.25) selects a specific frequency range to pass and attenuate any frequencies outside that range. This filter can also be built by combining a low-pass filter and a high-pass filter. In this case, the high cutoff frequency is $f_H = 60/60$ Hz, and the low cutoff frequency is $f_L = 50/60$ Hz.

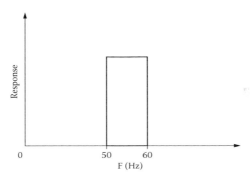

FIGURE 7.25 The ideal band-pass filter for temporal filtering.

Infinite Impulse Response Filtering

An IIR filter is designed to have an infinite response to an impulse function (a strong pulse input in a very short period). The filter's output contains the feedback from the previous outputs so that it can go on forever or for a period of time. The IIR filter can be designed numerically with a transform function, typically called the z-transform, which can generate the desirable response curve, including amplification gains, frequencies, and attenuation characteristics. Because of the IIR filter's capacities, it can be used for both color and motion amplification. The details can be found in an article available online.[149]

Ambient Diagnostic Applications

We can apply color and motion amplification to monitor people's pulses and subtle movements, creating affordable ambient diagnostic apps. To amplify color changes, we can combine the spatial and temporal filters to obtain results. To amplify motion

---

[149] http://people.csail.mit.edu/mrub/papers/vidmag.pdf

rather than color requires a more sophisticated filter such as IIR filter. The pseudo-code is as follows:

1. Use Gaussian blur filter
2. If it is color_amplification then use Ideal Band filter
3. If it is motion_amplification then use IIR filter

Here, let us test pulse detection using the color amplification method. We used the MATLAB code provided on the VIDMAG website (http://people.csail.mit.edu/mrub/vidmag/). We used a Canon digital camera to take a video at thirty frames per second. From the raw video, there are no obvious color changes on the subject's forehead (see Figure 7.26).

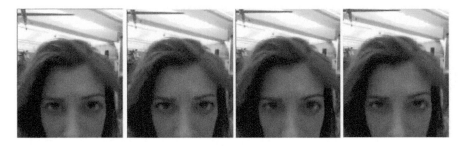

FIGURE 7.26 Original video.

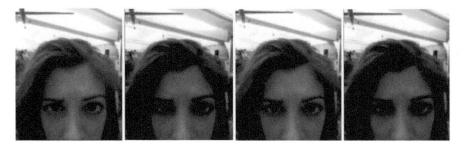

FIGURE 7.27 Color amplification for pulse detection, using R + B = Magenta, limited for y-axis = 100 pixels.

Let us apply the color amplification process to the video and obtain the results shown in Figure 7.27. We can observe the color changes on the subject's forehead now.

We can analyze the pulses by measuring the color values. Let us put a small box on the forehead of the subject as a measurement point (see Figure 7.28).

To have a better representation of the skin color, we take the sum of the red and blue values for 100 pixels vertically inside the box. Figure 7.29 shows that the pulse patterns are noisy in the original video. Figure 7.30 shows the significant improvement after the color amplification. We can clearly see the pulses.

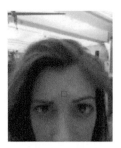

FIGURE 7.28 Selecting a pixel patch (10 × 10) on the subject's forehead.

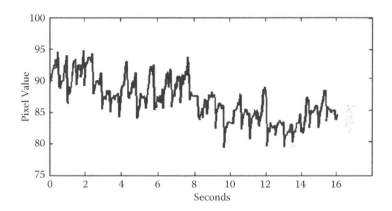

FIGURE 7.29 Original average color value in the patch on the forehead.

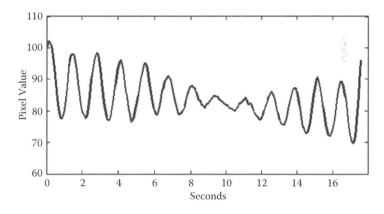

FIGURE 7.30 Color amplification result.

We can notice that there is a distorted waveform from the eighth to the thirteenth second. This was because of head movement during the videotaping. After the head returned to its original position, the pulse pattern recovered. The "drifting" problem can be solved by adding a head-tracking algorithm, for example, detecting the face in front of the camera and tracking the face during the measurement. There are plenty of face-tracking open sources online (e.g., OpenCV API for face detection).

7.8   SUMMARY

This chapter explored two groups of algorithms: intuitive video summarization and simple video analysis.

Video summarization is easy to implement and intuitive to understand. The methods include time lapse, thumbnails, superimposition, scanning line, MEI, and MHI. By all means, these intuitive methods should be used before more complicated methods.

Video analytics starts with blob extraction, assuming the camera is fixed. The approximate median filter performs better than frame subtraction and advanced models such as the GMM, which overspends computational resources just to build a perfect background model.

Object tracking can be helpful in ambient diagnoses such as gesture tracking and face tracking for measurements. However, compared to the Kinect, it is less robust because of the sensitivity to lights, skin color, and environments.

Color and motion amplification unleashes the potential of a regular camera to be a sophisticated pulse and breathing sensor, providing a wonderful case for ambient diagnosis.

PROBLEMS

1. Read thirty frames from a video file. Create thirty thumbnails in one image.
2. Use thirty frames from a video sequence to create a superimposed image.
3. Use thirty frames from a video sequence to create a heat map.
4. Add a red box to a sequence of images and write to a video file.
5. Draw your daily activities in symbols and compose thirty images. Write the thirty images to a video file to animate the sequence. Adjust the frame rate or duplicated frames to make an impressive visualization.
6. Extract moving objects from a video and compare the results of frame subtraction and approximate median filter.
7. Based on the results of Problem 6, plot the contours for the extracted objects.
8. Based on the results of Problem 6, plot the convex hulls for the extracted objects.
9. Based on the results of Problem 6, plot the MEI.
10. Based on the results of Problem 6, plot the MHI and compare the results of MEI.
11. The polar coordinate profile is effective in representing contour shapes. However, for some values of angle θ, there may exist a number of different values of the radial distance r. Write an algorithm to solve the problem and test it on ten images of subjects, including humans, cars, and dogs. Discuss the advantages and disadvantages of the method.
12. Use MHI to recognize sign language for the letters A, B, and C.
13. Use the mean-shift method to track a moving hand in a video. You may manually enter the bounding box to initiate the tracking target.

14. Write an algorithm that tracks a moving hand without manual initiation of the target. Hint: you have to detect the hand first.
15. Develop a demonstration for tracking faces and compare the results from the Kinect-based face tracking.
16. Integrate face tracking and a color amplification method to measure the facial pulse patterns in the video. Compare the results between with tracking and without tracking.

8 Fatigue Detection

> The strongest have their moments of fatigue.
>
> —Friedrich Nietzsche

8.1 INTRODUCTION

In Chapter 7, we explored video analytics for ubiquitously monitoring human pulse patterns, gaits, and activity level. Here, we go further to address how to evaluate fatigue over time. Human fatigue is a state of capacity reduction in mental or physical performance caused by work, stress, disease, therapy, or other factors. For decades, the prevailing clinical methods for evaluating fatigue were questionnaires, which are subjective and intrusive.[150] They cannot be used for real-time and continuous evaluation, or so-called online monitoring. This chapter covers two types of objective fatigue evaluation methods useful in ambient diagnostics: the vigilance clock test and fatigue facial expression recognition. The vigilance clock test is a cognition test well known to experimental psychologists but is not widely used in medical diagnosis; it is an interactive but off-line evaluation. Fatigue facial expression recognition is a video-based evaluation; it is nonintrusive and can be used for online evaluation.

8.2 DISEASE-RELATED FATIGUE

Fatigue signals can be used for ambient diagnoses and be related to diseases and treatment. For example, fatigue is one of the initial signs of diabetes. When the human body develops insulin resistance, it is unable to turn the ingested sugar in the body to the energy needed. The resulting fatigue is an indicator of high glucose levels, a sign of prediabetes. Other symptoms of diabetes, such as dehydration from increased urination, can also contribute to feeling tired all the time.[151]

Studies show that there is a possible correlation between fatigue and depression. When people are depressed, they often have symptoms similar to sleep deprivation. Therefore, a ubiquitous fatigue detection method might shed light on depression, which is hard to detect and even hard to clearly define.[152]

---

[150] Martha Davis et al. *The relaxation and stress reduction workbook*, 4th ed. New Harbinger, Oakland, CA, 1995.

[151] http://prediabetescenters.com/fatigue-and-diabetes/?utm_source=facebook&utm_medium=cpc&utm_term=fatigue&utm_content=tired-of-being-tired&utm_campaign=symptoms-fatigue

[152] D. Ebert, R. Albert, G. Hammon, B. Strasser, A. May, and A. Merz. Eye-blink rates and depression. Is the antidepressant effect of sleep deprivation mediated by the dopamine system? *Neuropsychopharmacology* 15(4):332–339, 1996.

Fatigue is also a common symptom of some cancers.[153] Patients describe fatigue as feeling tired and weak. Fatigue in cancer patients may be called cancer fatigue, cancer-related fatigue, and cancer treatment-related fatigue, such as with chemotherapy, radiation therapy, and biologic therapy.[154]

8.3   VIGILANCE THEORIES

Unlike material science, human fatigue is often viewed as a subjective state in which one feels tired or exhausted. There is no well-defined fatigue measurement in the context of health and illness simply because fatigue depends on a variety of factors,[155] including therapeutic treatment, culture; personality, lifestyle, the physical environment (e.g., weather, light, noise, vibration), social interaction, diseases or disorders, and the type and duration of work or exercise.

To scientifically measure fatigue, we may gain some insight from cognitive theories such as *vigilance*. Vigilance is the ability to sustain attention and alertness for a prolonged period of time. Since World War II, monitoring tasks have become overwhelming to operators. For instance, keeping operators alert in radar operation, long-distance flight, or driving can be a challenge because they are required to perform the same task over long periods of time. The vigilance theories that are related to health boil down to two: the attention resource theory and the theory of signal detection (TSD).

Attention Resource Theory

Attention is the ability to focus and maintain interest in a given task or idea while avoiding distractions. Attention is a scarce resource. Due to our limited perception, memory, and reaction capacities, our attention spans are limited.

Vigilance is closely related to attention; it is often described as a quality or state of alertness or watchfulness. Several concepts related to attention and vigilance have been developed in the past decades, including:

Covert attention is the instinctual use of senses (vision, hearing, smell, etc.) to focus on a particular stimulus source to gather more information. For example, when we smell burning, we often direct our attention to the source of the smell.

Selective attention involves focusing on a specific stimulus while ignoring other stimuli. It can be conscious or subconscious. For example, when a driver pays attention to the road up front, he or she may not pay attention to the scenery on either side.

Sustained attention is the ability to focus on specific stimuli for a long period of time.

---

[153] http://cancer.gov/cancertopics/pdq/supportivecare/fatigue/Patient

[154] M. O. Davis and D. Walsh. Mechanism of fatigue. *Journal of Supportive Oncology* 8:164–174, 2010.

[155] Linsey M. Barker. Measuring and modeling the effects of fatigue. Dissertation, Virginia Polytechnic Institute and State University, 2009.

Divided attention refers to limited attention resources being taken up by multiple tasks,[156] which in fact may cause a lot of stress and lead to depression and diseases, such as hypertension and heart attack.

Theory of Signal Detection (TSD)

The TSD was originally developed by electrical engineers and adopted by psychologists. Assume an operator detects a weak signal from background noise. The TSD specifies four possible measurable results: correctly detected ("hits"), false alarm, missed ("miss"), and correctly rejected.

According to the TSD, when an operator performs a task for a long period of time, the number of hits will decrease and the reaction time will increase after a long period of vigilantly performing the task. This is because of (1) the decrement of the skills to perceive a sensory stimulus (e.g., the ability to distinguish signs and signals); and (2) the shift of the decision criteria (e.g., thresholds).

Figure 8.1 shows the proportion of signals detected in a period of time, represented as a percentage.

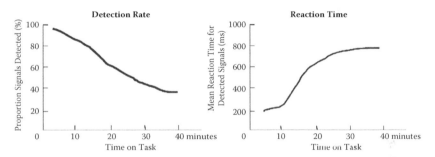

FIGURE 8.1 Signal detection rate (left) and the mean response time for detected signals (right), over a period of time.

8.4 THE VIGILANCE CLOCK

The vigilance clock, also known as the Mackworth clock, is a tool in experimental psychology for studying the effects of long-term vigilance on signal detection. It was originally created by Norman Mackworth to simulate long-term monitoring by radar operators in the British Air Force during World War II.[157]

Assigned the task of determining why motivated and skilled airmen were missing signals, Mackworth devised the "vigilance clock" with a large black clock

---

[156] A. D. Fisk and W. Schneider. Controlled and automatic processing during tasks requiring attention: a new approach to vigilance. *Human Factors* 23:737–750, 1981.

[157] N. H. Mackworth. The breakdown of vigilance during prolonged visual search. *Quarterly Journal of Experimental Psychology* 1:6–21, 1948.

hand on a large circular background, similar to an analog clock (Figure 8.2). The clock hand moves in short jumps, like the second hand of an analog clock, approximately every second. At infrequent and irregular intervals, the clock hand makes a double jump in a random interval (e.g., six times every sixty seconds). Whenever the clock hand makes a double jump, the subject is instructed to press a button.

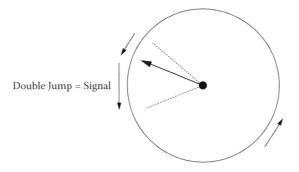

FIGURE 8.2 A vigilance clock, or Mackworth clock, is a simulation of the radar screen. Whenever the hand jumps twice in an interval, the subject is expected to press the button.

IMPLEMENTATIONS OF THE VIGILANCE CLOCK

The vigilance clock can be implemented on a desktop computer or a mobile phone (Figure 8.3). It is an animated clock hand with random jumps. The program tracks the detection rate and reaction time until the end of the experiment.

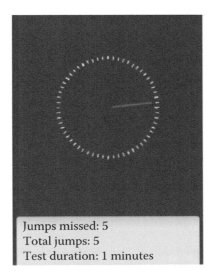

FIGURE 8.3 The graphical user interface of the vigilance clock on an Android phone.

The pseudocode for the vigilance clock is as follows:

1. Input data to set minutes
2. While minutes is not 0 then do:
3.   If random jump is true, then double_jump
4.   else single_jump
5.   Update event (tapped the button)
6.   If double_jump is true and tapped is true, then detected_counter + 1
7.   If double_jump is true and tapped is false, then missed_counter +1
8.   If double_jump is false and tapped is true, then false_alarm +1
9. End while
10. Display results

Experiment with the Vigilance Clock

How does the program run? First, a user must open the app and enter the test period (in minutes). Then, the user watches the moving clock hand that normally moves one unit a time but sometimes jumps two units at a time. When the double jump is found, the user clicks the screen. The app records the user's feedback on the screen in the background. Once the test is over, the app displays the detection rate and response time.

Experiments can be designed to show the effect of time on tasks and attention. The subjects were asked to watch the vigilance clock and detect the critical signal (the double jump of the clock hand) and to ignore the noncritical signal (the single jumps). The factor that affects performance the most in a vigilance task is the rest-to-activity ratio.

In the first experiment, we want to show the decrement of the detection rate and increment of the response speed over time. Figure 8.4 shows the results of ten subjects for sixty minutes. Figures 8.5 and 8.6 show the false alarm result for nonsignals and the response time for detected signals, respectively.

In the second experiment, the impact of rest on vigilance was tested. The user monitored the clock for twenty minutes and took twenty minutes rest. The user then

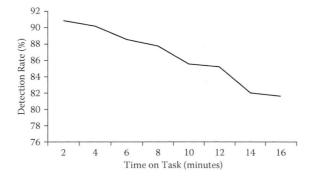

FIGURE 8.4 Vigilance clock app experimental results: detection and false alarm rates.

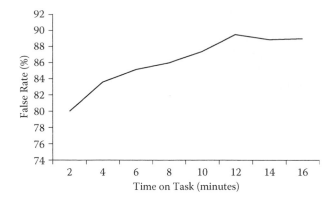

FIGURE 8.5   Vigilance clock app experimental results for false alarm for non-signals.

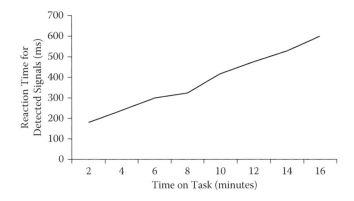

FIGURE 8.6   Vigilance clock app experimental results for the response time for detected signals.

repeated this four times. Then, we repeated the same experiment, but this time the rest/activity ratio was 10/10, ten minutes of test and ten minutes rest. Figure 8.7 shows the experimental results for both scenarios.

We can see that a short-rest activity cycle (ten minutes of activity/ten minutes of rest) was better than a long-rest activity cycle (twenty minutes activity/twenty minutes of rest).[158] We can concentrate more and put more attention on shorter activities. Our capacity and vigilance detector did not decrease as fast as long periods of test.

In the third experiment, we wanted to see the impact of the time of the day on detection rate and response time. The subjects were tested with the vigilance clock during the day and at night, and then results were compared. Figure 8.8 shows subjects' performance at 10 a.m. and 8 p.m.

---

[158] N. H. Mackworth. *Researches in the measurement of human performance*. MRC special report 268. HMSO, London, 1950.

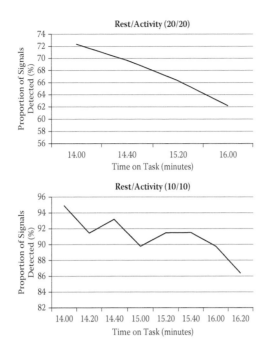

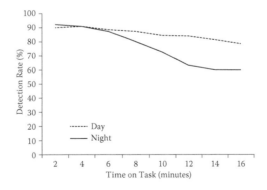

FIGURE 8.7   Impact of rest on signal detection rate.

FIGURE 8.8   Impact of the time of day on signal detection rate.

8.5   FACIAL FATIGUE DETECTION

Studies show that there is a correlation between eye-blink rate and fatigue. For example, patients with sleep deprivation or depression normally have a significantly higher rate of blinking. Blinking rate and yawning are two indicators of fatigue. To measure the blinking rate, we need to detect the eyes and track the open and closed states; to detect yawning, we have to detect the location of the mouth and track its open and

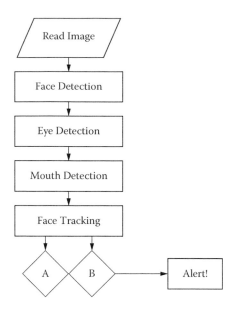

FIGURE 8.9   Facial fatigue detection flowchart.

closed states. Figure 8.9 illustrates the flowchart of the process. There are two main groups of technologies for detecting them: passive sensing and active sensing.

Passive sensing technologies use normal lighting and a regular digital camera. Active sensing technologies, on the other hand, use special illumination such as infrared lights.

8.6   PASSIVE FACE DETECTION

The vigilance clock is a disruptive and lengthy test method for testing for fatigue in lab settings. In the real world, it is desirable to have a nondisruptive method that can continuously and ubiquitously monitor a person's state of fatigue by using the indicators of blinking and yawning in passive face detection.[159]

To detect facial expressions, we first need to detect the face and its components: the eyes and mouth. The Viola-Jones object detection framework is the most popular algorithm for real-time object detection.[160] Although it has been widely used for detecting the entire face, it can be trained to detect a variety of object classes, including eyes and mouths.[161,162]

[159] Linda J. Vorvick. Yawning—excessive. January 31, 2011. http://www.nlm.nih.gov/medlineplus/ency/article/003096.htm

[160] Paul Viola and Michael J. Jones. Robust real-time object detection. *International Journal of Computer Vision* 57(2): 137–154, 2001.

[161] Cognitics: Resources for cognitive robotics. How face detection works. http://www.cognitics.com/opencv/servo_2007_series/part_2/sidebar.html

[162] Z. Zhiu and Q. Ji. Robust real-time eye detection and tracking under variable lighting conditions and various face orientations. *Computer Vision and Image Understanding* 98(1):124–154, 2005.

The Viola-Jones object detection algorithm has been implemented in OpenCV MATLAB and the Python-based SimpleCV library.

Haar-Like Features

The Viola-Jones algorithm uses the "Haar-like" features as discussed in Chapter 2 (Figure 8.10). How these features are calculated? The eyebrows are typically darker than the cheeks, and the bridge of the nose is typically brighter than the two sides of the face around it. A feature is essentially all of the pixels in one area of the image added together minus the pixels in another area added together. The lower-level classifier, or so-called weak classifier, takes the value and classifies it as "feature" or "not feature" based on a threshold and a polarity. For example, if the threshold is fifty and polarity is "greater than," the weak classifier will classify an image as a feature if the sum of the intensity in one area minus the sum of the intensity in another is greater than fifty.

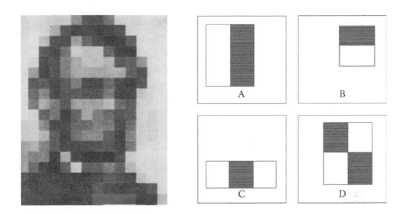

FIGURE 8.10   Haar-like features.

Cascade Decision Making

The Viola-Jones algorithm aims to find multiple rectangular features to detect an object in an image. It uses cascade decision-making architecture to combine the weak feature classifiers and their weighted errors to make a strong classifier (Figure 8.11).

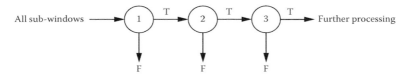

FIGURE 8.11   Cascade decision making.

The cascade architecture has interesting implications for the performance of the individual classifiers because the activation of each classifier depends entirely on the behavior of its predecessor. The Viola-Jones algorithm is fast at detection. However, it has a few weaknesses. For example, it is very sensitive to lighting conditions and works best when the portraits are well lit, like in a passport photo (Figure 8.12). It is also sensitive to the training objects, such as skin color, poses, and so on. The algorithm is sensitive to scaling, rotating, and sheering.

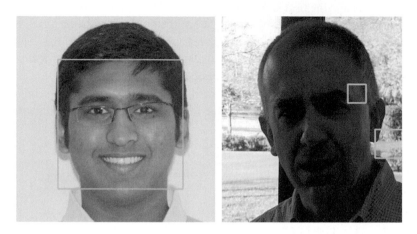

FIGURE 8.12   Face detection under good and bad lighting conditions.

While detection speed can reach real time, the algorithm's training process is horribly slow and can take an order of days or weeks. This is essentially a brute-force approach for learning all possible combinations of feature, polarity, and threshold. Assume we have 100,000 possible features, 10,000 object and nonobject training images, and 100 weak classifiers to search for; it could possibly require 100 billion operations to perform the training process.

8.7   PASSIVE FACE TRACKING

Active Shape Model

The active shape model (ASM)[163,164] tracks a face shape by aligning a facial template to images using several specific landmark points. The template can be deformed by iteratively modifying landmark points to fit the local neighborhood. The process is similar to matching a rubber mask to a face. Figure 8.13 shows a typical template, and Figure 8.14 shows how the template is gradually made to fit the face. (Note that the term *active shape* here is different from the term *active sensing*; the first is about

---

[163]   T. F. Cootes, C. J. Taylor, D. H. Cooper, and J. Graham. Active shape models—their training and application. *Computer Vision and Image Understanding* 61:38–59, 1995. http://www.mathworks.com/matlabcentral/fileexchange/26706-active-shape-model-asm

[164]   Active shape model (ASM) and active appearance model (AAM). http://www.mathworks.com/matlab-central/fileexchange/26706

actively moving landmark points, and the second is about actively illuminating a spectra light to an object.)

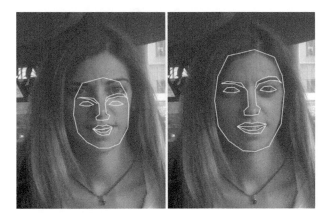

FIGURE 8.13   The facial template is deformed until it fits the face.

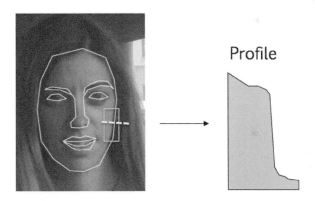

FIGURE 8.14   The intensity profile at each landmark point is extracted.

Iterative template fitting is implemented by moving those landmark points. For each landmark point, we draw a line along the perpendicular to the boundary line and then extract the gray-level profile along the line. The extracted profile is used to check whether the errors are in the allowable range compared to the stored expected profile. If not, the landmark point locations can be moved until the profiles match.

For a two-dimensional (2D) image, we can represent the n landmark points (x_i, y_i) as the $2n$ element vector x, where

$$x = \left(x_1, \ldots, x_n, y_{1,} \ldots y_n \right)^T \tag{6.1}$$

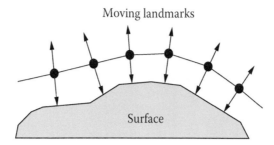

Moving landmarks

Surface

FIGURE 8.15   The landmark points are moved along the intensity profile to search for the best fit.

The ASM model is trained from manually drawn contours in training images. It then finds the main variations in the training data using principal component analysis (PCA), which reduces data dimensions to t.

Given the transformation matrix P with eigenvector t, the mean shape $\bar{x}$, and a vector of weight b, the active shape landmark coordinates x can be estimated as

$$x = \bar{x} + P \cdot b \qquad (6.2)$$

After creating the ASM, an initial contour is deformed by finding the best intensity profile match for the control points. Apply global transformation T to the image, including scaling, translation, and rotation. This is an iterative process in which the control points are moved along the profile to search for the optimal locations (Figure 8.15):

$$\arg\min_{T} \left| x - T\left(\bar{x} + P \cdot b\right)\right|^2 \qquad (6.3)$$

Implementations of the software are already available. The simplest way to experiment with ASM is to obtain the MATLAB-based ASM package, available from Visual Automation Limited. This provides an application that allows users to annotate training images, to build models, and to use those models to search new images. In addition, the package allows limited programming for its MATLAB interface.

STASM is a C++ software library for finding features in faces. Users give it an image of a face and it returns the positions of the facial features. It also allows users to build their own ASMs. The source code is provided under the GPL (General Public License).[165]

ASMLIB is an open source implementation of ASM with OpenCV (2.0 or higher)[166] written in C++. It can be run on Linux, Windows, Mac OS X, and Android.

---

[165] S. Milborrow and F. Nicolls. Locating facial features with an extended active shape model. *ECCV*, 2008. http://www.milbo.users.sonic.net/stasm

[166] http://code.google.com/p/asmlib-opencv/

Blink Detection

Similar to face detection, eye detection can be learned from cropped eye image samples using the Viola-Jones algorithm (Figure 8.16). An eye detection algorithm was tested on 450 images from the California Institute of Technology database. The successful detection rate was nearly 86%. The algorithm failed when lighting was poor, when there were multiple faces in the background of images, and when the person was too far from the camera.

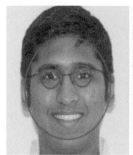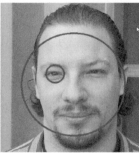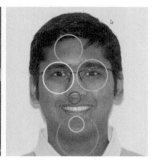

FIGURE 8.16   Eye and face detection under good lighting (left), eye detection failure due to small eye opening (middle), and mouth detection failure (right).

Yawn Detection

The Viola-Jones algorithm does not work well with yawn detection due to the variations and dynamics of the mouth. Here, we need to use the ASM to detect and track the mouth when it opens and closes passively.

For yawn detection, we need up to twelve landmark points to map the contour of the mouth. When the mouth is closed, these landmarks competently detect a mouth lining, but when the mouth opens beyond a certain threshold value, the landmarks become skewed. Replicating this skew over a number of frames is used to detect the occurrence of a yawn.

To conduct this process, we can use the Viola-Jones detection algorithm to locate the face to initiate the origin for the ASM template. A set of sixty-eight landmarks should be enough to model the expressions of the face. We then train the model with an ample number of face images. The landmark points of these images are registered manually or tracked automatically from previous frames. The landmarks are detected and assigned coordinate values relative to the origins that have just been marked. The values of these landmarks are then compared to the sample set, the image in the sample set that is the closest match is chosen as the mapping image, and the landmarking of that image is replicated in this image.

The training images that are chosen are such that no image represents the case where the mouth is open to an extent equivalent to a yawn; thus, the presence of a yawn will skew the landmarking. A utility that is provided as a part of the STASM package, called STASM, generates a log file of the landmarks of a certain image that is passed to it (Figure 8.17). Thus, if we divide each video into frames and we

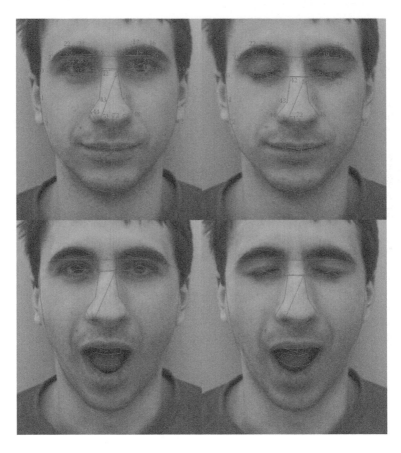

FIGURE 8.17 Facial landmark tracking using the active shape model (STASM package).

pass each frame to STASM, it generates a log file for each frame. From this log file, we can look at the values of two specific landmarks. For instance, number 51 and number 57 correspond to the upper lip of the image and the lower lip of the image, respectively (Figure 8.18). By measuring the vertical distance between the two land-mark points (P_{51} and P_{57}), we can detect the presence of a yawn.

The algorithm's effectiveness was measured by testing the process with real-time video processing under different conditions, such as inside a car at nighttime, inside a car during the day, and in front of the laptop (Table 8.1).

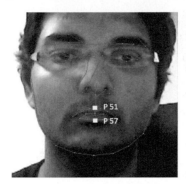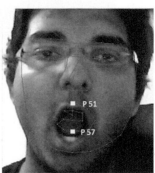

FIGURE 8.18   Yawn detection from the vertical distance between upper lip and lower lip.

TABLE 8.1 Blinking and Yawn Detection Results *

Detection	In Car (Day)	In Car (Night)	Laptop
Face	70% (VJ)	50% (VJ)	100% (VJ)
Blink	25% (VJ)	<10% (VJ)	86% (VJ) 60% (ASM)
Yawn	80% (VJ)	70% (VJ)	100% (ASM)

* VJ = Viola-Jones method, ASM = Active Shape Model

From the lab experimental results, we can see accuracy for the face detection, blinking and yawning detection are adequate. Although the blinking detection accuracy is rather low, the Viola-Jones detection algorithm is better than the ASM algorithm. All the detection results become worse when lighting is poor (e.g., in the car or in a dark area). To improve iris detection accuracy, we can combine active sensing technologies, such as near-infrared (IR) lighting sources.

8.8   ACTIVE SENSING FOR DETECTING BLINKING AND YAWNING

Active sensing technologies, on the other hand, use special illumination such as IR light sources to detect blinking and yawning. The pupils show distinct spectral or reflective properties under near-IR illumination (Figure 8.19). This property can be used for locating the eyes by thresholding. Active eye detection techniques are generally more accurate than passive techniques. However, they require a special light source as an input, and results can be distorted by ambient light.

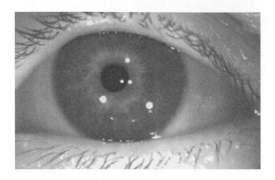

FIGURE 8.19   Reflections of the near-IR light in the eye.

Kinect is also an active sensor that emits structured near-IR light dots to create a three-dimensional model of a surface in front of it. Detecting yawning with Kinect is straightforward because of the unique cavity on the face. By thresholding the depth value of the mouth, we can detect the mouth when it is open or closed and for what duration in real time (Figure 8.20).

From the two examples, we may conclude that active sensing can detect eye blinking and mouth opening in a simple and elegant way without substantial modeling and programming. This can be implemented on the Kinect using its IR light source and the IR camera. However, the Kinect is designed for remote control. It might cause some problems if the distance between the eyes and the IR source is too close because it is not in the designated safe range. More studies should be done to ensure the safety of the device.

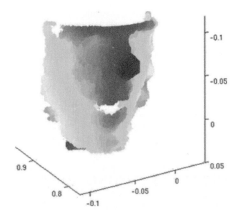

FIGURE 8.20   Mouth detection with Kinect (the white area).

8.9 SUMMARY

Diseases, depression, therapy, and work can cause fatigue, which is often viewed as a subjective matter. In this chapter, we explored objective measurements for fatigue evaluation. The vigilance clock is an off-line test method from a cognitive background. It is simple and easy to test. However, it is time consuming because watching the clock itself is a task. It may not totally reflect the nature of fatigue. The facial fatigue detection includes eye blinking and yawning detection. With the Viola-Jones and ASM model, facial landmark tracking can reach a fairly good level of accuracy, showing potential for continuous and passive fatigue evaluation from a webcam. It is worth noting that active sensors such as the Kinect can detect eye blinking and yawning in a rather simpler and more robust way.

The technologies discussed here are useful not only for ambient diagnosis but also for other applications, such as "smart truck" that can sense drivers' level of fatigue and take control of the car or advise the driver to pull off the road.[167]

PROBLEMS

1. Download the vigilance clock.[168] Perform the vigilance experiment. Test the detection rate for five minutes and then work on a computer for one hour and test the detection rate again. Plot the chart and discuss the results.
2. Discuss fatigue detection for drivers and compare the pros and cons of various methods.
3. Use the Kinect to detect yawning. Analyze the results with a confusion matrix. Discuss the sensitivity and specificity.
4. Discuss the safe wavelength and distance for pervasive IR-based active sensing for fatigue detection.
5. Discuss the feasibility of fatigue detection from voices on a cell phone. Collect samples and plot spectrograms to support your design.
6. Prototype an eye-blinking detection system with ASM (e.g. STASM). Find minimal landmarks for fatigue expression detection.
7. Define a biorhythmic variable for predicting fatigue (e.g., number of courses, online time, assignment load, exams, work, exercises, parties, and so on). Draw a pie chart to illustrate the contributing factors.
8. Write an essay about fatigue and depression. Discuss the potential of detecting depression.
9. Use the vigilance clock to study the relationship between detection errors and task duration. Plot the chart to summarize your finding.
10. Discuss how to embed the fatigue detection in video games so that it would display a warning message when the system detects the player's fatigue.

---

[167] J. Healey and R. Picard. Smart car: detecting driver stress. In *Proceedings of the 15th International Conference on Pattern Recognition*, Barcelona, Spain, 4:218–221, 2000.
[168] http://www.millisecond.com/download/library/MackworthClock/

Section 3

Pervasive Sensors

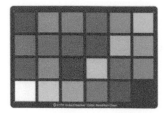

Figure 5.14

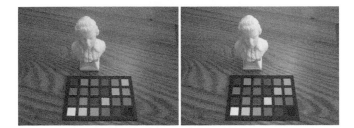

Figure 5.15

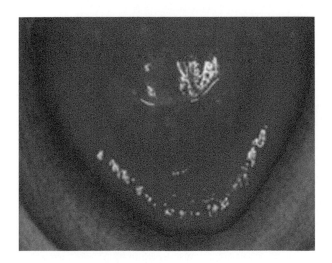

Figure 5.16

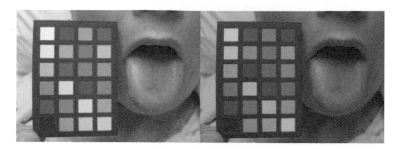

Figure 5.17

Original Image

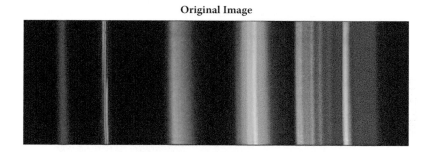

Image Gray Spectrogram [using weighted sum] vs wavelength

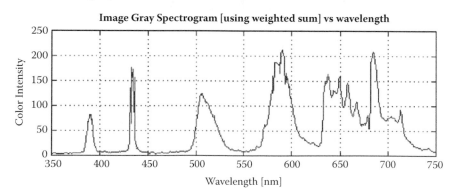

Figure 12.16

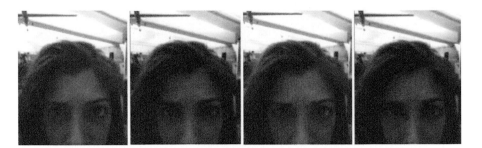

Figure 7.27

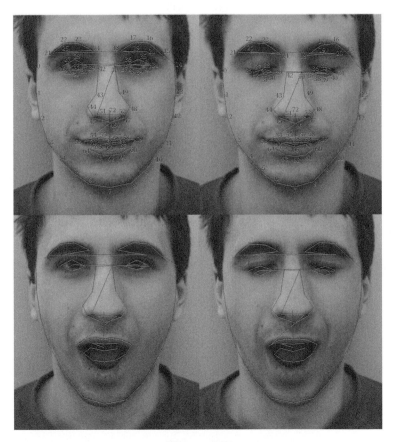

Figure 8.17

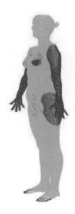

Figure 13.13

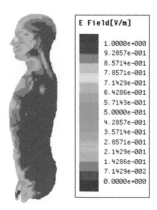

Figure 13.14

9 Mobile Sensors

> Computers in the future may weigh no more than 1.5 tons.
>
> —Popular Mechanics, 1949

9.1 INTRODUCTION

Microelectromechanical system (MEMS) devices truly bridge the gap between electrical and mechanical engineering, and their design involves contributions from industrial, materials, mechanical, electrical, biomedical, chemical, computer, and software engineers. Developers have unprecedented access to the underlying hardware on a mobile device. In addition to hardware such as the camera, the Android and iOS operating systems have a variety of application programming interfaces (APIs) for accessing low-level hardware features on the handsets, including

- Accelerometers
- Gyroscopes
- Near-field communication (NFC)
- Magnetic sensors
- Touch sensors
- Environmental sensors
- GPS, Wi-Fi (wireless fidelity), and Bluetooth sensors
- Apps for accessing sensor data

This chapter explores those mobile sensors, their potential for ambient diagnostics, and applications in activity classification for elderly care at home. Finally, we walk through available apps for collecting mobile sensing data.

9.2 ACCELEROMETERS

Accelerometers measure acceleration in three dimensions. They are already standard components in air bags. Accelerometers are also widely used in personal mobile devices, such as smartphones and fitness products.

A MEMS accelerometer can be visualized as masses on springs. They jiggle when we shake them, and they pick up just about every kind of movement. There are different ways to make an accelerometer. For example, the piezoelectric method turns motion into a current. Here, we just focus on the most popular way to make an accelerometer: by sensing changes in capacitance. Why? In most micromachining technologies, it takes minimal processing to make movable microscopic capacitances, and they are insensitive to temperature changes.[169]

A typical MEMS accelerometer is composed of a movable plate that are attached through a mechanical suspension system to a reference frame, as shown in Figure 9.1. Movable plates and fixed outer plates represent capacitors. The deflection of the movable plate is measured using the capacitance difference. The free-space capacitances between the movable plate and two stationary outer plates are functions of the corresponding displacements and the movable plate displacement results due to acceleration (Figure 9.2).[170]

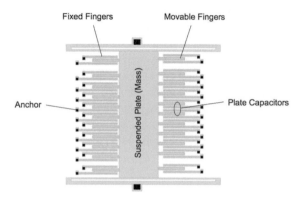

FIGURE 9.1 Accelerometer MEMS sensor structure. The movable plate is attached through springs at substrate. It can only move up and down. Movable and fixed plates construct capacitors.

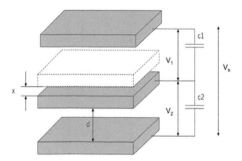

FIGURE 9.2 Parallel plate capacitive circuit in which the middle plate moves a distance x.

[169] Matej Andrejašić. MEMS accelerometers. http://mafija.fmf.uni-lj.si/seminar/files/2007_2008/ MEMS_accelerometers-koncna.pdf

[170] S. E. Lyshevski. *MEMS and NEMS: systems, devices and structures.* CRC Press, Boca Raton, FL, 2002.

Assuming that the outer two electrodes are fixed and the inner electrode is free to move in a parallel direction toward the top plate, the gap between the top plates and the moving plate will decrease, and the gap between the moving plate and the bottom one will increase.[171] If the gap distance d and the center electrode are moved by a distance x, then the relationship between the differential output voltage and the deflection is given by

$$V_x = V_1 - V_2 = V_s \cdot \frac{x}{d} \tag{9.1}$$

According to Hooke's law, an ideal spring exhibits a restoring force F_s that is proportional to the displacement Δx. Thus, $F_s = k_s x$, where k_s is the spring constant. From Newton's second law, $ma = k_s x$. The acceleration, as a function of the displacement, is

$$a = \frac{k_s}{m} x = \frac{k_s \cdot d}{m} \cdot \frac{V_x}{V_s} \tag{9.2}$$

Here, we find that the acceleration is proportional to voltage output. For MEMS accelerometers, the measurements are rather small. The mass of the movable plate mentioned is approximately 0.1 µg, the smallest detectable capacitance change is about 20 aF, and gaps between capacitor plates are approximately 1.3 µm. This is the simplest example of a one-axis accelerometer. Its capacitance changes due to changes of distance d between capacitor plates. If one includes sets of capacitors turned in perpendicular directions, one can obtain a two-axis or three-axis accelerometer (Figure 9.3).

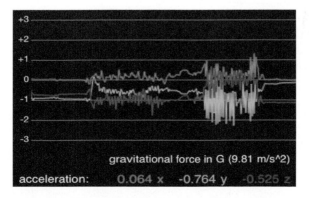

FIGURE 9.3 Three-axis accelerometer data from SensorLog on iPhone 4: sitting, walking, and then running.

---

[171] http://cgs.unimap.edu.my/flashxml/2012/10/2-A-Review-of-MEMS-Capacitive-Sensing-Technique-and-Capacitive-Sensor.pdf.

Gravity Component

A three-axis accelerometer sensor provides a three-value array: a_x, a_y, and a_z. All values are in SI units (meters/second squared). In particular, the force of gravity always has an influence on the measured acceleration (Figure 9.4).

Gravity   Free Fall   Linear Acceleration

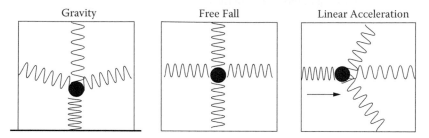

FIGURE 9.4   Gravity effect on the three-axis accelerometer in resting, free fall, and linear acceleration.

For this reason, when the device is set on a table (and obviously not accelerating), the accelerometer reads a magnitude of $g = 9.81$ m/s². However, when the device is in free fall and therefore dangerously accelerating toward the ground at 9.81 m/s², its accelerometer reads a magnitude of 0 m/s². The reason is that gravity pulls both on the mass in the middle and on the frame of the accelerometer. So, there is no relative movement between the mass and the frame.

How do we remove gravity? This can be done in two ways: We can move the accelerometer horizontally to create a linear acceleration or subtract gravity digitally (Figure 9.4).

Coordinate Systems

Accelerometers in a device have a default coordinate system called the device coordinate system (Figure 9.5). For the Android phone platform, the x-axis is horizontal and points to the right, the y-axis is vertical and points up, and the z-axis points toward the outside of the front face of the screen. In this system, coordinates behind the screen have negative z values.

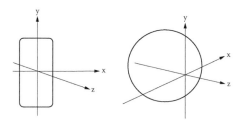

FIGURE 9.5   Device coordinate system and global coordinate system.

It is worth noting that this coordinate axes are not swapped when a device's screen orientation changes, while the phone position may vary. The data from the sensor may not reflect the actual condition. Therefore, we need to transform any vector from the device's coordinate system to the global coordinate system, where z points toward the sky, y points toward the magnetic North Pole, and x points east.

The transform can be done by multiplying it by the rotation matrix. For the Android platform, we can obtain the rotation matrix from getRotationMatrix(). A quick tutorial about how to access the accelerometer data is available.[172]

9.3   GYROSCOPE

A gyroscope is a device for measuring orientation, based on the principles of conservation of angular momentum. Mobile phones such as the iPhone and Android HTC Sensation utilize an MEMS gyroscope.

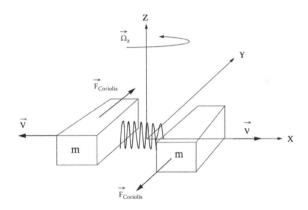

FIGURE 9.6   Coriolis effect in MEMS gyroscopes.

MEMS gyroscopes use the Coriolis effect to measure the angular rate, as shown in Figure 9.6. When a movable plate m is moving in direction v and angular rotation velocity is applied, then the mass will experience a force in the direction of the arrow as a result of the so-called Coriolis force.[173] The Coriolis acceleration is

$$a = -2\vec{\Omega} \times \vec{V} \tag{9.3}$$

where a is the acceleration of the particle in the rotation system. The symbol represents the cross-product operator. The resulting physical displacement caused by the Coriolis force is then read from a capacitive sensing structure, similar to the accelerometers.

---

[172] http://www.techrepublic.com/blog/app-builder/a-quick-tutorial-on-coding-androids-accelerometer/472

[173] http://www.electroiq.com/articles/stm/2010/11/introduction-to-mems-gyroscopes.html

Most available MEMS gyroscopes use a tuning fork configuration. Two masses oscillate and move constantly in opposite directions. When angular velocity is applied, the Coriolis force on each mass also acts in opposite directions, which results in capacitance change. This differential value in capacitance is proportional to the angular velocity Ω and is then converted into output voltage for analog gyroscopes or bits for digital gyroscopes.

When linear acceleration is applied to two masses, they move in the same direction. Therefore, there will be no capacitance difference detected. The gyroscope will output a zero-rate level of voltage or least significant bits digitally, which shows that the MEMS gyroscopes are not sensitive to linear acceleration such as tilt, shock, or vibration.

Gyroscopes measure how quickly an object rotates. They are the only inertial sensors that provide accurate, latency-free measurement of rotations without being affected by any external forces, including magnetic, gravitational, or other environmental factors. This rate of rotation can be measured along any of the three axes: x (roll), y (pitch), and z (yaw).[174] Adding gyroscopes to the sensor mix allows algorithm designers to take advantage of a pure measurement of angular velocity that cannot be delivered by compasses or accelerometers. This measurement allows for accurate pitch and roll measurements when combined with an accelerometer, and these measurements can be used to more accurately compensate for the tilt.

The sensitivity of MEMS gyroscopes is usually in millivolts/degrees per second, so the output of the oscillator (in millivolts) divided by the sensitivity (millivolts/degrees per second) provides the angular rate applied to the package in degrees per second. Figure 9.7 shows log data from an iPhone's gyroscope.

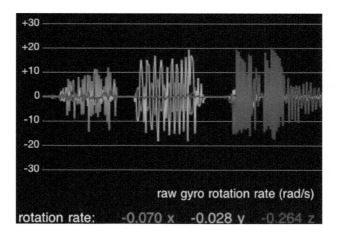

FIGURE 9.7   Three-axis gyroscopic data from SensorLog on iPhone 4: pitch (red, left), roll (green, middle), and yaw (blue, right).

MEMS gyroscopes can be embedded in mobile devices such as smartphones for sensing subtle angular movements. They can also be mounted on people's arms and legs for body tracking and monitoring. A gyroscope-based gait-phase detection

---

[174] http://mobiledevdesign.com/tutorials/motion-processing-next-breakthrough-070110/

sensor is used to help people with a dropped-foot walking dysfunction.[175] The sensor can be embedded in the shoe insole and detects in the four walking phases during the gait cycle: stance, heel off, swing, and heel strike. The gyroscope in the shoe insole measures the angular velocity of the foot. The signal can be recorded in the embedded microprocessor and downloaded for off-line gait analysis, for example, walking dysfunction and fall risk assessment. The gyroscopic signal can also be transmitted in real-time to the electrical stimulator attached to the affected muscles, providing a feedback control loop for gait correction. The electrical stimulations induce muscle contractions in the paralyzed muscles, leading to a more physiological motion of the affected leg. Figure 9.8 shows the foot positions during the swing phase.

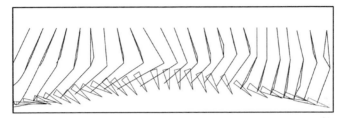

FIGURE 9.8 The foot positions of a patient with a dropped-foot walking dysfunction during a gait cycle.

9.4 MAGNETIC FIELD SENSOR

A magnetic field sensor measures magnetism in three dimensions. The geomagnetic field sensor and orientation sensor return multidimensional arrays of sensor values for each sample, measuring geomagnetic field strength along the x-, y-, and z-axes in microtesla (μT). Why do we need three axes? In theory, if we know how the user holds the compass, we can just use two axes instead of three. However, as we usually do not know the orientation of the compass, we need to use a three-axis system in addition to the input from the accelerometers to obtain the orientation data. Furthermore, Earth's magnetic field does not exactly point north, so we need GPS data to know the location and where the magnetic north is.

How does the magnetic field sensor work? In MEMS technology, it does not need a spinning needle. Current is sent through a wire and is deflected by the Hall effect if there is a magnetic field presence (Figure 9.9). The Hall effect was discovered by Edwin Herbert Hall in 1879.[176] Hall found that electrons moving through a conductor will migrate to one side of the conductor in the presence of magnetism. The resulting charge separation is induced voltage. In modern electronics, semiconductor-based Hall effect devices (HEDs) sense the presence and magnitude of a magnetic field. Since signal levels are very low (typically micro- to millivolts) from the actual HED sensor, a HED is coupled with an electronic amplifier, comparator, voltage

[175] I. P. I. Pappas, T. Keller, and S. Mangold. A reliable gyroscope-based gait-phase detection sensor embedded in a shoe insole. *IEEE Sensors Journal* 4:268–274, 2004.

[176] http://www.driveforinnovation.com/build-a-magnetic-sensing-hall-effect-sensor-interface/

references, and an output driver in the same package to make it easier to use for a variety of applications. Now, compasses can actually be created with just pure silicon electronics without ferromagnetic material for them.

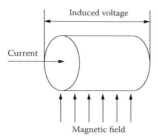

FIGURE 9.9   The Hall effect occurs when charged particles move in the presence of a magnetic field, resulting in an inducted voltage.

9.5   ORIENTATION SENSOR

An orientation sensor measures a device's orientation (Figure 9.10). The orientation sensor is software based and derives its data from the accelerometer and the geomagnetic field sensor. The orientation sensor provides pitch, roll, and yaw (or azimuth) values during a single sampling interval in degrees.

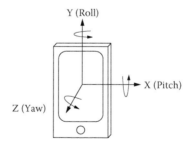

FIGURE 9.10   Orientation sensor: azimuth (z), pitch (x), and roll (y) axes.

Pitch (rotation around the x-axis). This value is positive when the positive z-axis rotates toward the positive y-axis, and it is negative when the positive z-axis rotates toward the negative y-axis. The range of values is 180 degrees to −180 degrees.

Roll (rotation around the y-axis). This value is positive when the positive z-axis rotates toward the positive x-axis, and it is negative when the positive z-axis rotates toward the negative x-axis. The range of values is 90 degrees to −90 degrees.

Yaw or azimuth (rotation around the z-axis). This is the angle between magnetic north and the device's *y*-axis. For example, if the device's *y*-axis is aligned with magnetic north, this value is zero, and if the device's *y*-axis is pointing south, this value is 180 degrees. Likewise, when the *y*-axis is pointing east, this value is 90 degrees, and when it is pointing west, this value is 270 degrees.

9.6 TOUCH GESTURE SENSORS

In the world of touch screen devices, the use of gestures such as multiple swipes of the finger in different directions on the screen enables the device to capture complex patterns (Figure 9.11). Many touch screens these days are also pressure sensitive, with the pressure proportional to the size of the touch area. A touch screen can capture strokes and compare them with the gesture data in the gesture library. The output includes a score and name, with the score indicating the closeness to the named gesture within the library.

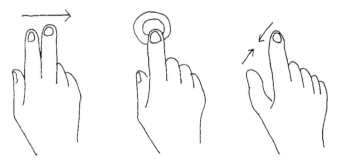

FIGURE 9.11 Multitouch tactile gestures on a touch screen.

Touch Gesture Feature Vector

The basic anatomy of a gesture consists of multiple gesture stroke objects, and each object is made up of gesture points, including *x* and *y* spatial coordinates and a single timestamp indicating when the point was generated. When a gesture is stored in a gesture library, it is keyed with a name. Using the order of points as the timestamp for each gesture, we can acquire an equal-length vector in the form of $(x_1, y_1, t_1, x_2, y_2, t_2, \ldots, x_n, y_n, t_n)$. For $N = 16$, it allows a 48-element vector for each gesture, which is enough resolution for feature extraction and classification. We can also convert the points from a Cartesian coordinate system to a polar coordinate system (ρ_i, θ_i, t_i). Using a polar coordinate system enables orientation-invariant analysis. For example, we can align the gesture with a closest alignment of the eight major orientations (Figure 9.12).[177]

---

[177] https://www.lri.fr/~anab/teaching/M2R-2011/5-gestures/protractor-chi2010.pdf

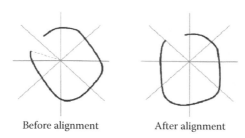

Before alignment   After alignment

FIGURE 9.12   For orientation-sensitive cases, we can align the gesture with a closest alignment of the eight major orientations.

Tremor Evaluation

Tremors are common among people with Parkinson's disease, people who have had a stroke, or people with other brain diseases. Another disorder called "essential tremor" is common among older adults and occurs twenty times more often than Parkinson's disease. Unlike Parkinson's, essential tremor is not due to an underlying disease and does not lead to serious complications. Shaky hands can also be due to anxiety, but to reach this diagnosis, a physician must first rule out physical causes. In addition to essential tremor and Parkinson's, shaky hands may be caused by thyroid disease, drug side effects, or heavy metal poisoning.

Measuring hand coordination is essential to the diagnosis of tremors. This can be done by showing the user one of the training gesture samples and letting the user repeat the gesture as close as possible on the touch screen. The algorithm assesses the similarity of the sample and the user input. The similarity can be calculated using Euclidean distance or cosine angle similarity between the two vectors (Chapter 2).

Measuring the tremor frequency and magnitude adds more quantitative descriptions to the diagnosis. Given a sequence of the recorded gesture points, we can use following pseudocode:

1.   Input the gesture data.
2.   Convert the data from Cartesian coordinate system to polar coordinate system.
3.   Process fast Fourier transform (FFT).
4.   Compute periodicity of the gesture.
5.   Plot the periodicity curve and find the peak of the frequency.

Gesture Recognition

Gesture recognition is designed to recognize the gesture from the gesture library and user defined gestures. It has two modes: training and recognition. During training, users record the gestures. For this purpose, each intended gesture is to be performed several times. This allows the system to learn the gesture and internally generate a code for it. During recognition, the system tries to identify the gesture that has just occurred by computing which of the training gestures have the best fit for the performed gesture and reports this. The user may then trigger a desired function accordingly.

Let us assume the user draws a square on the touch screen (Figure 9.13). Since different users perform this task in different ways, we have to make sure that the system recognizes squares in a reliable way as well as a robust way. Thus, telling the system only once what a square is will not be sufficient. Users have to train it repeatedly to obtain reliable results for a great range of users. In the system, training is a recording process. Repeating this whole procedure further trains the system and, by that, makes it more likely that a gesture is correctly identified during the later phase of recognition.

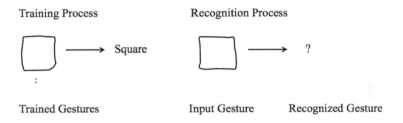

FIGURE 9.13   Gesture classification for touch screen.

Recognition can be implemented using k-nearest neighbor to find the closest training samples and vote for the classification result. More sophisticated methods can be found from the citations, such as $1, $N,[178] and Protractor.[179]

$1 does templates are matched by $1; it compares an articulated candidate unistroke to a set of stored templates. The template closest to the candidate is the recognition result, where "closeness" is determined by the average Euclidean distance between corresponding points.

$N is similar to $1, but $N is much more versatile by recognizing gestures comprising multiple strokes, automatically generalizing from one multistroke template to all possible multistrokes with alternative stroke orderings and directions, recognizing one-dimensional (1D) gestures such as lines, and providing bounded rotation invariance.

Protractor uses cosine angle similarity to measure the similarity between two gestures and adds an orientation-invariance function to improve the speed and robustness of the recognition.

[178] http://depts.washington.edu/aimgroup/proj/dollar/ndollar.html
[179] Y. Li. Protractor: a fast and accurate gesture recognizer. In *Proceedings of the ACM Conference on Human Factors in Computing Systems (CHI '10)*, Atlanta, GA, April 10–15, 2010. ACM Press, New York, pp. 2169–2172.

9.7   ENVIRONMENTAL SENSORS

Many smartphone platforms provide sensors for monitoring various environmental properties, including ambient light, ambient relative humidity, ambient pressure, and ambient temperature near the device. All environmental sensors are hardware based and are available only if a device manufacturer has built them into a device.

The ambient light sensor measures brightness of the environment. It is useful not only for controlling camera flashes but also for other virtual sensors, such as the proximity sensor.

Unlike most motion sensors and position sensors, which return a multidimensional array of sensor values for each sample interval, environmental sensors only return a single sensor value for each data event, such as light in lux, temperature in degrees centigrade, pressure in hectopascals or millibars, and relative humidity as a percentage. Similarly, unlike motion sensors and position sensors, which often require high-pass or low-pass filtering, environmental sensors do not typically require any data filtering or data processing. If a device has both a humidity sensor and a temperature sensor, we can use these two data streams to calculate the dew point and the absolute humidity.[180]

9.8   PROXIMITY SENSOR

The proximity sensor measures the distance from the device to a point in space. The proximity sensor is common on most smartphones with touch screens. This is because the primary function of a proximity sensor is to disable accidental touch events. An example of this is an ear contacting the mute button on a touch screen while on a call.

Common proximity sensors are often implemented using a light sensor. The distance value is measured in centimeters. Most proximity sensors return the absolute distance in centimeters, but some proximity sensors only support a binary "close" or "far" measurement. When the ear is close to the smartphone, the ambient light around the light sensor slowly drops below the threshold, and the sensor switches the state from FAR to NEAR. The thresholding is done on the light measurement in lux value.

For the Android platform, the proximity sensor is implemented similarly to the other sensors, but with one critical exception: The proximity sensor is interrupt based as opposed to poll based. All the other sensors are polled at regular intervals. This means that we have a proximity event only when the proximity changes.[181]

9.9   NEAR-FIELD COMMUNICATION SENSORS

Near-field communication (NFC) is a short-range (up 20-cm) wireless communication technology. It is an extension of the radio-frequency identification (RFID)

---

[180] http://developer.android.com/guide/topics/sensors/sensors_environment.html
[181] http://thecodeartist.blogspot.com/2011/01/proximity-sensor-on-android-gingerbread.html

standard because it combines the interface of a smartcard and reader into a single device. This enables a mobile phone to be a contactless reader for sensors (such as RFID tags), a smartcard, and a data interface to another NFC device. NFC works in two modes:

Passive communication mode. The initiator device provides a carrier field. The target device may draw its operating power from the initiator-provided electromagnetic field, thus making the target device a transponder.

Active communication mode. Both initiator and target device communicate by alternately generating their own fields. A device deactivates its radio-frequency (RF) field while it is waiting for data. In this mode, both devices typically have power supplies.

Compared to other wireless channels, such as Wi-Fi and Bluetooth, NFC is more private and location sensitive and consumes less energy. The NFC sensor platform can be integrated with low-cost, disposable skin patches, or "smart tattoos,"[182] that are directly readable with NFC-enabled mobile phones (Figure 9.14). Applications for NFC skin patch technologies include using them with mobile phones to monitor fever onset at home, patients in hospitals, or the well-being of elderly relatives or friends remotely. The technology also applies to skin health and can be combined with printable, passive sensors that work without batteries to monitor glucose, ultraviolet (UV) light exposure, pressure, or biomarkers.

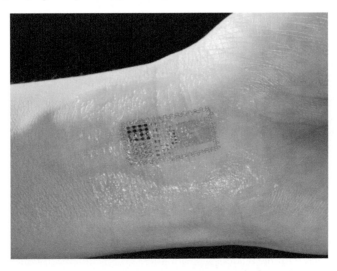

FIGURE 9.14 The low-cost, passive, NFC-enabled smart tattoo can communicate with mobile phones with the NFC app in one-tenth of a second without manually pairing. Courtesy of MC10, Inc. <http:// www.mc10inc.com>

---

[182] http://www.gentag.com/applications.html

NFC and Bluetooth are both short-range communication technologies that are integrated into mobile phones. NFC operates at slower speeds than Bluetooth but consumes far less power and does not require pairing. NFC sets up more quickly than standard Bluetooth but has a lower transfer rate than Bluetooth Low Energy. Instead of performing manual configurations to identify devices, the connection between two NFC devices is automatically established quickly—in less than a tenth of a second. The maximum data transfer rate of NFC (424 Kbps) is slower than that of Bluetooth V2.1 (2.1 Mbps). With a maximum working distance of less than 20 cm, NFC has a shorter range, which reduces the likelihood of unwanted interception.

9.10 GPS SENSORS

Location sensors help calibrate magnetic field sensing data and can track people's activities, such as their jogging distance. Most smartphones provide location data by calling a simple function from the GPS tracker, where we can enable GPS to get latitude and longitude data.

9.11 WIRELESS FIDELITY SENSING

Mobile applications with appropriate permission can access the built-in Wi-Fi sensor on a device by using the API calls. The Android SDK (software development kit) provides a set of APIs for retrieving information about the available Wi-Fi networks to a device as well as Wi-Fi network connection details. This information can be used to track signal strength, find access points, or perform actions when connected to specific access points. For the Android platform, the API is WiFiManager object, and the permission flags are ACCESS_WIFI_STATE and CHANGE_WIFI_STATE. We can retrieve an instance of WiFiManager using the getSystemService method.[183] It is worth noting that the emulator on a personal computer (PC) does not emulate Wi-Fi support, so we need to perform all testing of Wi-Fi on a device.

Many existing information systems may also be used as empathic sensor webs. A wireless local network, for example, can provide a serendipitous user positioning system. Based on the received signal strength indication (RSSI) in an indoor wireless environment, the system can estimate the distance between the access point and the wireless device. The triangulation of the user's location can be calculated from multiple access points. However, in many cases, only one access point is actively connected. Indoor furniture information and the Bayesian model are used to improve positioning accuracy with physical constraints and historical ground truth data. Figure 9.15 shows a screen capture of the wireless laptop positioning output. With mobile sensors such as RFID tags and multiple readers, a positioning system can be configured in addition to the Wi-Fi system. Combined with multimodal sensors (e.g., RFID, sound, infrared, and magnetic signals), the positioning accuracy can be further improved.

This widely distributed open sensory system also raises serious concerns about data privacy. Figure 9.15 shows an output from a wireless device positioning system

[183] L. Darcey and S. Conder. *Android application development*. Sams, Indianapolis, IN, 2012.

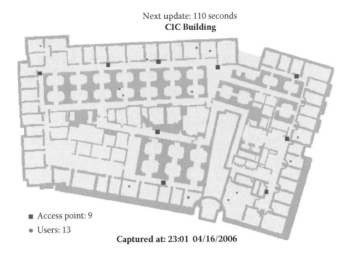

FIGURE 9.15   Screen capture of the real-time wireless positioning system.

at a building, where the location of wireless users and access points are visible on the Internet. The identity of users is replaced with a dot to preserve individuals' privacy.

9.12   BLUETOOTH SENSING

Bluetooth is a short-range device-to-device communication interface and an industrial standard. It originated in Europe and was named after an ancient Danish emperor nicknamed Bluetooth. Most smartphones have a Bluetooth interface by which one can scan for Bluetooth-enabled devices, pair them, and transfer data. By measuring the strength of a Bluetooth signal, we can estimate the distance between the two Bluetooth devices.

For Bluetooth RSSI, we can read RSSI for connected devices or perform a Bluetooth discovery to check the RSSI for nearby devices. Basically, a Bluetooth discovery is a broadcast to all stations within range to respond back. As each device responds back, Android fires off an ACTION_FOUND intent. Within this intent, we can getExtra EXTRA_RSSI to obtain the RSSI. Note that not all Bluetooth hardware supports RSSI.[184]

9.13   SENSORY FUSION

Sensory fusion is to make sense out of multiple sensory channels using registration, filtering, and decision-making methods.

---

[184] For Android: short rssi=intent.getShortExtra(BluetoothDevice.EXTRA_RSSI, Short.MIN_VALUE)

A pedestrian navigation system requires accelerometers, compass, and gyro-scope. The accelerometers are used for long-term measurements of pitch and roll and for pedometer algorithms; the compass is used for long-term measurements of yaw; and the gyroscope is used as the underlying measurement of angular velocity. The gyroscope can also help the accelerometer to separate out gravitational and linear acceleration components, the compass can distinguish Earth's magnetic field from ambient magnetic noise, and the sensors update their calibration parameters. Therefore, a sensory fusion algorithm is needed. Figure 9.16 illustrates a nine-axis sensor fusion algorithm (three-axis gyroscope, three-axis accelerometer, and three-axis digital compass).

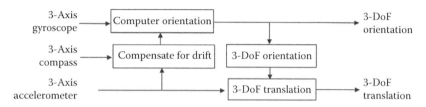

FIGURE 9.16 Nine-axis sensor fusion algorithm. Information from a gyroscope, acceler-ometer, and digital compass is integrated to generate motion information with six degrees of freedom (DOF) (three-axis orientation and three-axis translation).

Now, let's think about where to put the sensors on our body. Many successful pedestrian navigation systems are bolted to some known reference frames. For example, they are worn on the belt; this ensures that the heading of the compass is equivalent to the heading of the user, with only a fixed angular offset depending on the location of the sensors on the belt. Others have been designed with the sensors attached to the user's foot. While foot movement is more complicated than hip move-ment, foot-mounted systems have the advantage that the foot is known to be motion-less whenever it hits the ground, allowing for a zero-velocity update.

9.14 MOTION CLASSIFICATION

There has been an increasing demand for detecting elderly people's state of health at home. There are many solutions for detecting a fall, such as passive sensor networks and active sensor networks. Motion classification is needed in the detection process. In this case study, we investigate how to detect a fall from the wireless sensor net-work. The sensor platform is MICA2, made by Crossbow. These sensors are able to sense temperature, x and y position, light, sound, and x and y acceleration. The sensory nodes can be programmed in TinyOS, an open source operating system for ad hoc wireless networks. The experimental setup is shown in Figure 9.17, with the base station connected to a computer and the sensor node attached to the subject.

This, of course, can be extended to include multiple nodes all over the body as well as all over the house. By using these tiny sensors, our goal was to determine, in the most accurate and nonintrusive way possible, if someone had fallen down

(Figure 9.18). The algorithm must be able to process data quickly and to distinguish a fall from other daily activities, such as sitting, lying down, bending over, and so on.

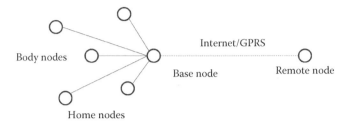

FIGURE 9.17   The sensor web test bed.

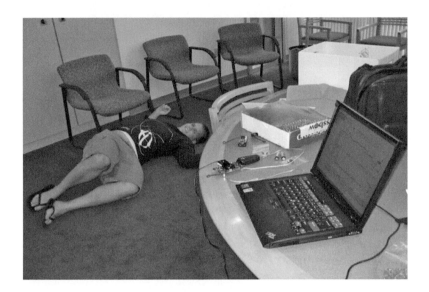

FIGURE 9.18   Lab environment for simulated falls.

Sampling Rate and Sensor Placement

When choosing a sampling rate for the sensor, it is important to determine how fast a person falls and how fast the sensor could reliably send data back to the base node. Assume the sensor's sampling rate is set as one data point every four seconds. With this slow sampling rate, one could see that the person was standing and then fell, but it is hard to find where the initial fall was. If the sampling rate is increased to four times per second, then the system is able to see the change as the person falls. Four times per second allows the sensor to generate enough data for the model to determine a fall but not create too much network traffic.

Where to place the sensor on the body is another important factor (Figure 9.19). The objective is to make the sensor invisible to the user, yet still functional. There are several potential locations to consider: the knee, the belt, the shoulder, and the

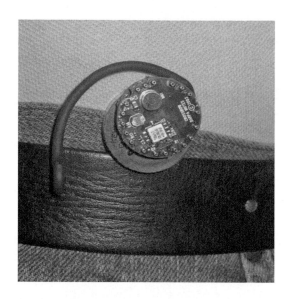

FIGURE 9.19   Example of node placed on body.

forehead. When the sensor is placed on these different parts of the body, it gives very different readings due to the different movements of each particular body part. We want to pick the location that gives us the cleanest readings. Although test results showed that the belt and the forehead locations are the best, it is more realistic to put the sensor on the belt. Figure 9.20 shows the sensor responses to falls when the sensor is placed on different parts of the body.

When a person falls, the body orientation changes from vertical to horizontal. This causes the x and y acceleration to switch values, making it a very good indicator that someone has fallen. When the sensor is placed on the belt, there are few times that a person changes xy-orientation at that speed. So, we need to train a novel classifier for detecting drastic changes in the xy-orientation of the subject (Figure 9.21). The "lazy man's" classifier k-Nearest Neighbor can take all the training data as a model and tries to find the closest sample to the classification result.

We then can train each model using two walking samples, two falling samples, two fallen samples, and two getting up samples, for a total of eight training samples for the classifier. We want to develop a way to keep analyzing data as it comes into the database while comparing it to previous data. We can set up a window of ten measurements at a time. As soon as a new signal came in, we can put all ten values through neural networks and read the results. If the resulting value that came from the neural networks is above a certain threshold, the system will count that as a *fall*. Once a person had fallen, they could not fall again, yet the data continued to indicate that they had fallen until they got up. This problem can be easily solved with the inclusion of a flag that is set when someone fell and reset when they got up. As long as the flag is set, they can not fall again until it is reset.

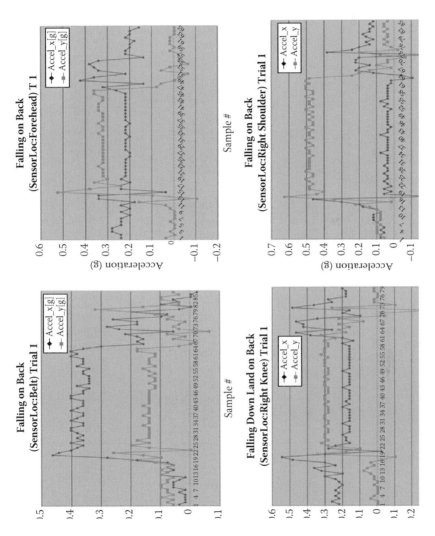

FIGURE 9.20 Differences in fall when sensor was placed on different parts of the body: on belt (top left), forehead (top right), knee (bottom left), and shoulder (bottom right).

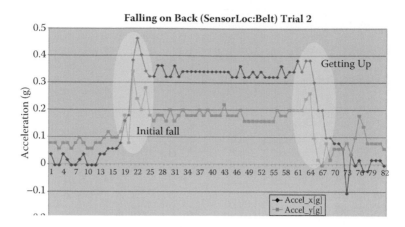

FIGURE 9.21 Example of data received from a fall. The point where the person fell is indicated.

Real-Time Database

The system needs to log all the data received from the nodes into an SQL-compliant database. The reason for this is so that the data is kept in a place that can be easily accessed by programs or hospitals that need to check all of the data to see if there are changes over time in various areas. Also, if all of the data is in a database, the programs can be set up to run from anywhere in the world as long as there is Internet access. This means that the programs could be run from a hospital or a caretaker's home, making it easier to report anomalous behavior. Using TinyOS, it is possible to set up a program that simply reads data packets received from the nodes, parses them into relevant data, and logs them into an SQL database for us to a defined format.

Detection Results

The algorithm was tested with data received from placing the node on different parts of the body. The results are summarized in Table 9.1.

TABLE 9.1 Results of Detecting the Fall

Sensor Position	Identified Correctly (%)	Identified Incorrectly (%)	Missed (%)	Total Trials
Belt	90	5	5	21
Forehead	81	14	5	21
Right shoulder	71	19	10	21
Right knee	62	29	9	21

The model developed in this study is not adequate for detecting all the conditions. Patients with diabetes, for example, often collapse slowly when their blood sugar is low. In this case, a combination of motion sensors with other sensors or interfaces would be desirable, such as a digital watch that sends a beep to the user after detecting a motionless event. The user would push a button if everything were okay. Otherwise, the wearable device will send the alarm to the network after a few inquiries.

9.15   ACCESSING SENSORS ON MOBILE PHONES

There are apps for logging sensor data on mobile phones (e.g., SensorLog for the iPhone platform).[185] The app can save the sensor log data into an ASCII file and analyze it on computers.

For developing new sensor applications, we need to access the sensor APIs. Let us see how to access Android sensors (Figure 9.22). We can use SensorManager to access the device's sensors.[186] We then register the sensor event in the class called sensorEvent that holds information such as the sensor's type, the timestamp, accuracy, and sensor data. Then, we configure an EventListener for receiving notifications or "callbacks" from the SensorManager when sensor values have changed.

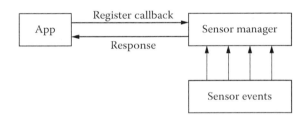

FIGURE 9.22   Android sensor event management.

Because there is only one interface for multiple types of sensors, listening to multiple sensors requires switching on the type of event or creating separate listener objects, forcing registration at the same rate per listener.

It is worth noting that the system will not disable sensors automatically when the screen turns off, which can drain the battery quickly. Therefore, one must always make sure to disable sensors when the activity is paused.

In Appendix A, readers can find the sample code SimpleSensorLog for logging sensor data (Figure 9.23). The sample Android app displays the sensor values on the screen live. The sensor values displayed include accelerometers and orientation for all the three dimensions. Also, the app has the ability to log the sensor data onto a file so that one can analyze it later.

---

[185] https://itunes.apple.com/us/app/sensorlog/id388014573?mt=8
[186] http://developer.android.com/reference/android/hardware/SensorManager.html

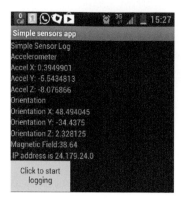

FIGURE 9.23   The screenshot of the app SimpleSensorLog on Android phone

9.16   SUMMARY

The sensors discussed in this chapter are just a portion of existing MEMS sensors available in smartphones, cameras, GPS devices, watches, and laptops. "Sensor-rich computing" means there exists an abundance of sensor power that creates opportunities to compose systems, similar to a spectrum of colors on a painter's pallet. It is worth noting that the combination of sensors and communication interfaces creates innovative solutions such as NFC to read and write data to smart skin systems and elderly fall detection systems. On the other hand, simple and novel apps have great potential in ambient diagnostics, such as tremor detection from touch screen sensors and finger gesture recognition and analysis. With accelerometers, we can sense user's handshaking patterns and assess the level of tremors. The apps can be embedded into video games so that the ambient diagnosis can be a part of a video game. Chapter 14 explores video game applications further.

PROBLEMS

1. Download the sensor log demo app SimpleSensorLog for Android phones or SensorLog for iPhones. Run the log for one minute and save the data to a file. Plot the log data in Excel or MATLAB.
2. Based on Problem 1, plot the curves for the following cases and discuss the results: (A) move the phone horizontally; (B) move the phone upward; (C) free fall onto a bed.
3. Based on Problem 1, log the sample data from accelerometers for walking, running, sitting, and dancing. Save the sample data files. (A) Develop a classification model to recognize the activities. (B) Use a confusion matrix to analyze the results.
4. Based on Problem 1, log the sample data from gyroscopes for walking, running, sitting, and dancing. Save the sample data files. (A) Develop a

classification model to recognize the activities. (B) Use a confusion matrix to analyze the results.

5. Based on Problems 3 and 4, log the sample data for both accelerometers and gyroscopes for walking, running, sitting, and dancing. Save the sample data files. (A) Develop a classification model to recognize the activities. (B) Use a confusion matrix to analyze the results.

6. Based on the previous problems, discuss how to obtain reliable classification when the phone is in different orientations.

7. The signal strength emitted from a Bluetooth headset can be used for measuring the proximity and speed of the user. Some intelligent transportation systems have already used the Bluetooth signal strength to detect the vehicle speed. Here, let us develop a demonstration for sensing a home user's status based on Bluetooth signal strength. (A) Plot the signal strength in a two-dimensional map. (B) Analyze the signal patterns and correlation to the location and activities. (C) Cluster the data using k-means. (D) Recognize the patterns using k-nearest neighbor or other methods. (E) Summarize your findings in a report.

8. Use two phones to test NFC by sending and receiving a message. Report the distance and the content of the messages sent and received. Discuss the potentials for ambient diagnosis.

9. Use the mouse to simulate touch screen handwriting gestures and capture the mouse movement data. Develop a training sample dataset for writing the numbers 0 through 9. Use k-nearest neighbor with Euclidean distances to recognize the gestures.

10. Similar to Problem 9, recognize the gestures but use the cosine angle similarity to measure the distances between the gestures.

11. Design the hand tremor data recording and analysis system using the three-axis accelerometer, three-axis gyroscope, and three-axis compass to build a three-axis translation and three-axis orientation sensory system. Develop a demo and summarize your findings in a report.

10 Body Media

> I've got you under my skin.
>
> —Frank Sinatra

10.1 INTRODUCTION

Inspecting the human body like a parasite has often been a subject in science fiction novels and movies. In *Fantastic Voyage*, a 1966 film, scientists developed technology that could miniaturize matter by shrinking individual atoms. Agents used the miniaturized submarine *Proteus* to remove a blood clot in a scientist's brain. Today, this vision has been in part implemented in the real world. This chapter explores sensors that can be swallowed, attached to the skin, and worn as a headset or shoes. These wearable sensors are called body media, and they represent a revolution in personal and affordable diagnostics. The areas covered in this chapter are just a few snapshots of a big wave in wearable sensors, including

- Body-area networks (BANs)
- Brain-computer interfaces (BCIs)
- Epidermal electronics
- Capsule cameras, or pill cameras

10.2 EMERGING WEARABLE SENSORS

A number of wearable health sensors have come into our lives: pedometers, Fitbit activity sensors, and eWatches. They are inexpensive, simple, and fitness oriented. Here, we focus on more advanced ambient diagnostic systems.

A BAN[187] is a wireless network of wearable sensors that are attached to the body. In particular, the network consists of physiological sensors, low-power processors, and wireless communication. BANs are designed for monitoring physical activities, diseases, and telemedicine. BANs are moving from connecting single vital sign sensors to connecting nonvital bioinformatics data with smartphones.

Brain-computer interfaces are commercially available in reduced capacities, but the distance between those products and clinical ones is narrowing. The dual-use markets of those products enable makers to massively produce the systems with affordable costs.

Epidermal electronics have started a new era of smart fiber, smart skin, and smart tattoos. These move clinical labs from well-shielded rooms to individual homes,

---

[187] http://en.wikipedia.org/wiki/Body_area_network

vehicles, and swimming pools. They also create technical challenges (e.g., how to shield the noise in daily environments).

Wireless capsule cameras provide a unique way to check abnormities in patients' bodies with a fraction of the cost for regular endoscopies, creating valuable alternatives for healthcare.

Figure 10.1 shows an overview of the wearable body media in terms of data collection cycles against the information complexity. We can see the trends in body media.

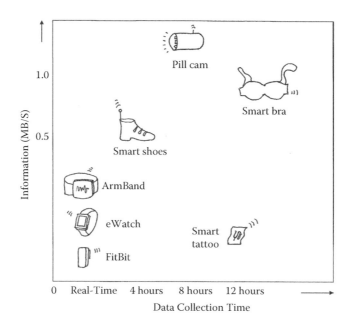

FIGURE 10.1   Clustering analysis of wearable sensors.

10.3   BODY-AREA NETWORKS

With rapid growth of broadband services and smartphone connectivities, BANs could allow inexpensive and continuous health monitoring with real-time updates of diagnostic data through the Internet. The objective of the BAN is to continuously monitor and log vital parameters of patients suffering from chronic diseases such as diabetes, asthma, and heart issues. A BAN network on a patient at home, by measuring changes and rates of changes in the vital signs of multiple channels (Figure 10.2), can alert the hospital even before the patient has a heart attack.

The Federal Communications Commission (FCC) has approved a 40-MHz spectrum allocation for medical BAN low-power, wide-area radio links at the 2,360- to 2,400-MHz band. This will allow off-loading BAN communication from the already-saturated standard Wi-Fi spectrum (25 GHz) to a special band. Ironically, the FCC-approved BAN spectrum has not been used much because most vital signal monitors are still based on wired connectivity. Few consumer products are using the approved band except Armband™ by BodyMedia.

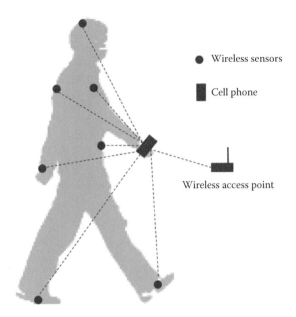

Wireless sensors

Cell phone

Wireless access point

FIGURE 10.2   Body-area network.

On the other hand, more and more fitness products have emerged. For example, Fitbit and eWatches use existing wireless connectivity to smartphones such as Bluetooth, Wi-Fi, and near-field communication (NFC) interfaces for nonvital health data transmissions such as workout logs, dietary logs, blood pressure logs, and glucose logs. Using common wireless bandwidth enables makers to use off-the-shelf components and code to communicate with the growing number of smartphones, which are data hubs between body-borne sensors and cloud data servers.

Linked to the standard wireless band is also a survival strategy for popular fitness products. Personal fitness device is a competitive market; it is hard for a product alone to survive. It had better be connected to other products, such as in GNC stores, fitness clubs, and sports stores.

Perhaps, the most interesting connection is the online gaming: linking health monitoring systems to social media for sharing progress, competition, network games, and group therapies. Online social game platforms such as Second Life and OpenSim have provided interfaces to analog or digital devices, such as pressure sensors. The borderline between the virtual world and the physical world has blurred. More details about this topic are discussed in Chapter 14, "Gaming for Diagnoses."

10.4   BRAIN-COMPUTER INTERFACE

Earphones and headsets are perhaps the most popular prostheses so far in the digital age. People use them for listening to music and for phone conversation. Some people may not even take them off during working hours.

The Japanese company Neurowear released the product Necomimi,[188] which is designed to free the user from having to select songs and artists, allowing users to encounter new music just by wearing the device. *Neco* in Japanese means "cat," and *mimi* means "ears." Neco and mimi are very popular in Japanese culture. The Neco system is made of two parts: earphones and an application that resides in a smartphone. The earphones detect brain waves through sensors on the user's forehead. They automatically analyze the user's brain condition and search for music that best matches the user's mood: focused, drowsy, stressed, and so on. Neco provides a new experience, or so-called music serendipity, by detecting users' subconscious minds through their brain waves (Figure 10.3). The product also has a robotic display on the artificial ears, reflecting the user's mood by turning the ears up and down.

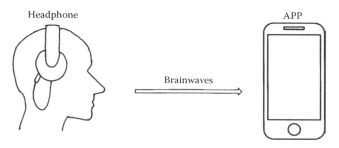

FIGURE 10.3   The Neco headphone can detect the user's brainwaves (EEG) and control the music selection application.

How can brain waves be detected? For decades, electroencephalography (EEG) has been provided by special equipment hidden behind the walls of labs, hospitals, and universities. EEG utilizes metal electrodes attached to a human subject's scalp, measuring tiny electrical potentials that reflect the brain's electrical activity.

Figure 10.4 shows five types of brain waves that are associated with brain states: excited (gamma, 40+ Hz); focused (beta, 13–40 Hz); relaxed (alpha, 8–12.9 Hz); daydreaming (theta, 4–7.9 Hz); and deep sleep (delta, 0.2–3.9 Hz). The bottom line is that whenever the brain activities increase, the frequencies of EEG increase.

Most clinical EEG devices use the International Federation 10–20 system of electrodes (Figure 10.5), which uses a matrix of 21 or more electrodes on the scalp. This method was developed to ensure standardized reproducibility so that a subject's studies could be compared over time and subjects could be compared to each other. This system is based on the relationship between the location of an electrode and the underlying area of brain tissue. The "10" and "20" refer to the distances between adjacent electrodes: either 10% or 20% of the total front-back or right-left distance of the skull.[189]

---

[188] http://www.thecreatorsproject.com/blog/smart-headphones-determine-your-mood-and-choose-your-music-for-you
[189] http://en.wikipedia.org/wiki/10-20_system_(EEG)

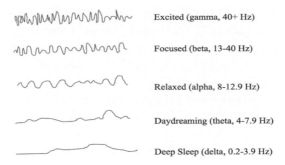

FIGURE 10.4   Brainwaves: excited, focused, relaxed, daydreaming and deep sleep.

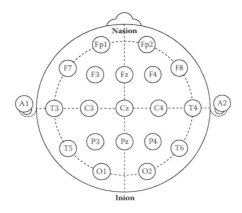

FIGURE 10.5   EEG 10–20 system electrode layout. (From 10–20 system (EEG). Wikipedia, 2013. http://en.wikipedia.org/wiki/10-20_system_(EEG).)

We use a letter to identify each electrode's lobe and a number to identify the hemisphere location. The letters F, T, C, P, and O stand for frontal, temporal, central, parietal, and occipital lobes, respectively. Even numbers (2, 4, 6, 8) refer to electrode positions on the right hemisphere, whereas odd numbers (1, 3, 5, 7) refer to those on the left hemisphere. In addition, the letter codes A and Fp identify the earlobes and frontal polar sites, respectively.

We also use two landmarks for the essential positioning of the EEG electrodes: first, the nasion, the distinctly depressed area between the eyes, just above the bridge of the nose; second, the inion, the lowest point of the skull from the back of the head.

Necomimi, the commercial entertaining device, only has two electrodes (one on the nasion and the other on the earlobe), generating a single-lead EEG wave. This is the same for NeuroVigil, which provides a single-channel EEG to the phone application.[190]

---

[190] http://www.imedicalapps.com/2011/10/neurovigil-eeg-open-wireless-window-brain/

Emotiv EEG,[191] another commercial product used for game control and wheelchair navigation, has fourteen EEG channels plus two references, offering optimal positioning for more accurate spatial resolution (Figure 10.6). The fourteen EEG channel names, based on the International 10–20 locations, are AF3, F7, F3, FC5, T7, P7, O1, O2, P8, T8, FC6, F4, F8, and AF4. Emotiv EEG has it own chip for speeding up EEG signal processing and incorporates a gyroscope generating optimal position information for cursor and camera controls. Emotive EEG was originally designed for game control, but now it has been used in a broad range of applications, including neurotherapy, biofeedback, and BCI. For researchers, Emotiv provides test bench software and a software development kit (SDK) to obtain the proprietary software tool kit. The Emotiv EEG Neuroheadset connects wirelessly to personal computers (PCs) running Windows, Linux, or MAC OS X. It is worth noting that due to the massive production of the device, Emotiv EEG's price is a fraction of clinical EEG devices. The differences could be on the order of one or two magnitudes.

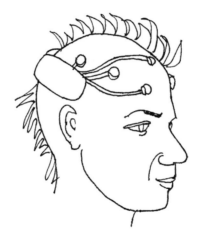

FIGURE 10.6   Emotiv EEG 14-channel brain-computer interface (BCI).

As we know, for a clinical-grade EEG, we need at least 21 electrodes for better spatial resolution. Emotiv EEG's 14-electrode system is not far from the 21-electrode system, which generates multiple-lead EEG waves, similar to the music notes of a symphony orchestra. Doctors have to read the waves in parallel to compare the location, timing, frequencies, and voltages. The dynamic patterns of EEG are spatial and temporal, which can be roughly interpolated as a surface and displayed as a topological spectrogram that changes over time like a movie montage. The topological map montage can be generated by the fast Fourier transform (FFT).

Figure 10.7 shows a topographic map of brain activity while listening to an audiobook.[192]

---

[191] http://www.emotiv.com/eeg/features.php
[192] http://www.qeeg.com/qeegfact.html

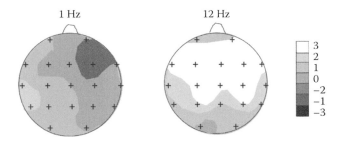

FIGURE 10.7 Topological heat map visualization of the EEG of the brain activities when listening to an audiotape.

The EEG can be used not only for mood detection but also for locating tumors and for finding abnormal spiking waves originating in diseased brain tissue that might predispose one to epileptic attacks. Once such a focal point is found, surgical excision of the focus often prevents future epileptic seizures.[193] Some abnormal patterns may occur with a number of different conditions, not just seizures. For example, certain types of waves may be seen after head trauma, strokes, or brain tumors. A common example of this type is called "slowing," in which the rhythm of the brain waves is slower than would be expected for the patient's age and level of alertness.[194]

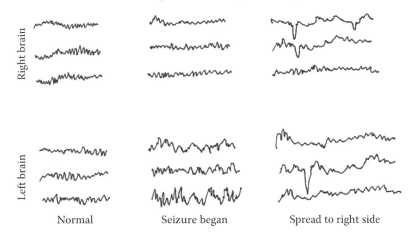

FIGURE 10.8 Brain waves of a seizure.

As we can see in Figure 10.8, the EEG waves went wild when a seizure started in the left temporal lobe and then spread to the right side as well. Wearable EEG devices provide the potential for affordable biofeedback for patients at home or at work. For example, the EEG device sends real-time brain wave data through a wireless link to either a phone or a laptop. The phone or laptop then performs signal

---

[193] J. G. Webster. *Medical instrumentation*, 2nd ed. Houghton Mifflin, New York, 1992.
[194] http://www.epilepsy.com/epilepsy/testing_eeg

processing and pattern recognition and generates real-time audiovisual feedback to patients. Figure 10.9 is a diagram of the biofeedback system.

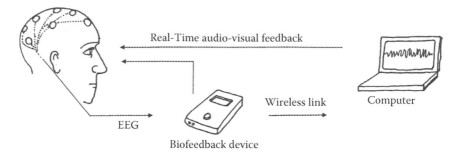

Real-Time audio-visual feedback

Wireless link

Computer

EEG

Biofeedback device

FIGURE 10.9   Biofeedback using EEG signals.

Figure 10.10 shows a 16-channel ambulatory EEG seizure monitor, made by the Chicago-based software company Wave Technology Group,[195] proposing to replace these legacy systems with a lightweight, minimally invasive, and most important, affordable solution. On the patient side, data is captured via body-worn sensors, which interact wirelessly with a smartphone application via Bluetooth, and is sent to the cloud, where it is processed and transferred to a clinician-side application for real-time remote patient monitoring.

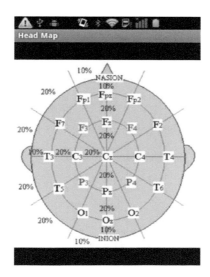

FIGURE 10.10   Mobile 16-channel EEG for ambulatory seizure monitoring.

---

[195] http://www.imedicalapps.com/2011/10/wave-technology-group-unveils-screenshots-ambulatory-eeg-seizure-monitoring-app-2/

Both EEG and magnetic resonance imaging (MRI) can do brain imaging. Relatively, EEGs have better temporal resolution than MRIs. On the other hand, MRIs have better spatial resolution than EEGs. Size-wise, EEGs are definitely smaller and more portable than MRIs. Finally, EEGs are orders of magnitude less expensive compared to MRIs. Nevertheless, an EEG is a mature diagnostic tool that can be used alone or as a complementary source of MRI diagnoses.

To build an EEG device for an unshielded home is a nontrivial task. The household electrical interferences are the main issues. Electrical power in a house is the main interference of EEG signals. Electrical power lines use sinusoidal voltages with a frequency of 50 or 60 Hz. The alternating current (AC) line power voltage is typically 110 or 220 volts and thus exceeds the EEG's 50 to 100 microvolts by a factor of 2×10^6. Therefore, AC power line interference is ubiquitous in EEG recordings, especially if taken outside specially equipped, shielded lab rooms. EEG amplifiers usually provide a so-called notch filter that suppresses signals in a narrow band around the AC frequency in question. Amplifier notch filters are designed to suppress a certain amount of household AC power line interference (or power line interference).

The second interference source is from muscular electromyographic (EMG) activities, such as eye blinking and eye movements (Figure 10.11). EMG activity effects can completely obscure any frequency analysis. The most common sources of EMG are the muscles that lift the eyebrows and those that close the jaw. Studies suggested that keeping the mouth slightly open (or the tip of the tongue between the foreteeth) is a good strategy to avoid jaw-generated EMG.[196]

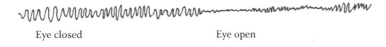

Eye closed   Eye open

FIGURE 10.11   EEG wave when eyes are open and closed.

10.5   EPIDERMAL ELECTRONICS (SMART FIBER)

Smart Bra

Thermal imaging measures surface temperatures associated with blood supply, inflammation, estrogen stimulation, and benign or cancerous cells. Figure 10.12 shows thermal images; the dark pixels indicate higher temperature. These images show patients with a 2-mm cancerous tumor in the lower left breast, in an area where we can see extensive blood supply.[197] Studies show that thermal imaging can catch breast cancer at early stages, even 8–10 years earlier than other methods, such as mammograms, which are minimally effective with dense breast tissue and are only able to detect an abnormality once it is large enough to image.

---

[196] http://www.bci2000.org/wiki/index.php/User_Tutorial:EEG_Measurement_Setup
[197] http://www.thermogramcenter.com/Images.htm

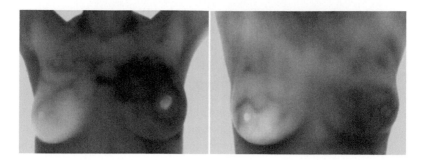

FIGURE 10.12 Thermal images of patients with breast cancer on the left side (images provided by the Breast Health and Prevention Center: BetterBreastHealthforLife.com).

Current breast cancer screening procedures overlook or misdiagnose approximately 30% of the breast tissue abnormalities and cancers. In X-ray imaging, for example, cancerous cells are white, and the density of breast is also white. So doctors are seeing white-on-white, leaving a lot of room for errors.

Thermal imaging is an alternative to using X-rays for early-stage breast cancer diagnosis. However, clinical thermal imaging devices are rather expensive, and it is less possible for a patient to obtain one for continuously monitoring the surface temperature at home. Is it possible to obtain an affordable thermal imaging device in the same manner as a blood pressure meter?

The First Warning System™ [198] (FWS) released the smart bra for breast thermal imaging, costing around US$200, pending approval by the Food and Drug Administration. [199] The system uses 16 temperature sensors placed under a bra to collect 12 hours of breast surface temperature data (Figure 10.13).

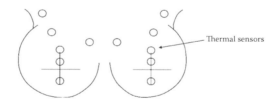

FIGURE 10.13 The layout diagram of the 16-channel thermal sensors (illustrated from US Patent US 8231542 B2).

Due to the movement, the contact between the sensors and the skin is often interrupted. A low-pass filter can be used to remove the drastic temperature values (Figure 14). All of the generated temperature data can be stored in a mobile device such as a smartphone these days. The sensors are placed on the locations on the breast by using a sensor placeholder, as shown in Figure 10.13. The sensor placeholder is lobate aligns with the glandular regions of the breast where cancers are most likely

[198] http://www.firstwarningsystems.com/technology.html
[199] http://chicago.cbslocal.com/2013/02/22/breast-cancer-detecting-bra-could-be-new-option-for-women/.

to develop.[200] The temperature data is then analyzed by a machine learning-based classifier; its input are sixteen temperature sensors and four output classes: normal, benign, cancer, and suspected cancer (Figure 10.15).

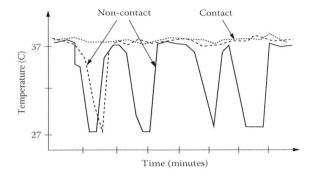

FIGURE 10.14 Temperature readings for three sensors plotted versus time, showing abnormal temperature readings (illustrated from US Patent Application US 2010/0056946 A1).

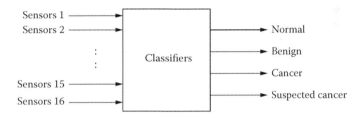

FIGURE 10.15 Diagram of the pattern recognition system (16-channel input and four output).

As we can see, after the multiple-channel sensory data are collected, a smart bra problem becomes a classification problem. Conventional classifiers, such as GMM (Gaussian Mixture Model), RBF (Radial Basis Functions), or SVM (Support Vector Machine),[201] can be easily implemented with standard libraries, such as the MATLAB neural network toolbox, and so on. Many machine learning-based algorithms are inclined to over-fit the training data. So a well-designed evaluation process is required. Here, let us focus on ways to evaluate the classification results. According to U.S. patent application U.S. 2010/0056946 A1,[202] a few common classifiers, GMM, RFB, and SVM, have been tested with 5,000 training samples and 1,000 testing samples. GMM had the highest percentage of correct classifications, 90.6%, whereas RBF and SVM had 86.1% and 85.6% accuracy, respectively.

How to evaluate results from machine learning is essential to the technology. Two indices are recommended: sensitivity and specificity, as discussed in Chapter 2.

---

[200] Holmes, J. System for analyzing thermal data based on breast surface temperature to determine suspect conditions. US 20100056946 A1, May 27, 2010.http://www.google.com/patents/US20100056946

[201] https://docs.google.com/a/google.com/viewer?url=www.google.com/patents/US8185485.pdf

[202] https://docs.google.com/a/google.com/viewer?url=www.google.com/patents/US20100056946.pdf

Sensitivity of a test is the proportion of people with the disease who have a positive test result: the higher the sensitivity, the greater the detection rate and the lower the false-negative (FN) rate. The specificity of the test is the proportion of people without the disease who have a negative test result: the higher the specificity, the lower the false-positive rate (FP) and the lower the proportion of people who have the disease who will be unnecessarily worried or exposed to unnecessary treatment.

The receiver operator characteristic (ROC) curve[203] is a plot of sensitivity against 1-specificity (normalized to 1). Sensitivity refers to the probability that a test result was positive when the disease was present. The area under the ROC curve indicates the performance of the classifier across the entire range of cutoff points. Conventionally, the area under the ROC curve must range between 0.5 and 1 (Figure 10.16). If the area is closer to 1, it shows that the classifier has better accuracy in the testing. The area under the ROC curve is a good indicator for the classifier's performance with regard to the misclassification rate and the measure of risk based on confusion and loss matrices. In short, an ROC plot is able to provide a holistic way of quantifying the diagnostic accuracy.

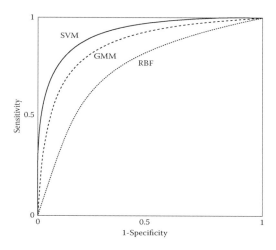

FIGURE 10.16 ROC curves of three classifiers: SVM, GMM, and RBF (illustrated from US Patent Application US 2010/0056946 A1).

According to the patent document (US 2010/0056946 A1), the SVM classifier shows the highest specificity, 90%, followed by both GMM and RBF classifiers, which has the same specificity, 78%.

Now, let's look at the area under the ROC curve, which is an important parameter as it determines the overall classification accuracy for the classifiers. The ROC curves for each of the classifiers show that the SVM has the largest area under the curve (0.872), followed by GMM (0.864) and RBF (0.834). The SVM classifier is the most accurate classifier in this case due to its area under the ROC curve being

---

[203] http://www.medicalbiostatistics.com/roccurve.pdf

closer to 1. In the statistical analysis of ROC curves, the SVM classifier is considered the best for the 16-channel thermal sensory data, even though the GMM classifier achieved the highest sensitivity. This result is based on the two performance indices, for which the SVM classifier attained the best result in three of these indices: SVM has the greatest specificity, sensitivity and attained the largest area under the ROC curve, which implies its accuracy. Therefore, the SVM classifier is considered to be the optimal choice for the classifier.

Three topics are worth further investigation: *signal filtering, sample diversity, and dynamic modeling.* First, a low-pass filter is needed for removing the drastic temperature drops due to loss of contact between the skin and the sensors.

Sample diversity is critical to any machine learning algorithm and it is perhaps the most vulnerable factor. A common practice is to split a single sample into many small pieces for training and testing, showing more homogeneous patterns than heterogeneous ones. The benefits of this approach include higher classification success rates, economy in data collection, and meeting the minimal requirement to run some classification models; for example, GMM needs at least thirty samples. However, splitting samples may result in over-fitting the model, leaving a vulnerable spot in the system. It is recommended to feed the machine-learning model with fresh samples that are not any part of training samples.

It is worth noting that the classification models in the case of SVM, RBF and GMM do not consider the time variable and ignore the dynamic temperature-changing and moving patterns that would have been helpful for diagnostics. This requires spatial and temporal data-mining methods, which are part of a rapidly growing area in machine learning. As a preliminary study, thermogram animation is a useful visualization method to show the spatiotemporal patterns.

Smart Shoes

Chapter 9 discussed how to use accelerometers to detect falls. The problem of this approach is that when the sensor detects the fall, the damage has already been done. It is desirable to detect the warning signs before the fall happens. Smart shoes have been developed to provide gait- and balance-related data.[204] A typical smart shoe system combines embeddable sensors, batteries, and a communication interface. For example, the mobile phone application for the Smart Shoes Nike Lunar Hyperdunk+, released in 2012, uses a Bluetooth wireless connection to communicate with the application on a smartphone. Although it was developed for sports, the product can also be used for elderly balance checks. Its US$250 price is steep at this moment, but it could decrease as the market grows. Figure 10.17 shows a screenshot for the smart shoe application with a smartphone.

By monitoring walking behaviors, we can observe balance abnormality patterns. The fall risk assessment model can be built in two ways: developing an expert system, using the heuristic rules derived from geriatric motion study experts; or machine learning from collected experimental data to discover the correlations between balance abnormality and extracted features.

---

[204] http://cs.ucla.edu/~ani/publications/SmartShoe-2008-eScience-.pdf

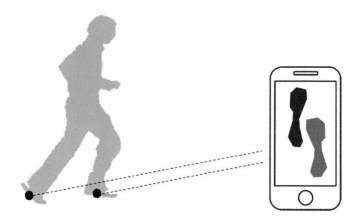

FIGURE 10.17   The mobile phone application of the Smart Shoes, with Bluetooth wireless connection to the application on a smartphone.

Future development would differentiate if the user is walking on a flat surface or a hilly surface and if he or she is walking uphill or downhill.

Perhaps a logical next step is to connect the pressure sensors with the power generated from the shoe itself. Walking or running applies a first force deforming a piezoelectric actuator, thereby generating electrical energy. An energy storage circuit stores electrical energy generated by the piezoelectric actuator for the sensing, recording, and wireless transmitting (Figure 10.18).[205]

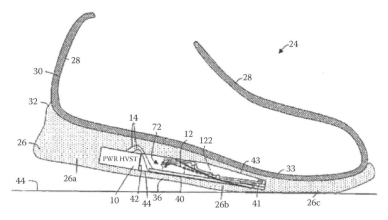

FIGURE 10.18   Piezoelectric energy-harvesting system. (U.S. patent application 2006/0021261 A1.)

---

[205] http://www.gizmag.com/piezoelectric-generator-shoes/14945/

Smart Tattoos

Smart tattoos are thin, stick-on sensor patches. In contrast with traditional micro-electronics that depended on rigid silicon materials, smart tattoos are based on stretchable and transparent polymers such as silicone. Smart tattoos can be applied to human skin for monitoring heart rate, temperature, motion, respiration, and skin moisture.

Like all electronics, smart tattoos need electrodes and wires to connect signals between the parts. How can one make the circuit stretchable yet conductive? There are three state-of-the-art approaches: patterned wires, liquid metal, and nanoparticle coating (Figure 10.19).

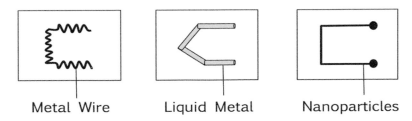

Metal Wire   Liquid Metal   Nanoparticles

FIGURE 10.19 Three approaches for stretchable sensor patches: patterned wires, liquid metal, and layer-by-layer nanoparticles on a stretchable polymer material.

Patterned gold wires can be embedded in the thin stretchable polymer film in tortuous zigzag or spring-like patterns. The gold wires are just a few hundred nanometers thick, much thinner than a human hair. Therefore, they are flexible enough to be embedded into stretchable polymers, such as silicone, an implantable material for plastic surgery. The thin polymer protects the electronics from water and scratches. On the other side, the polymer can be attached to the skin with electrodes and the conductive bounding gel. When the polymer stretches, the electrodes and wires stretch as well. The gold wires work well when pulled to twice their length. The electrodes can act like a sensor for measuring electrical impedance to detect the temperature of the wearer and hydration levels on the skin.

The liquid metal approach consists of carving tiny tunnels inside an extremely elastic polymer and filling the tunnels with a liquid metal alloy of gallium and indium, which is an efficient conductor of electricity. These conductive wires can be stretched up to eight times their original length while remaining conductive.[206]

Spherical nanoparticles can be embedded in elastic polyurethane by building the thin film layer by layer (LBL). When stretching, the nanoparticles align themselves into a chain form to maintain the conductivity. The chain-forming tendency of nanoparticles exists in many materials, such as semiconductors and metals, which make excellent conducting pathways. A recent study shows that without stretching, the LBL material with five gold layers has a conductance of 11,000 siemens per centimeter (S/cm). When it is stretched a little more than twice its original length,

---

[206] http://video.techbriefs.com/video/Ultra-Stretchable-Wires

its conductivity is sustained at 2,400 S/cm, enough for some sensory devices.[207] Although stretchability and electrical conductivity of the nanoparticle approach are still humble compared to liquid metals, the approach does have its advantages, including simplicity, universality, and most important, potential as electrodes for smart tattoo patches and implantable sensors.

As discussed in Chapter 9, many smartphones have an NFC chip inside. If we hover the smartphone over the patch, we can wirelessly transmit information to and from the patch. Since it is bound directly to the skin, it can withstand activities such as showering and swimming. With the new three-dimensional (3D) printed miniature batteries shown in Chapter 1, the smart tattoo may last even longer. The so-called *epidermal electronics* era has arrived.

10.6 PILL CAMERAS

Pill cameras seem like they come directly from the movie *Fantastic Voyage*. The digital cameras are capsulized to the size of a pill with 4 to 6 LED (light-emitting diode) lights and take at least four images per second. Pill cameras are used to detect internal bleeding, colon polyps, and other digestive diseases. They are noninvasive and affordable tools—an alternative to the colonoscopy, an invasive procedure in which a plastic tube with a tiny closed-circuit or fiber-optic camera is inserted into a patient's anus and passed up through the colon.

The cost of a pill camera is around US$250, an order of magnitude lower than colonoscopy procedures. It can go into small intestinal areas where normal scopes are unable to go. Using it does not require anesthesia. However, it requires similar preparation as colonoscopies (e.g., twelve hours of fasting and cleaning the colon). Pill cameras have their weaknesses; for instance, they cannot perform biopsies, and their orientation and speed cannot be controlled *in vivo*.

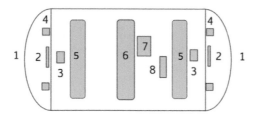

FIGURE 10.20 Anatomy of Givenimaging's PillCam: 1) optical dome; 2) lens holder; 3) optical lens; 4) light-emitting diodes; 5) CMOS imaging sensor; 6) batteries; 7) ASIC transmitter; and 8) antenna. PillCam's dual-camera design enables the system to inspect the back of the folds in the colon more efficiently than regular endoscopes without increasing the scope's size or operational area (to bend the scope head 180 degrees in order to look backward).

---

[207] Yoonseob Kim, Jian Zhu, Bongjun Yeom, Matthew Di Prima, Xianli Su, Jin-Gyu Kim, Seung Jo Yoo, Ctirad Uher, and Nicholas A. Kotov. Stretchable nanoparticle conductors with self-organized conductive pathways. *Nature* 500:59–63, 2013.

Figure 10.20 shows the internal structure of the pill camera. As you can see, the batteries occupy a large space inside the capsule. Normally, the batteries only last for eight hours, but it takes twenty-four hours for a pill to go through the body. Therefore, a timer is used to turn on the camera and LEDs during the last eight hours.

Image Feature Extraction

A color PillCam image is a snapshot of the digestive tract taken at rate of four images or more per second for at least eight hours. That is a lot of color images. Doctors may only view a small portion of the collected images. To use a computer to assist doctors in diagnosis, we must translate the image content to numerical features. Figure 10.21 shows the pill camera images from a colon.

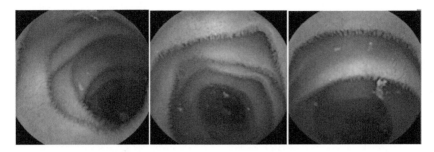

FIGURE 10.21 Typical images captured by capsule camera at different locations. (From Yingju Chen and Jeongkyu Lee, *Diagnostic and Therapeutic Endoscopy* Article ID 418037, 9 pages, 2012. Courtesy of Hindawi Publishing Corporation.)

The popular features include (1) color, (2) texture, and (3) shape features. Let us take a closer look at each of these features:

Color is the first feature to consider. Because it is totally dark inside the human body, pill cameras use white light LEDs for illumination. Toward the end of its trip, the battery of a capsule weakens, and therefore so does the intensity of the light. To make the color representation less sensitive to the changes in illumination, we want to find color spaces that decompose the illumination factor from color factors. We can use either International Commission on Illumination (CIE) L*a*b* or hue saturation value (HSV), by which we can eliminate the illumination factor (Chapter 5). By computing a color histogram, certain features can be detected, such as bleeding, the presence of stool, and so on. The visual appearance of bleeding images is bright red. However, depending on the lifetime of blood, it could be black or tarry. Figure 10.22 shows a bleeding area located by the computer.

Texture is how surface structures reflect the light with pixel intensity variation distributions. The texture feature is in fact sensitive to image resolution, lighting changes, and focus length; however, texture is assumed to be invariant to rotation and grayscale transformation. A common texture model is gray-level co-occurrence matrices (GLCM), which describe spatial relationships between the reference and neighboring pixels within a local neighborhood.[208]

Shape is the final feature to consider. Shape-based features are often used in polyp and tumor detection, in which we want to find a bump-like shape.[209] Figure 10.23 shows a polyp shape captured by the PillCam. Shape features can also be used to detect artifacts such as stool and folds. Edge detection is the first step for extracting shape outlines. The orientation of lines can be modeled by Gabor filters, which are defined by harmonic functions modulated by a Gaussian distribution. Since frequency and orientation representations of Gabor filters are similar to those of the human visual system, a set of Gabor filters with different frequencies and orientations is useful for texture-based region segmentation of an image.[210]

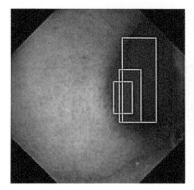 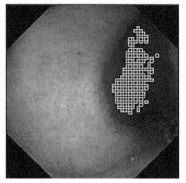

FIGURE 10.22 Bleeding detection based on color histogram. (From Y. J. Chen, W. Yasen, J. Lee, D. Lee, and Y. Kim, in *Proceedings of the Medical Imaging: Computer-Aided Diagnosis, Proceedings of SPIE*, Orlando, FL, Vol. 7260, February 2009. Courtesy Hindawi Publishing Corporation.)

Polyp Detection

The preliminary use of capsule endoscopy is to find the source of bleeding and abnormality in the small intestine.[211] The new generation PillCam II is designed for colon inspection for abnormalities such as polyps or precancerous growths. The polyp detection algorithm starts with preprocessing, the input frame image that includes

[208] R. M. Haralick, Statistical and structural approaches to texture. *Proceedings of the IEEE* 67(5):786–804, 1979.

[209] Sae Hwang, JungHwan Oh, Wallapak Tavanapong, Johnny Wong, and Piet C. de Groen. Polyp detection in colonoscopy video using elliptical shape feature. In *International Conference on Image Processing, 2007. ICIP 2007.* 2:465–468, 2007.

[210] J. G. Daugman. Uncertainty relation for resolution in space, spatial frequency, and orientation optimized by two-dimensional visual cortical filters. *Journal of the Optical Society of America A* 2(7):1160–1169, 1985.

[211] Alexandros Karargyris and Nikolaos Bourbakis. Detection of small bowel polyps and ulcers in wireless capsule endoscopy videos. *IEEE Transactions on Biomedical Engineering* 58(10):2777–2786, 2011.

image segmentation, enhancement or adjustment, and denoising. Image segmentation focuses only on regions of interest. The major part of the detection algorithm lies in feature extraction, including shape, curvature, color, luminance, and texture. After extracting the features, we can locate polyps according to the values of the features we extracted. A combination of the features can be used to determine if a location has a possible polyp candidate. Each feature will be weighted differently so that more common or efficient features play a more important role in polyp location. Figure 10.24 shows a basic flow of the polyp detection algorithm.

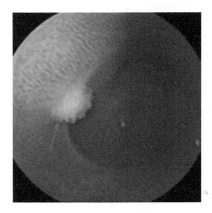

FIGURE 10.23   The small jejunal sessile polyp captured by PillCam SB. (Courtesy of West Penn Health System.)

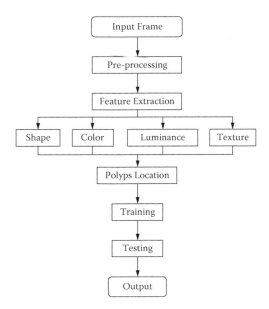

FIGURE 10.24   Polyp detection algorithm.

Curvature-Based Polyp Detection

Curvature is the most significant feature in the detection because of the unique shape of polyps. The challenge is distinguishing the curvature of a polyp versus colon folds or normal mucosa.

Let's first extract shape features. The way we detect shape is by detecting the edge of polyps. As opposed to the way we detect ellipses, we detect the curve of polyps. By observing the images, we found that most tend to be red in color. Therefore, we compare different color channels of images, and the result proves that the red channel image gives better edge information for shapes.

We then perform contrast enhancement as preparation for edge detection (see Figure 10.25, left). But, this introduces more noises as well. Therefore, we have to apply a Gaussian blur after contrast enhancement. The blurred image is shown on the right side of Figure 10.25.

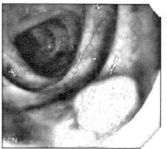 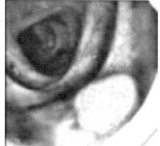

FIGURE 10.25   Contrast-enhanced image (left) and blurred image (right).

Then, we apply Canny edge detection on the blurred image. The Canny detector is chosen because it gives more detailed edge detection results than other edge detectors, such as Sobel or Prewit. Besides, it provides more continuous edge detection results that are better for detecting an edge as a whole rather than separate edge segments. The drawback of Canny edge detection is that it is too detailed, so even very small edges can be detected. To deal with this, let us add one step of noise removal after Canny edge detection. Go through every connected region that is regarded as an edge curve and delete those with a number of pixels less than a threshold. Figure 10.26 shows the result of Canny edge detection and the result after removing some of the small edges.

As seen in Figure 10.26, there are still edges that needed to be eliminated to have only the polyp edge left. Consider deleting two kinds of edges; first are those that are too close to the center of the colon or rectum. As shown in Figure 10.27, the center of a colon/rectum is usually a very dark area, so not much information can be provided by these areas. Second are those edges where the variance of distance from each pixel to the center is too large since these edges are more likely to be the edge of folds of colon/rectum.

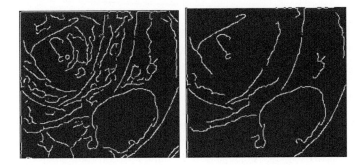

FIGURE 10.26   Result of Canny edge detection (left) and result after noise removal (right).

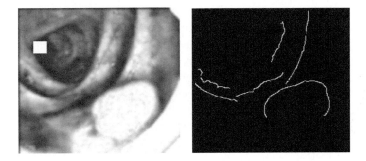

FIGURE 10.27   The center is labeled with a white square (left), and the result after deleting the two kinds of edges is shown (right).

FIGURE 10.28   The circular center is labeled as a small grey block (left), result after deleting pixels with a large angle (middle), and the result of polyp edge detection (right).

To do this, we first detect the center of a colon/rectum that we define as the darkest area in an image. The center is labeled as a white square in Figure 10.27 (left). The result of the edge detection is shown on the right in Figure 10.27.

To eliminate the remaining the non-polyp fold edges, we would like to detect the circumcenter of each pixel on the edge and two other pixels near it. In Figure 10.28 (left), the circumcenter is labeled as a red (grey) block; the two lines are the line between the pixel and the center of the colon or rectum and the line between the pixel and the circumcenter. Then, we calculate the angle between the two lines. As the angles of pixels on the fold edge will be small, we can separate the fold edge from the polyp edge. Figure 10.28 (middle) shows the result after deleting pixels that have a large angle value. Let us adjust the threshold for the curvature angle so that only the polyp edge remains. See the right side of Figure 10.28 for the final rersult.

10.7 SUMMARY

Body media involve a network of wearable sensors. In this chapter, we overviewed three types of technologies: BCIs, smart fiber (epidermal electronics), and pill cameras.

The BCIs have escaped from research labs and hospitals and entered individuals' homes. The products range from single-electrode EEGs for entertainment, to 14-electrode EEGs for game control, to the near-professional 16-electrode EEG systems for emergency responses and biofeedback. Their applications in ambient diagnosis are endless (e.g., a biofeedback cap for patients with seizures, sleep disorder diagnosis, brain injury assessment, and so on).

Smart fibers (epidermal electronics) have great potential in the consumer market, including a smart bra for cancer detection, smart shoes for walking pattern recognition, and smart tattoos for temperature, moisture, and electrical potential sensing.

Pill cameras have been a breakthrough in endoscopic diagnoses. Automated image interpretation algorithms are meaningful because doctors are not able to review all the frames. The case study in this chapter is just a small portion of the capacity of an automated diagnostic algorithm. The good news is that the manufacturers of the products and medical professionals have created open source databases so that the knowledge about captured images and diseases can be used worldwide.

It is worth remembering that body media are more powerful if they are connected with the network, such as passive NFC with a smartphone. Compared to the conventional body media of several years ago, the new mode of NFC can reduce the cost by an order of magnitude.

PROBLEMS

1. Compare the three methods for sleep disorder diagnosis (BCI, smartphone-based accelerometers, and sound analysis) in terms of principles, costs, and usability.
2. Discuss the usage of Wi-Fi, Bluetooth, and NFC in hospitals in terms of safety, privacy, and bandwidth issues.
3. What are the safety requirements for BCIs? List your sources and provide supporting data in your report.
4. Redraw Figure 10.8 in two-dimensional heat maps (i.e., render the intensity in gray scale to show the signal strength in the left brain and the right brain in multiple frames). Make a flip-book from the frames to show the animation.
5. What are the differences between thermal imaging and the smart bra in breast cancer detection?

6. Research 3D printing technology and discuss its potential applications in smart bra design. Google the 3D printed bra for the starting point. Discuss feasibility, costs, and limitations.

7. Improvise a method with your available components to record your walking patterns in shoes.

8. Study the walking imbalance patterns using accelerometers, Kinect, and webcam.

9. Compare battery solutions for smart shoes. List options, costs, and pros and cons.

10. Smart tattoos can transmit data to smartphones with the NFC mode. Write a pseudocode about the communication protocol.

11. Design a battery-powered smart tattoo with the 200-μm 3D printed battery. Estimate the power needed and design the layout of the battery.

12. Assume the pill camera can only operate for eight hours, but it takes twenty-four hours for the pill camera to exit. Say we want to inspect the small intestine. How can we solve this problem?

13. If a pill camera does not use a white light, what spectrum lights would you recommend? List justifications, sources, and pros and cons for each alternative.

14. Assume the pill camera can view a colon from both the front and back ends. Discuss its advantages and disadvantages compared to conventional colonoscopies.

15. Draw a map between the colon diseases and related image samples. Discuss the semantic gap between visual features and verbal descriptions. Find online data to support your points.

16. Replot the chart in Figure 10.1 with more accurate and updated data. Summarize the trend in the next five years in your report.

11 Pocket Microscopes

> Why has not Man a microscopic eye?
>
> —Alexander Pope, 1733

11.1 INTRODUCTION

The purpose of microscopes is to magnify extremely small objects that cannot be seen by the naked eye (Figure 11.1). They are incredibly valuable to medical diagnoses, including blood cell counting, bacteria detection, tissue analysis, and disease classification. This chapter discusses

- History of microscopes
- Microorganism sizes
- Mobile phone microscopes
- Time-lapse videos
- Laser holography
- Virtual microscope
- Image stitching
- Cell-labeling algorithm

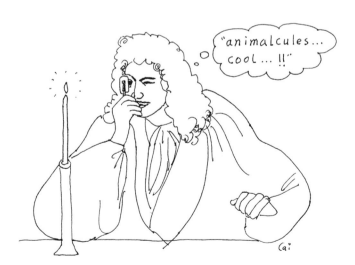

FIGURE 11.1 Using handmade microscopes in the 1700s, Dutch businessman Antoni van Leeuwenhoek was the first to observe and describe bacteria, which he originally referred to as animalcules.

11.2 THE AMATEUR EXPERT

Looking back on the history of microscopes, many extraordinary discoveries were made by curious amateurs using simple devices. For example, Antoni van Leeuwenhoek was a cloth merchant and amateur scientist who lived in the seventeenth and eighteenth centuries in the Netherlands. Leeuwenhoek is known to be the first to observe and describe bacteria, microphages, red blood cells, sperm cells, and other microorganisms (Figure 11.2). Almost all of Leeuwenhoek's instruments were simple magnifying glasses, not compound microscopes of the type used today. Compared to modern microscopes, these are extremely simple devices, using only one lens, mounted in a tiny hole in the brass plate that made up the body of the instrument. Leeuwenhoek's craftsmanship enabled him to build microscopes that magnified over 200 times, with clearer and brighter images than the compound microscopes of his time.

Today, microscopes are much more powerful and affordable, but they are mainly locked inside the walls of labs and operated by professionals. This chapter liberates the microscopy technologies and reveals their potential for affordable personal diagnostic purposes. For example, we can use a modified mobile phone to enable

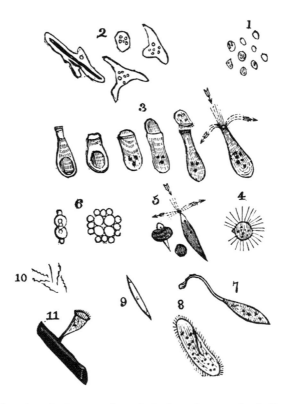

FIGURE 11.2 Samples of microorganisms Antoni van Leeuwenhoek discovered. Can you name the microorganisms in the figure?

individuals to perform *in situ* analysis by turning the phone into a microscope and looking at cells in a sample.

Currently, doctors often have a nurse draw a sample of blood, label it, and send it to a lab for analysis. This takes coordination, correct sample preparation, good labeling, fast shipping, and careful handling and analysis at the lab so the sample is not contaminated, all of which cost money and a large amount of time. Alternatively, a new mobile phone device could allow a patient to smear a sample of blood on a glass slide, shine a light on it, and take a picture of it with a mobile phone. The mobile phone or a computer could then do the analysis or send the image, not the sample, to doctors for further analyses. The results would be as accurate as sending the sample to a lab, similar to the personal glucose meters used today.

11.3   SIZES OF MICROORGANISMS

The smallest objects that the unaided human eye can see are about 0.1 mm long.[212] That means that, under the right conditions, we might be able to see the largest bacteria known to us, the *Thiomargarita namibiensis,* at 0.75 mm, a human egg at 0.1 mm, and a louse egg at 0.8 mm without using magnification.

Smaller cells are easily visible under a light microscope. It is even possible to make out structures within the cell, such as the nucleus, mitochondria, and chloroplasts. Most bacteria range in size from 0.15 to 4 µm. A micrometer is 0.001 mm. The smallest worm eggs visible using the cell phone in our experiments would be 40–60 µm in diameter. The average yeast cell is 4 to 12 µm long. The measurements for the diameter of a yeast cell are diverse because there are about six hundred different species of yeast in the world. Each type of yeast comes in different sizes; as a result, the diameters are just estimates of some of the more common yeasts.[213]

Light microscopes use a system of lenses to magnify an image. The power of a light microscope is limited by the wavelength of visible light, which is about 500 nm. The most powerful light microscopes can detect bacteria but not viruses.[214]

To see anything smaller than 500 nm, we will need an electron microscope. Electron microscopes shoot a high-voltage beam of electrons onto or through an object, which deflects and absorbs some of the electrons. Resolution is still limited by the wavelength of the electron beam, but this wavelength is much smaller than that of visible light. The most powerful electron microscopes can see molecules and even individual atoms. Figure 11.3 shows a spectrum of different sizes of microscopic objects.

---

[212] http://learn.genetics.utah.edu/content/begin/cells/scale/

[213] http://hypertextbook.com/facts/2000/JennyNg.shtml

[214] A light microscope, even one with perfect lenses and perfect illumination, simply cannot be used to distinguish objects that are smaller than half the wavelength of light. White light has an average wavelength of 0.55 µm, half of which is 0.275 µm. Any two lines that are closer together than 0.275 µm will be seen as a single line, and any object with a diameter smaller than 0.275 µm will be invisible or, at best, show up as a blur. To see tiny particles under a microscope, scientists must bypass light altogether and use a different sort of "illumination," one with a shorter wavelength.

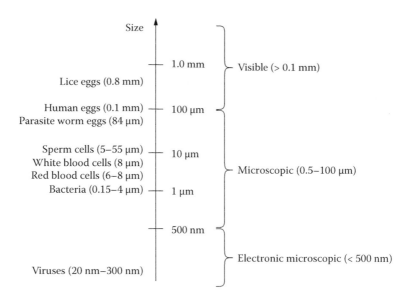

FIGURE 11.3   Sizes of microscopic specimens in logarithmic scale.

11.4   MOBILE PHONE MICROSCOPES

This section discusses mobile phone microscopes.[215,216,217]

Snap-On Microscope

Off-the-shelf mobile phone microscopes have amplification powers ranging from ×10 to ×100. They normally have two light-emitting diode (LED) white lights. Some even have an ultraviolet (UV) light, which is good for skin imaging. Figure 11.4 shows two popular models of the snap-on microscopes for iPhones.

Phone Case as an Interface

The snap-on case for cell phones is an affordable adaptor for microscopes or other sensors (Figure 11.5). These are normally regular phone cases with the addition of a thin-threaded hole at the camera area, where a microscope can be screwed on. This

[215] D. N. Breslauer, R. N. Maamari, N. A. Switz, W. A. Lam, and D. A. Fletcher. Mobile phone based clinical microscopy for global health applications. *PLoS ONE* 4:e6320, 2009.

[216] Z. J. Smith, K. Chu, A. R. Espenson, M. Rahimzadeh, A. Gryshuk, M. Molinaro, D. M. Dwyre, S. Lane, D. Matthews, and S, Wachsmann-Hogiu. Cell-phone-based platform for biomedical device development and education applications. *PLoS ONE*, 6(3), 2011. PMID: 21399693.

[217] Isaac I. Bogoch, Jason R. Andrews, Benjamin Speich, Jürg Utzinger, Shaali M. Ame, Said M. Ali, and Jennifer Keiser. Short report: mobile phone microscopy for the diagnosis of soil-transmitted helminth infections: a proof-of-concept study. *American Journal of Tropical Medicine and Hygiene* 12-0742; published online March 11, 2013.

enables users to attach and detach the microscope easily and provides a stable support for the microscope and related pieces.

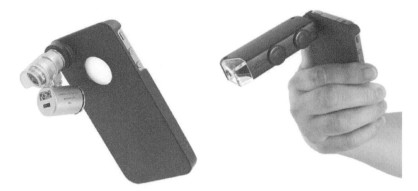

FIGURE 11.4 An X60 microscope with white light and UV light (left) and X100 microscope with white light for Apple iPhones.

The snap-on phone case is indeed an effective interface between sensors and phones. However, most manufacturers make phone cases that are only usable with particular microscopes. There is no compatibility between phone models as the dimensions of phones are varied and always evolving. The new three-dimensional (3D) printing technology would bring a solution to the problem. For example, the case interface design can be translated into the 3D printer executable code in stereolithographic (STL) format and stored online. Users could download, modify, and run the code for a particular brand of phone that contains a standard threaded hole on the case. It would not be impractical for someone to print an entire set of microscope parts, minus a lens.

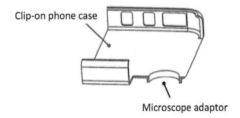

FIGURE 11.5 Snap-on phone case with microscope interface.

Do-It-Yourself Ball Lens

To increase the magnification ratio and reduce the size of the microscope, researchers have developed ball lens designs as illustrated in Figure 11.6, which is similar to Antoni van Leeuwenhoek's microscope from the 1700s. Now, there is a renaissance for simple DIY (do-it-yourself) microscopes.

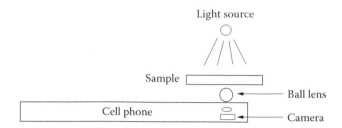

FIGURE 11.6   Ball lens microscopy. (Adapted from Z. J. Smith, K. Chu, A. R. Espenson, M. Rahimzadeh, A. Gryshuk, M. Molinaro, D. M. Dwyre, S. Lane, D. Matthews, and S. Wachsmann-Hogiu. *PLoS ONE*, 6(3), 2011. PMID: 21399693. Courtesy of PLOS ONE.)

According to the laws of optics, we can increase magnification by using multiple lenses (compound microscope) or a smaller ball lens. For example, a 3-mm ball lens can magnify 100–200 times the actual size and a 1-mm ball lens can magnify 200–350 times. Figure 11.7 shows designs of the attachments to an iPhone.

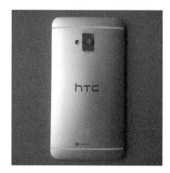

FIGURE 11.7   Ball lens microscopes (the lens is inserted in a hole on the rubber sheet that is taped to the cell phone).

The mobile phone-based microscope has been shown to have a resolution of 1.5 μm in the center of its field of view. Although the image quality rapidly degrades in a raw image due to the use of a single ball lens, the images can still be used to accurately diagnose a variety of blood diseases.

It would be possible to create a robust program that could take individual frames of a movie recorded by a phone and stitch those images together into a single image where the whole field of view would be well focused. Through motion tracking and image fusion algorithms, the overall burden on the experimenter would be reduced, and a high-quality image could be obtained without needing to carefully mount or hold the sample with respect to the phone.[218]

Furthermore, mobile phone microscopes can be used to find the red cell count of a blood sample imaged by a mobile phone camera. The CellC algorithm or one similar

---

[218] W. Huang and Z. Jing. Evaluation of focus measures in multi-focus image fusion. *Pattern Recognition Letters* 28:493–500, 2007.

could be used to report morphometric parameters that could enable an approximate complete blood count (CBC), discriminating cells into several blood cell classes.

However, it takes skillful craftsmanship and patience to obtain a meaningful image. For example, the imaging results are sensitive to the distance between the light source and the sample because the focus plane is delicate. For high-power magnification, subtle hand shaking can make a big difference. In addition, the way samples are prepared is critical. These issues create more degrees of freedom (DOF) for errors.

11.5 DIGITAL MICROSCOPES

With digital camera prices constantly dropping, digital microscopes are becoming more affordable to individuals (Figure 11.8). The low-end products fall into three categories: (1) adding a webcam or a digital camera to the conventional analog microscope, (2) stand-alone digital microscopes, and (3) dual-use digital microscopes. The analog-to-digital microscope produces good-quality images. However, these microscopes are usually not portable. The stand-alone digital microscopes are pocket size, but they are mainly used for nonbiomedical applications such as currency checking and electronic circuit debugging. Dual-use digital microscopes have a regular slide support and dark-field and bright-field lighting and allow users to detach the pocket-size scope from the base for traveling. The dual-use digital microscopes appear to be an optimal selection in terms of cost-effectiveness in portable applications.

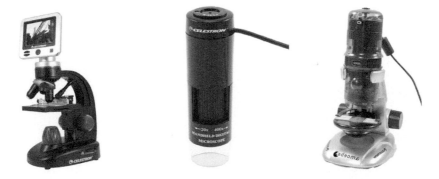

FIGURE 11.8   Digital microscopes: analog-to-digital, stand-alone, dual-use designs.

Microscope Lighting

Unfortunately, most snap-on microscopes are designed for inspecting currencies, coins, and diamonds, and they are not intended for biomedical applications. Lighting is a problem. Microscopes usually use backlighting, but the snap-on microscopes use front lighting, and they do not have the dark-field or bright-field lighting options. Dark-field lighting produces a hollow cone of light that is scattered by the sample. In contrast, bright-field lighting produces a solid cone of light that enters the sample directly. Figure 11.9 shows the difference between the two modes.[219] Other lighting methods, such as holographic focus grid illumination, may also enhance the images.

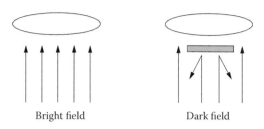

FIGURE 11.9 The bright-field lighting (left) and dark-field lighting (right).

11.6   SPECTRUM LIGHTING

Mobile phones can be used as photonics hardware in ambient diagnoses. Phones with a color screen can generate the light source for a fluorescence microscope setup. For example, there is a free downloadable app on the Android market called color flashlight for spectral control on Android smartphones. Figure 11.10 shows the human skin and the bread yeast under the UV light, captured by the cellphone microscope at the scale of 40 times.

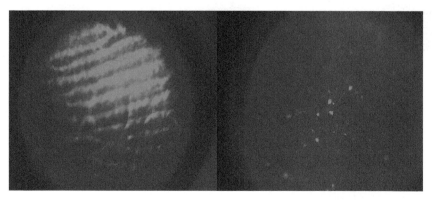

FIGURE 11.10 Human skin and bread yeast under the UV light, captured by the cell phone microscope at X40.

Researchers believe that a custom app would raise the signal intensity and allow rapid modulation for fluorescence decay measurements. In addition, modifying the

[219] J. Wu, X. Cui, G. Zheng, Y. M. Wang, L. M. Lee, et al. Wide field-of-view microscope based on holographic focus grid illumination. *Optical Letters* 35:2188–2190, 2010.

setup to use the phone's own camera will further simplify the device, raising its potential for use in remote areas.[220]

11.7   OBSERVING YEAST CELLS

Shall we do some experiments with your pocket microscopes? We can start with the yeast that is commonly used for baking bread. Let us obtain a blank slide and coverslip; check to make sure that they are clean. Place one drop of water-diluted yeast solution on the center of the slide (Figure 11.11). Since the yeast is alive, it may make air bubbles as it sits on the slide (Figure 11.12).

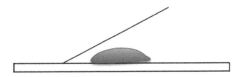

FIGURE 11.11   Microscopic slide preparation for yeast observation.

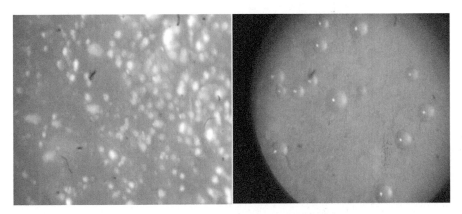

FIGURE 11.12   Microscopic views of yeast cells recorded on iPhone.

Start from low-power magnification. Observe yeast cells under ×40 and ×100 and observe the detail of one good representative yeast cell under ×400. When we carefully focus up and down with the fine adjustment, we can observe that these cells are three dimensionally fairly oval in shape. Yeast cells do have a thin cell wall and clear cytoplasm. The nucleus cannot be seen unless special staining techniques are used. If you see a round object (or several) with a broad, black ring around the outside, it is an air bubble.

---

[220] John Canning et al. Measurement of fluorescence in a rhodamine-123 doped self-assembled "giant" mesostructured silica sphere using a smartphone as optical hardware. *Sensors*, 11:7055–7062, 2011; doi:10.3390/s110707055.

11.8 OBSERVING PARASITIC WORMS

Worms that infect human intestines, such as roundworms and hookworms, or soil-transmitted helminths, have harmed nearly two billion people worldwide. In remote regions of developing nations, rates of disease from worms are particularly high and can result in chronic malnutrition and anemia in children. For some hospitals, a real microscope is too expensive, especially in remote areas of Africa. However, in many of these places, it is still possible to find mobile phones.

New technologies are being developed to use mobile phones to spot parasitic worm eggs in intestines with a microscope (Figure 11.13).[221] The DIY microscope includes a 3-mm diameter ball lens, two segments of double-sided tape, and a flashlight. Ball lenses are normally used in the telecommunications field in coupling with optical fiber cable. They are inexpensive, generally costing US$8 to US$10. They can even be made for free if one manages to take the glass ball out of a used CD drive. The entire setup can be developed for US$15 in addition to the cost of the phone.

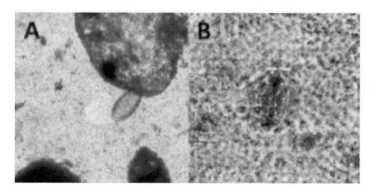

FIGURE 11.13 Parasitic worm egg images from a (a) standard microscope and from the (b) cell phone-based microscope. (From iPhone microscope helps detect parasitic worm eggs. *Medgadget* March 14, 2013. http://www.medgadget.com/2013/03/iphone-microscope-helps-detect-parasitic-worm-eggs.html. Courtesy of *American Journal of Tropical Medicine and Hygiene* with copyright permission.)

Researchers compared this cheaper solution to a proper microscope while diagnosing children in rural Tanzania and have shown that, for some nematodes, the phone microscopes were sufficient in detecting worm eggs; for others, they were not.[222] iPhone microscopy has a sensitivity of about 70% for detecting the eggs of helminths.

In the Tanzanian study, researchers found that mobile phone microscope sensitivity was dependent on the type of worm and the strength of the infection. For example, the mobile phone found 81% of giant roundworm (*Ascaris lumbricoides*) infections and 54% of roundworm (*Trichuris trichiura*) infections. However, it only

---

[221] O. Mudanyali, C. Oztoprak, D. Tseng, A. Erlinger, and A. Ozcan. Detection of waterborne parasites using field-portable and cost-effective lensfree microscopy. *Lab Chip* 10:2419–2423, 2010.
[222] Bogoch et al., Short Report.

detected 14% of all hookworm infections; the researchers said that this was due to the much smaller number of eggs present than with the other parasites. Studies showed that it was quite successful at detecting moderate-to-heavy infections, but not very good at detecting mild infections for which there might be only a few eggs in the sample.

11.9 TIME-LAPSE VIDEO

The beauty of digital microscopes is their ability to record time-lapse video without extra cost. Time-lapse videos help us to understand the momentum, trajectories, and interactions of microorganisms. Fortunately, there are many free or inexpensive mobile phone applications for time-lapse video capturing. For example, HD Video for iPhone[223] allows user to capture images in the interval from 0.1 seconds to 1 hour. Figure 11.14 shows a sequence of frames from a time-lapse video of yeast cells when they were activated to generate CO_2 bubbles.

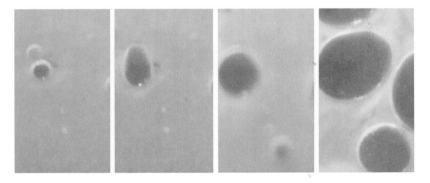

FIGURE 11.14 Time-lapse video frames of the activated yeast cells recorded from an iPhone microscope.

11.10 LASER HOLOGRAPHY

Laser holography is not as mysterious as it sounds. A simple demonstration can be set up with office supplies. All that is needed is a 250-mW green laser pointer, a paper clip bent to form a tiny loop to hold a water drop, and a binder clip for supporting the laser pointer and the bent paper clip.[224] Shining the laser light through a hanging drop of water from a pond produces a simple laser microscope that projects shadows of the microflora on the wall so one can watch them flitter about with the bare eye[225] (see Figures 11.15 and 11.16).

The 3D models can be constructed from the laser holography. When the light passes through the test section, some of it hits objects and deflects, but some passes straight through. The combination of the direct light (this is called the reference

[223] Teravolt.org. Time-lapse video capture app for iPhone.

[224] http://blog.makezine.com/2010/12/13/ultra-minimalist-laser-microscope/

[225] http://blog.makezine.com/2010/10/07/laser-drop-of-water-microbial-movie/.

beam) and the deflected light hitting our eyes or the CCD (charge-coupled device) chip creates an "interference pattern," which is similar to the shining reflections we often see from oil spilled on pavement. Any other objects, such as dust on the lens, will also deflect the light and appear in the image.[226] Interested readers can download DigiHoloWin to try the algorithm.[227]

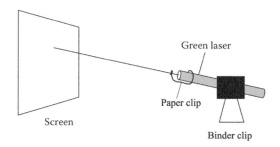

FIGURE 11.15   A laser projector can be made from a green laser pointer, a paper clip, and a binder clip.

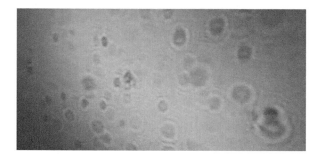

FIGURE 11.16   Live bacteria projected by the green laser pointer.

11.11   VIRTUAL MICROSCOPY

In microscopy, one can only see a very small portion of a slide. A large number of fields of view are required to capture a complete slide. For pocket microscopes, the focused field of view is even smaller. Image stitching is an important technology to produce a panorama or larger image by combining several images with overlapped areas. In much biomedical research, image stitching is highly desirable to acquire a panoramic image that represents large areas of certain structures while retaining microscopic resolution. With a digital microscope, we can take many images or videos to create frames for the stitching process.[228] We call it "virtual microscopy."

[226] D. Tseng, O. Mudanyali, C. Oztoprak, S. O. Isikman, I. Sencan, et al. Lensfree microscopy on a cellphone. *Lab Chip* 10:1787–1792, 2010.

[227] http://www.me.jhu.edu/lefd/shc/LPholo/DigiHoloWin.zip

[228] W. Bishara, T. W. Su, A. F. Coskun, and A. Ozcan. Lensfree on-chip microscopy over a wide field-of-view using pixel super-resolution. *Optics Express* 18:11181–11191, 2010.

Feature Extraction

For computerized stitching, we need to find landmarks, or so-called features or key points in the images. A common feature extraction method is the scale-independent feature transform (SIFT).[229,230] It generates feature points using the difference of Gaussian (DoG) model, which uses a Gaussian filter to blur the image at multiple levels and calculate the difference between images at different blurring levels. It then applies filters to remove the insignificant feature points, such as the points on the edge lines or low-contrast points. This reduces feature points to a manageable number.

To further describe the feature point, we take the gradients and orientations of pixels around the key point into consideration. SIFT takes a 16 × 16 window of "in-between" pixels around the key point. It then splits that window into sixteen 4 × 4 windows. From each 4 × 4 window, it generates a histogram of eight bins of directions. Each bin corresponds to 0–44 degrees, 45–89 degrees, and so on. Gradient orientations from the 4 × 4 are put into these bins. Finally, we obtain the normalized 128 numbers to form the "feature vector." The key point is uniquely identified by this feature vector. Figure 11.17 shows the definition of the feature vector, and Figure 11.18 shows a sample of the extracted feature points.

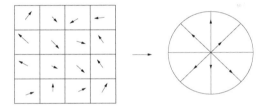

FIGURE 11.17   From each 4 × 4 window, the SIFT generates a histogram of eight directions.

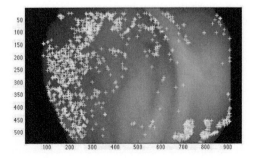

FIGURE 11.18   Sample key points in an image.

[229] David G. Lowe. Object recognition from local scale-invariant features. *Proceedings of the International Conference on Computer Vision* 2:1150–1157, 1999.
[230] U.S. Patent 6,711,293. Method and apparatus for identifying scale invariant features in an image and use of same for locating an object in an image, David Lowe's patent for the SIFT algorithm, March 23, 2004.

Image Registration

The SIFT features extracted from the input images are matched against each other to find k-nearest neighbors for each feature. These correspondences are then used to find m candidate matching images for each image. Homographies between pairs of images are then computed using random sample consensus (RANSAC) for verification. A homography is a geographic transform, including scaling, rotation, translation, and sheering. Figure 11.19 shows an example of the homographic transform in which the point p corresponds to p'. The two points are called corresponding points.

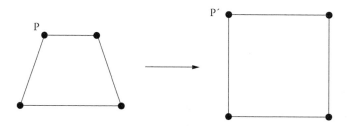

FIGURE 11.19   Homographic transform.

The main idea of RANSAC is to calculate a majority vote of the mapping directions as the consent direction to determine inliers or outliers of the key points.

Pseudocode for RANSAC for estimating homography is as follows:[231]

1. Select four feature pairs randomly.
2. Compute homographic transform.
3. Compute inliers where || original point – mapped point || < threshold
4. Repeat until all key points are covered.
5. Keep largest set of inliers.
6. Recompute optimal homographic transform for all the inliers.

The following is a toy problem to illustrate how the RANSAC algorithm works. Assume we have six pairs of key points (a, b, c, d, e, and f) that have corresponding points in another image: a', b', c', d', e', and f', respectively. We randomly start with four pairs a-a', b-b', c-c', and d-d' and find the homographic transform to map between the four pairs (Figure 11.20). Then, we add the e-e' pair and find it fits the current homographic transform well. In other words, the homographic transform can map e to e' within an allowable error. Next, we add f-f' and try the homographic transform again. However, let us say that in this case it does not fit well. As we have five inliers of six pairs that agree with the homographic transform, we can eliminate the "bad" (outlier) pair f-f'. Now, we recalculate the homograph again with the six inliers and find the optimal solution for the homographic transform that will be applied for stitching related images (Figure 11.21).

---

[231] http://saturday.csail.mit.edu/fa12/lectures/lecture13ransac/lecture13ransac.pdf

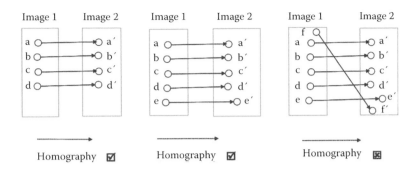

FIGURE 11.20 Example of corresponding points validation.

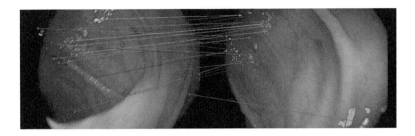

FIGURE 11.21 Homographic matching evaluation for image stitching.

SIFT is not sensitive to minor rotations (say, less than 30 degrees) or scaling, so it has been widely used in image stitching and object detection. However, SIFT is computationally expensive, and it depends on the complexity of the image. SIFT normally works well with "feature-rich" images such as an image of a centipede, but it does not work well with "feature-less" images such as blurred images or an image of bubbles without sharp corners or high-contrast spots.

There are several variations of SIFT. For example, sped-up robust features (SURF) are used to extract features from the images to be stitched with less time and higher repeatability. The histogram equalization (HE) method is employed to preprocess images to enhance their contrast for better feature extraction.

SIFT and SURF are open sources available for downloading. There are a few packages for using both in OpenCV and MATLAB. SIFT is patented, but SURF is not.

Superzooming Like Google Earth

After we register and stitch the microscopic images together to form a large one, we can add an interactive browser to navigate the details on a virtual slide image, similar to the geographical navigation experience of Google Earth. Virtual microscopy can be used for observing, exchanging, saving, and establishing a database of microscope images. Figure 11.22 shows a superzoom effect from 1% zoom-in to 100% zoom-in.

Before recent advances in virtual microscopy, various forms of film scanners were commonly used to digitize slides, and image resolutions were rarely above

5,000 dpi. Today, it is possible to achieve more than 100,000 dpi and thus resolutions approaching those that are visible under the optical microscope. This increase in scanning resolution in hardware comes at a high price. On the other hand, the software-based image stitching can increase the scanning resolution without additional costs. However, it is a time and resolution trade-off. Image stitching is a time-consuming process. To transmit a large image across the Internet would cause a network data traffic jam. A typical method is to cut the virtual microscopic image into many smaller patches, which allows the network to "breath" and maintain a stable data flow.

Those patches are streamed and reassembled "on demand." In other words, only those patches within the viewing area are downloaded.

FIGURE 11.22   Example of virtual microscopy while zooming into the onion bulb epidermis. Using a mouse or a multitouch screen on iPad, iPhone, or Android phone, the user can zoom, pan, and rotate the stitched panoramic image.

11.12   LABELING AND COUNTING

For automated image processing, we often need to label and count the objects we want to observe, such as blood cells, sperm cells, and parasitic worm eggs from microscopic images.[232,233,234] This can be done with binary morphology; a color or grayscale image is converted to a black-and-white binary image and then is processed. The targets appear as blobs in binary images, leading some to call the process "blobology," as discussed in the chapter on video analytics.[235]

Let us look at a toy problem. Figure 11.23 shows an image of yeast cells. On the top right, we can see the cell-splitting effect in action, called *budding*. This is a fairly easy problem because the image is sharp, and the background is clean. In the Appendix to this chapter, a MATLAB sample code is provided.

---

[232] J. Selinummi, J. Seppälä, O. Yli-Harja, and J. A. Puhakka. Software for quantification of labeled bacteria from digital microscope images by automated image analysis. *BioTechniques* 39:859–863, 2005.

[233] http://cdn.intechopen.com/pdfs/18389/InTech-Image_processing_methods_for_automatic_cell_counting_in_vivo_or_in_situ_using_3d_confocal_microscopy.pdf

[234] http://www.invitrogen.com/etc/medialib/files/Cell-Analysis/PDFs.Par.79060.File.dat/W-082494-Cell-Counting-Hemocytometer.pdf

[235] P. Soille. *Morphological image analysis: principles and applications*, 2nd ed. Springer-Verlag, New York, 2003.

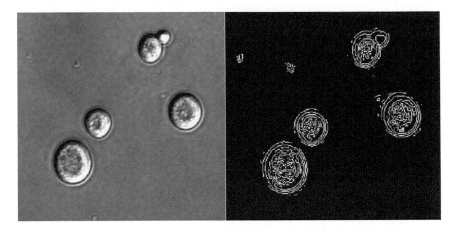

FIGURE 11.23   The original image of yeast cells (left) and result of edge detection (right).

Our first step is to read the image to a matrix and then detect edges. There are many filters for edge detection (e.g., the Sobel, Conney, and Robert). Let us try the Sobel filter.

After edge detection, let us dilate the edges to fill the area (Figure 11.24). The dilate algorithm adds layers of pixels around existing pixels. Note that too much dilation may change the shapes. In some cases, we can also use the "close" filter to close the borderlines. Then, we use the binary fill function to fill the interior gaps inside cells.

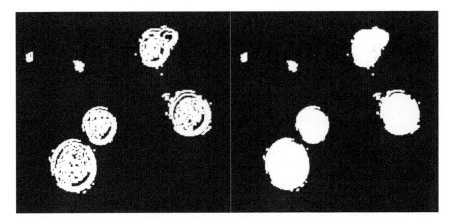

FIGURE 11.24   Results of dilation (left) and area filling (right).

Now, we can see the blobs. Using the erosion and smooth filters, we can remove the connected objects on borders and smooth the cell shape. Note that we used the dilation filter to make the shape fatter. We then use the erosion filter to make it thinner. In the end, the shape areas will stay approximately the same. This also

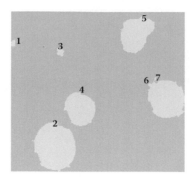

FIGURE 11.25 Results of labeling with numbers. The budding cell at 5 is missed, and the small blob 6 is counted as a cell. These errors can be corrected with advanced filters.

removes tiny objects that are smaller than a threshold. Then, we apply the binary labeling algorithm to mark individual blobs with numbers (Figure 11.25).

How does the labeling work? A simple way to label is to use the so-called flood fill algorithm that starts by finding a foreground pixel and then iteratively searching that pixel's neighbors to find the connected component.[236]

Now, let us look at a simple problem to illustrate the flood fill process. The left side of the matrix that follows is our binary image. Using four connected neighbors, the image has two connected components. The matrix on the right is going to become our label matrix when we are done. It is initialized to contain all zeros.

Pixel Values	Labeling Book
0 0 0 0 0	0 0 0 0 0
0 1 1 0 0	0 0 0 0 0
0 1 0 0 0	0 0 0 0 0
0 0 0 1 1	0 0 0 0 0
0 0 0 0 0	0 0 0 0 0

Step 1: Find a foreground pixel. Set the corresponding label matrix pixel to 1, which is the first label.

Pixel Values	Labeling Book
0 0 0 0 0	0 0 0 0 0
0 *1* 1 0 0	0 *1* 0 0 0
0 1 0 0 0	0 0 0 0 0
0 0 0 1 1	0 0 0 0 0
0 0 0 0 0	0 0 0 0 0

[236] http://blogs.mathworks.com/steve/2007/04/15/connected-component-labeling-part-4/.

Step 2: Set the pixels that were just labeled to 0 and then find all the nonzero 4-connected neighbors. Set the corresponding pixels in the label matrix to 1.

Pixel Values	Labeling Book
0 0 0 0 0	0 0 0 0 0
0 *0* *1* 0 0	0 *1* *1* 0 0
0 *1* 0 0 0	0 *1* 0 0 0
0 0 0 1 1	0 0 0 0 0
0 0 0 0 0	0 0 0 0 0

Step 3: Set the pixels that were just labeled to 0 and then find all the nonzero 4-connected neighbors. We have finished labeling object 1. Now, search for the next nonzero pixel. Set the corresponding pixel in the label matrix to 2, which is the next object label.

Pixel Values	Labeling Book
0 0 0 0 0	0 0 0 0 0
0 *0* *0* 0 0	0 *1* *1* 0 0
0 *0* 0 0 0	0 *1* 0 0 0
0 0 0 *1* 1	0 0 0 *2* 0
0 0 0 0 0	0 0 0 0 0

Step 4: Set the pixels that were just labeled to 0 and then find all the nonzero 4-connected neighbors. Set the corresponding pixels in the label matrix to 2.

Pixel Values	Labeling Book
0 0 0 0 0	0 0 0 0 0
0 *0* *0* 0 0	0 *1* *1* 0 0
0 *0* 0 0 0	0 *1* 0 0 0
0 0 0 *0* *1*	0 0 0 *2* 0
0 0 0 0 0	0 0 0 0 0

Step 5: Set the pixels that were just labeled to 0 and then find all the nonzero 4-connected neighbors. Set the corresponding pixels in the label matrix to 2.

Pixel Values	Labeling Book
0 0 0 0 0	0 0 0 0 0
0 *0* *0* 0 0	0 *1* *1* 0 0
0 *0* 0 0 0	0 *1* 0 0 0
0 0 0 *0* *0*	0 0 0 *2* *2*
0 0 0 0 0	0 0 0 0 0

To try the algorithm on real images, you may run this tiny blob-labeling code in MATLAB in Appendix A. Note the code calls the open source function vislabel(L) that can be downloaded from the MathWorks website.

ImageJ

ImageJ is an open source Java library for image processing.[237] The National Institutes of Health (NIH) originally funded it, so it has a broad impact on biomedical image analysis. ImageJ is written in Java, which allows it to run on Linux, Max OS X, and both 32-bit and 64-bit Windows modes. There are more than 500 plug-ins available.[238]

ImageJ has a cell counter plug-in library for manual cell counting and marking (Figure 11.26). After installing the plug-in, the user can open an image and count the cells with the cursor. Multiple colors can be used to mark different types of cells. When the user finishes counting, the plug-in will display a total for each cell type plus a grand total of all clicks. The results log can be copied and pasted and saved as an Excel spreadsheet.

In some cases, manual cell counting is almost impossible, so we need an automated counting algorithm. Fortunately, ImageJ comes with an automatic cell-counting

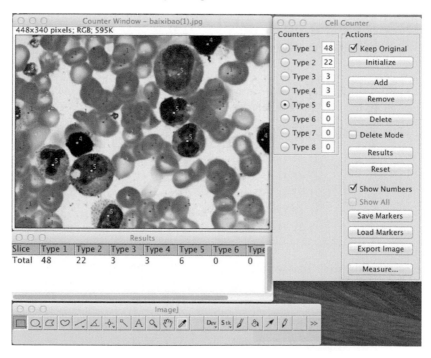

FIGURE 11.26   The ImageJ plug-in for manual cell counting and marking.

237 http://www.imageJ.org
238 http://www.unige.ch/medecine/bioimaging/tricks/imagejtutorials/CellCounting.pdf

function with a plug-in (Figure 11.27). The algorithm includes image segmentation, filtering, blob generation, labeling, and counting. ImageJ provides a window to list the intermediate results during the automated cell counting, enabling users to adjust thresholds and other parameters that are sensitive to the segmentation.

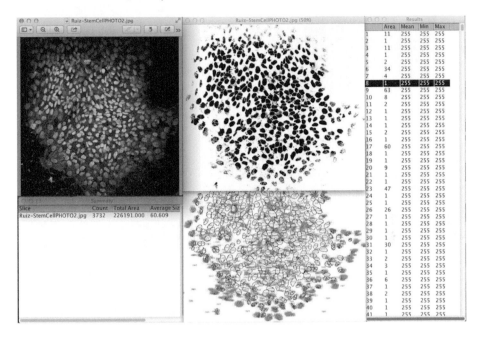

FIGURE 11.27 Cell counting with ImageJ enables automatic or manual processes; the original image is on the top left, blobs detected and filtered are in the top middle window, the mean pixel intensities are listed in the right window, and the numerically labeled and counted cells are outlined in the bottom windows.

CellC

CellC is the software for quantification of labeled bacteria by automated image analysis (Figure 11.28).[239,240] Many research groups around the world have used this tool for cell counting.[241]

11.13 USABILITY STUDY

The ability to build a microscope on one's own does not make anyone Antoni van Leeuwenhoek. It is worth noting that he was a specialist in lens making and devoted his entire life to observing microorganisms. Most DIY equipment introduced in this chapter is still in the early prototyping stage. Its usability is yet to be tested in the field in terms of sensitivity and specificity.

[239] https://sites.google.com/site/cellcsoftware/Home
[240] Selinummi et al., Software for quantification
[241] https://sites.google.com/site/cellcsoftware/articles-using-cellc

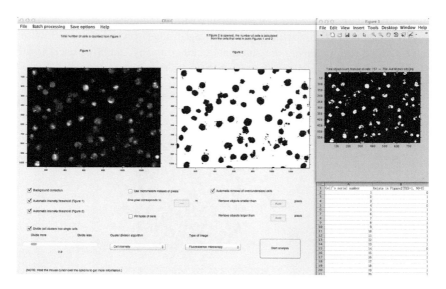

FIGURE 11.28 A screenshot of the CellC package for automated cell counting; the left windows are input and processed images, and the right shows the counting results.

There are many human factors involved in the development. For example, hand shaking is not ignorable in high-power lens microscopic imaging. A stationary slide holder or a snap-on accessory is necessary. The more human factors are removed from the process, the more consistent performance is. On the other hand, although automated cell counting is productive, it still has errors. Sometimes, manual inspection or adjustment is necessary. Semi-automated counting or manual counting with a computer's assistance can be more reliable than fully manual or totally automatic counting.

Economy also plays a critical role here. Many technologies use smartphones for prototyping DIY microscopes. An improvised lens from a used CD drive could save some money, but the smartphone itself and the time spent building it is rather expensive. We need to establish a utility function and quantitative measurement to evaluate multiattribute alternatives.

11.14   SUMMARY

This chapter explored how to acquire, analyze, and interact with microscopic images or videos. Microscopes are valuable in ambient diagnostics because of their ability to magnify objects that cannot be seen by the naked human eye. The cell phone-based microscopes not only enable ambient diagnoses in remote places but also provide computational power for image analysis, visualization, and pattern recognition.

The power of a light microscope is limited by the wavelength of visible light, which is about 500 nm. The most powerful light microscopes can resolve bacteria but not viruses. To see anything smaller than 500 nm, we will need an electron microscope.

Mobile phone microscopes can be made with snap-on lenses and glass ball lenses. The snap-on phone case can be standardized as an interface for many add-on optical sensors. 3D printing technologies make sense here for specific uses.

Digital microscopes provide more magnification power, better lighting, and stationary slide holders. The dual-use digital microscopes can be both portable and used in a lab.

Spectrum lighting can assist in seeing biomedical surfaces. Special lights can be generated from a phone application or add-on sources such as UV lights.

Time-lapse videos are a powerful tool in tracking cell movements, such as evaluating the vitality of sperm and the growth rate of bacteria.

Laser holography can be implemented with a simple green laser pointer, and it can be geared toward 3D holographic reconstruction of an object.

Virtual microscopes enable users to zoom and explore an entire sample slide or more with an interface much like that of Google Earth. This requires image stitching based on features. The process can be implemented using open sources such as SIFT or SURF.

Finally, labeling and counting objects in an image can be done manually or automatically, such as with ImageJ and CellC. A blob-labeling algorithm was introduced with a simple code in MATLAB.

PROBLEMS

1. Using microscopes that he made himself in the 1700s, Antoni van Leeuwenhoek was able to observe and hire an artist to draw the microorganisms he saw. How many microorganisms in Figure 11.2 can you recognize? Search for citations to support your answers.
2. Build your own microscope for your phone with the glass ball from a CD drive or online shop for snap-on products from Amazon. Estimate the magnification scale.
3. Prototype a laser holographic microscope with a green laser pointer, paper clip, and a binder clipper. Test it with the water sample from a fish tank. Record a video and summarize your findings in a report.
4. Following the instructions in the section, "Observing Yeast Cells," test your microscope with diluted yeast cells.
   a. Examine the cells under each power and record images about what you see.
   b. How much size variation can you see?
   c. Do you see any cells with reproductive buds attached?
   d. Were you surprised to see what the yeast looked like?
5. Take a video of what you see in your microscope while moving the sample slowly. Extract frames from the video. Use SIFT algorithms to stitch the images together.
6. For some microscopic images, SIFT performs poorly. What other features can be used for stitching? Demonstrate the results.
7. Given a stitched image larger than a screen size, design a virtual microscope interface so that you can zoom, pan, and rotate the image.
8. In the example in the section "Labeling and Counting," we generated edges and then dilated and filled holes. Discuss possible errors in this process.

9. Improve the labeling accuracy of the sample MATLAB code in Section 11.12. For example, you could include the budding cell and remove the noncell artifacts.
10. Given a 3D printer, make a ball lens holder for your phone. Use 3D modeling software such as SketchUp or AutoCAD to design the object and save as STL data format.

12 Personal Spectrometers

> This prism could be the spirit of the listener.
>
> —Arvo Part

12.1 INTRODUCTION

In 1666, Sir Isaac Newton experimented with a beam of sunlight passed through a glass prism (Figure 12.1). He discovered that the beam of light could be split into a continuous spectrum of colors. A spectrometer is an instrument used to quantify light energies generated by a light source, passed through a material, or reflected off a surface. It is a powerful tool for diagnostics. The ability to cheaply and rapidly record diffuse reflectance spectra or fluorescence spectra also has the possibility of helping with medical diagnosis. For example, the pulse oximeter, the needleless glucose meter, and noninvasive detection of tumors are all ways of improving medical diagnosis.[242,243] This chapter discusses the basic principles of spectrometers and explores medical applications. Topics include

- Beer's law
- Diffraction grating
- Do-it-yourself (DIY) spectrometers
- Spectrometer algorithm

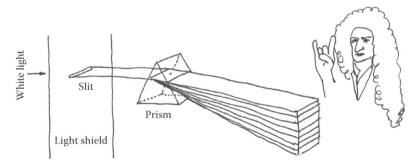

FIGURE 12.1 Isaac Newton discovered the beam of light could be split into a continuous spectrum of colors.

---

[242] L. Brancaleon, A. J. Durkin, J. H. Tu, G. Menaker, J. D. Fallon, et al. In vivo fluorescence spectroscopy of nonmelanoma skin cancer. *Photochemistry and Photobiology* 73:178–183, 2001.

[243] P. R. Bargo, S. A. Prahl, T. T. Goodell, R. A. Sleven, G. Koval, et al. In vivo determination of optical properties of normal and tumor tissue with white light reflectance and an empirical light transport model during endoscopy. *Journal of Biomedical Optics* 10:034018, 2005.

In addition, we study urine test and drink inspection cases and explore the potential applications in backlighting through tissues.

12.2   BEER'S LAW

In 1852, August Beer discovered that the concentration of a solution affects how much light the solution absorbs (Figure 12.2). For example, whole milk will absorb more light than skim milk with the same chemical content.[244] This can be expressed mathematically.

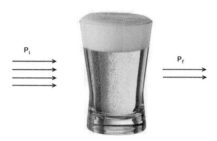

FIGURE 12.2   Light absorption.

If we let P_i stand for the initial amount or power of the light that is shining on a sample and P_f stand for the final amount of light left after it goes through the sample, then as the sample absorbs some of the light, P_f will be less than P_i. We can, then, talk about the amount of light that is transmitted (the amount that does get through). This is called the transmittance T, and these three numbers are related by the equation

$$T = \frac{P_f}{P_i} \tag{12.1}$$

The term *absorbance*, symbolized by A, which is equal to the logarithm of $1/T$, or

$$A = \log \frac{1}{T} \tag{12.2}$$

Absorbance is proportional to the length b, the concentration C, and the constant value for each kind of chemical K. This is called Beer's law.

$$A = b \cdot C \cdot K \tag{12.3}$$

Thus, if we keep b and C the same, then absorbance would be proportional to the constant value for the chemical. If we study various concentrations of solutions, then

---

[244] http://biology.clc.uc.edu/courses/biol111/Beerslaw%20Intro.htm

we might be able to predict the concentration of an "unknown" solution using the light absorbance values.

12.3   DIFFRACTION GRATING

A prism can diffract light to a spectrum, but prisms are too bulky and heavy to be built into a portable spectrometer. Alternatively, diffraction gratings can be used. A diffraction grating is a thin film of clear glass or plastic that has a large number of slits (lines) per millimeter drawn on it (Figure 12.3).

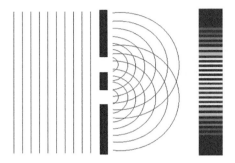

FIGURE 12.3   Diffraction grating.

When we shine a light through a diffraction grating, we can see bright and dark fringes appear on the screen. It is the constructive and destructive interference of light waves that causes such fringes. This simply verifies that light is a wave.

Constructive and Destructive Interference of Waves

When two waves have the same wavelength and are in sync with one another so that their highest and lowest peaks occur at the same time, they are called *coherent waves*. Coherent waves enhance each other's effect constructively and cause constructive interference, forming a bright fringe (Figure 12.4).

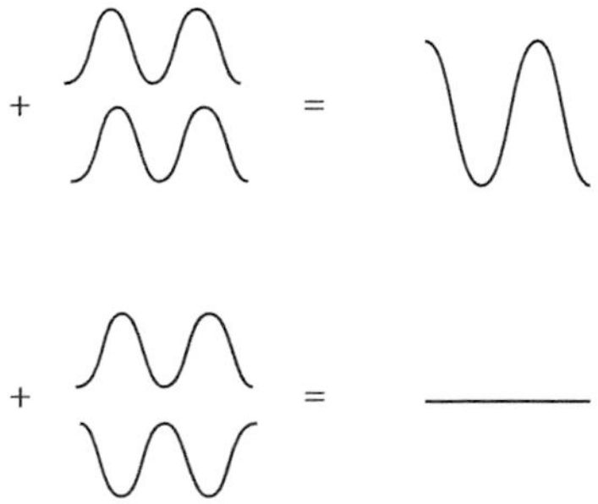

FIGURE 12.4   Constructive interference versus destructive interference.

On the other hand, when two waves are totally out of phase, they interfere destructively. For example, when one wave is at its maximum peak and another wave is simultaneously at its minimum peak, the waves work against each other, resulting in waves with the amplitude subtracted from one another, forming a dark fringe.

The bright and dark fringes follow the formulas here:

$$\textit{Bright Fringes:} \quad d\sin(\theta) = k\lambda \tag{12.4}$$

$$\textit{Dark Fringes:} \quad d\sin(\theta) = \left(k + 1/2\right)\lambda \tag{12.5}$$

where d is the distance between slits, θ is the angle of diffraction, λ is the wavelength of the light source, and k is the order number for the fringes. $k = 0, 1, 2, 3, \dots$.

Going from a dark or bright fringe to its next fringe changes the distance by ½ λ. If there are N lines per millimeter of the grating, then d, the space between every two adjacent lines, is

$$d = \frac{1}{N} \tag{12.6}$$

The diffraction grating formula for the principal maxima is

$$d\sin(\theta_k) = k\lambda \qquad k = 1, 2, 3, \dots \tag{12.7}$$

To find θ, measure the distance from the grating to the screen and the first-order distance and then, using trigonometry, calculate the angle (Figure 12.5).

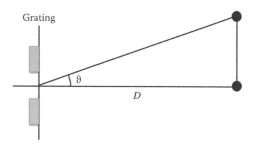

FIGURE 12.5 Diffraction grating calculations.

Holographic Diffraction Grating Film

Holographic diffraction grating film is used to break up white light into all the colors of the spectrum. It is an ideal choice for spectroscopy experiments since holographic gratings exhibit significantly sharper diffraction orders. This results in an increased ability to view absorption and emission lines, with higher spatial frequency gratings, for example, N = 1,000 lines/mm, or d = 1 μm.

By increasing the number of grooves per unit area, the angular dispersion of diffraction orders will be increased. Each variety of holographic gratings is normally available in sheets, rolls, or square cards. For example, the 1,000 lines/mm holographic diffraction grating film made by Edmund Optics[245] is a 6 × 12 × 0.003 inch clear polyester sheet with a 36° dispersion angle. The cost is US$10 per sheet. If we cut them into 72 pieces, the unit cost is US$0.14 each.

Creating Gratings from CDs and DVDs

We can make diffraction gratings from CDs.[246] Blank CDs work best. First, scratch the label from the surface of a CD, especially if the labels are painted. Then, use any sticky tape to peel off the label and reflective layers. Now, the CD is ready to use as a diffraction grating. Figure 12.6 illustrates the process.

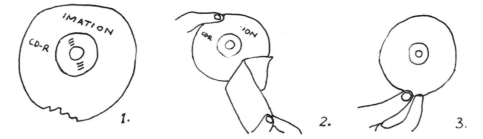

FIGURE 12.6   Making a diffraction grating from a CD.

We can also make diffraction gratings from DVDs. First, use a razor blade to split the two layers of a DVD along the outside edge. Next, use any sticky tape to peel off the reflecting layer. Third, separate the two polycarbonate layers. Finally, the transparent piece will act as grating. Figure 12.7 illustrates the process.

Now, let us do a simple experiment to estimate the distance between the track pitches on CD and DVD gratings (Figure 12.8). Assume we use a red laser pointer with λ = 650 nm and k = 1.

For the CD, we calculated the following:

$$x = 13.95 \text{ cm and } D = 29.5 \text{ cm}$$

$$\theta = \tan^{-1}(x/D) = \tan^{-1}(13.95/29.5) = 25.3°$$

$$d = (1)(650 \text{ nm})/\sin 25.3° = 1.52 \text{ μm}$$

---

[245] http://www.edmundoptics.com
[246] http://www.nnin.org/sites/default/files/files/Karen_Rama_USING_CDs_AND_DVDs_AS_DIFFRACTION_GRATINGS_0.pdf

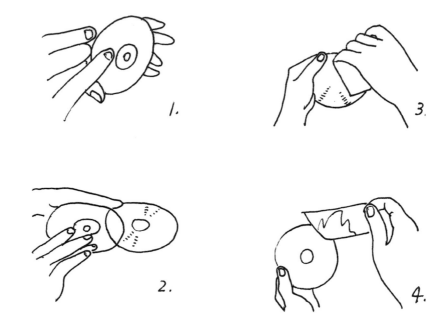

FIGURE 12.7   Making a diffraction grating from a DVD.

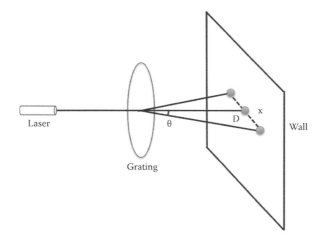

FIGURE 12.8   Test diffraction pattern with a laser and a grating disk.

For the DVD, we calculated

$$x = 42.5 \text{ cm and } D = 20 \text{ cm}$$

$$\theta = \tan^{-1}(x/D) = \tan^{-1}(42.5/20) = 64.8°$$

$$d = (1)(650 \text{ nm})/\sin 64.8° = 0.72 \text{ μm}$$

The actual track pitch of a CD is 1.6 μm (vs. the calculated value of 1.52 μm), and the actual track pitch of a DVD with 4.7 GB is 0.74 μm (vs. the calculated value of 0.72 μm). Therefore, our estimations are fairly close to the real values. The spacing of tracks in a DVD is about half of that in a CD, giving the DVD twice as many tracks per millimeter. This accounts for about a twofold gain in the capacity of a DVD relative to a CD.

As discussed, the grating spacing distance of the 1,000 lines/mm holographic grating film is 1 μm. The gap is smaller than on a CD but bigger than on a DVD.

12.4   DIY SPECTROMETER

There are several ways to build a DIY spectrometer.[247] Public Lab, a nonprofit organization, published step-by-step instructions about how to build DIY scopes from a webcam or a mobile phone. Other methods can be found on YouTube or other online sites.

Webcam-Based Spectrometer

Using a webcam and an old black VHS cassette box or black cardboard, we can easily construct a spectrometer. Detailed instructions about how to build it are available online.[248] Figure 12.9 shows a diagram of the webcam-based architecture.

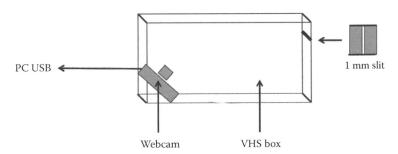

PC USB

1 mm slit

Webcam   VHS box

FIGURE 12.9   Webcam-based spectrometer.

To create a spectrometer from a mobile phone camera, we can use an old black VHS cassette box and a transmission grating between the slit and the camera lens. The grating splits the light into separate colors, much like a prism, while the original camera lens does all the focusing. This results in the spectrometer being able to detect colors in a range of 300 nm. For reference, human vision is defined as between 400 and 700 nm, so our eyes have about the same optical range as this camera spectrometer.

[247] Z. J. Smith, K. Chu, A. R. Espenson, M. Rahimzadeh, A. Gryshuk, M. Molinaro, D. M. Dwyre, S. Lane, D. Matthews, and S, Wachsmann-Hogiu. Cell-phone-based platform for biomedical device development and education applications. *PLoS ONE*, 6(3), 2011. PMID: 21399693.
[248] http://publiclaboratory.org/tool/spectrometer

The quality of resolution and light collection can be adjusted, with an increase in the quality of one negatively affecting the quality of the other. For example, widening the light aperture causes the overall light entering the system to increase at the expense of spectral resolution. On the other hand, reducing the aperture size increases the resolution. In addition, the system could be further improved by adding a lens. This is done at the expense of the depth of field, which is essentially infinite in the current system. The infinite depth of field arises by comparable means, as in the conceptually similar pinhole camera. In other words, one may think of the spectrometer described here as a pinhole camera's spectral analog.

Mobile Phone-Based Spectrometer

A mobile phone spectrometer provides a simple and inexpensive way to take a qualitative measurement of the energies of light in a given light "sample" that in current labs is done with equipment that costs thousands of dollars. Here, we can use a modified mobile phone to enable individuals to perform in situ analysis by turning the phone into a spectrometer. They can look at cells after injecting a dye in a sample. The setup is rather simple but yields excellent results. The phone used here can be just a phone with a good camera.

The schematic diagram of the system is shown in Figure 12.10. To characterize the performance of the mobile phone spectrometer, we can point the mobile phone at a fluorescent bulb featuring several narrow and intense peaks.

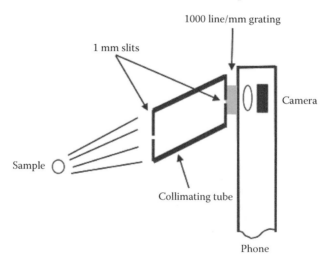

FIGURE 12.10 Mobile phone-based spectrometer. (Adapted from Z. J. Smith, K. Chu, A. R. Espenson, M. Rahimzadeh, A. Gryshuk, M. Molinaro, D. M. Dwyre, S. Lane, D. Matthews, and S. Wachsmann-Hogiu. *PLoS ONE*, 6(3), 2011. PMID: 21399693. With permission.)

The 1-mm slit (a narrow gap) size gives approximately 10-nm spectral resolution and allows enough light throughout to easily record a spectrum. Figure 12.11 shows the result from the work of Smith et al. compared to the commercial Ocean Optics spectrometer in terms of spectral accuracy, with peaks overlapping as expected after calibration.[249]

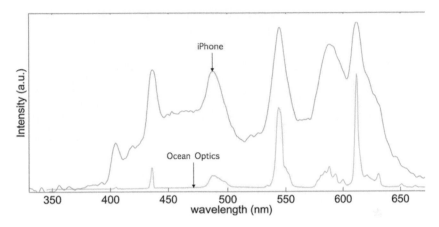

FIGURE 12.11   Image and spectrum of a fluorescent bulb. The cropped image of the spectrum and a comparison of the spectra of the same fluorescent light fixture taken with both the mobile phone spectrometer (top) and Ocean Optics spectrometer (bottom). (From Smith et al., *PLoS ONE*, 6(3), 2011, with permission.)

12.5   ANALYTICAL ALGORITHM

To analyze the spectrum image with an algorithm, we first read the image from the imaging camera and crop it to obtain the spectrum strips (Figure 12.12). Then we separate the color image into red, blue, and green channels. Each channel is in a grayscale image where the intensity of the pixel is between 0 and 255. The value 0 means the lowest level, and 255 means the highest level. Figures 12.13 through 12.15 show the red, green, and blue (R, G, B, respectively) channel images.

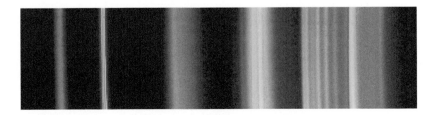

FIGURE 12.12   Sample of the captured color image from the camera.

[249] Smith et al., Cell-phone-based platform. PLoS ONE, 6(3), 2011

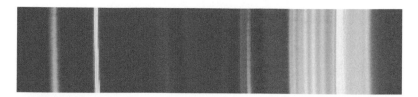

FIGURE 12.13   Red intensity channel.

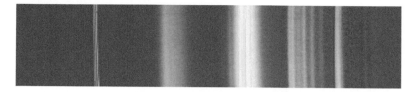

FIGURE 12.14   Green intensity channel.

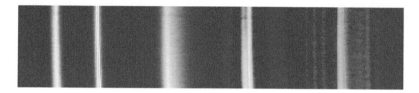

FIGURE 12.15   Blue intensity channel.

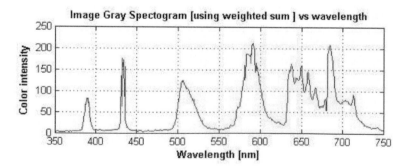

FIGURE 12.16   The DIY spectrometer output with the halogen light source.

To plot a spectrum response curve, we can combine the three primary color channels red, green, and blue into one gray-scale image. The easiest way to do this is to use the average of the three values, that is, (R + G + B)/3. However, this is not a good representation of the way humans respond to the color; for example, we respond to green or red more than blue. Therefore, here we use a weighted version of the equation (5.3) that produces a result more similar to true human color perception.

$$Y = 0.299 \cdot R + 0.587 \cdot G + 0.114 \cdot B \qquad\qquad 12.8$$

The visible color spectrum ranges roughly from 300 to 700 nm. After we mix the color sensors, we can plot a continuous curve across the spectrum in the wavelength from 350 to 700 nm, the visible color spectrum range. Figure 12.16 shows an example of the spectrometer output with the halogen light source.

The MATLAB code for the spectrum from RGB images can be found from Appendix A.

12.6   URINE SAMPLE TEST

Personal spectrometers enable people to monitor their bodies continuously. One possible way to do this is to analyze a urine sample (which can be easily collected in a bottle or Petri dish) with a personal spectrometer. That's why we call it "personal spectrometer." Here, we look at a simple experiment with a DIY spectrometer. The purpose of the experiment is to observe the color spectrum changes in urine in various conditions and at various times of day. The assumption is that the color of urine would change according to variations in activities and food, drink, and medicine intake. The eight sets of samples include:

- A1. Day 1, morning without food
- A2. Day 1, evening without food
- A3. Day 1, night, after dinner
- A4. Day 2, morning without food
- A5. Day 3, evening, after dinner
- A6. Day 4, evening, after dinner
- A7. Day 5, after dinner and a multivitamin pill
- A8. Day 6, after lunch and biking

The urine samples were held in Petri dishes above a webcam spectrometer. The laptop took the image from the webcam, which was analyzed by the previous algorithm. Here, we use A1, the sample data in the morning of day 1 without food as a baseline. All other data were compared to A1.

We found that the urine sample taken in the evening before dinner had more transparency than the sample in the morning. Both evening and morning samples had wavelengths between 610 and 700 nm (see Figure 12.17).

After dinner, the urine sample became less transparent, reaching down to the morning's level (see Figure 12.18).

At one evening, after having dinner and a multivitamin pill, the spectrometer output of the urine sample shifted toward the left, with more yellow color showing up in the sample (Figure 12.19).

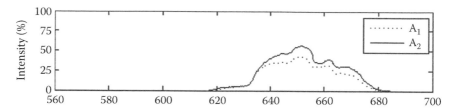

FIGURE 12.17 Evening spectrum without food (A2, solid line on top) versus morning without food spectrum (A1, dashed line at the bottom).

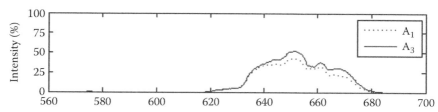

FIGURE 12.18 Night after-dinner spectrum (A3, solid line on top) versus morning without food spectrum (A1, dashed line at the bottom).

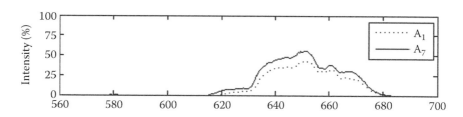

FIGURE 12.19 Evening after dinner and the multivitamin pill (A7, solid line on top) versus morning without food spectrum (A1, dashed line at the bottom).

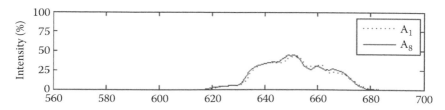

FIGURE 12.20 After lunch and biking (A8, solid line on top) versus morning without food spectrum (A1, dashed line at the bottom).

Finally, after having lunch and biking, the urine sample did not show a significant color change compared to the sample from the morning without food (Figure 12.20).

This analysis is just a simple example based on a rudimentary experiment and calculation. The purpose is to empirically prove the feasibility of a personal spectrometer at home, where we can measure samples more frequently and more privately.

12.7 CROWDSOURCING SPECTROMETER

The Internet enables DIY spectrometer users to share knowledge, algorithms, and most important, data. The nonprofit organization Public Lab was launched via Kickstarter, a crowd funding website, for the broader personal spectrometer community. The Public Lab website[250] provides instructions about how to build a personal spectrometer from a CD, webcam, or mobile phone. The site also hosts an online service for spectra analysis, called Workbench, where registered users can upload their spectra images and obtain analytical results, including plots of the spectrometer output, comparisons with known samples, and calibrations.

Public Lab is a perfect example of crowdsourcing for the personal spectrometer community. It has multiple benefits. First, it helps to standardize personal spectrometers. The Workbench provides utilities for users to upload calibration images and automatically calibrate their devices. The graphical user interface (GUI) also enables users to adjust the wavelength range and intensity level.

The shared spectra samples help online users acquire known sample properties, which help identify many unknown samples. Although the original purpose of the DIY spectrometer was for environmental monitoring, the same device can be used for public health monitoring as well (drink analysis, for example). As the publicly shared samples increase, the analytical method is expected to evolve rapidly.

Personal spectrometers create the potential for innovative diagnoses, such as for protein contents. As a rule of thumb, urine with lots of bubbles may have excessive protein in it. We expect new devices might be able to turn those health tips or heuristics into measurable indicators.

Let's look at how to use the Public Lab Workbench to analyze drinks, including milk (Figure 12.21) soda drinks and juices (Figure 12.22 - 12.24). Spectrometers can be used for drink inspection, e.g., the spectrometer distinguishes 1% milk, 2% milk, skim milk and whole milk, even though they appear the same to human eyes.

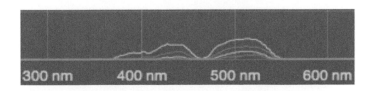

FIGURE 12.21 Spectrometer output of skim milk (top); 1% milk (second from top); 2% milk (third from top); and whole milk (bottom).

[250] http://www.publiclab.org

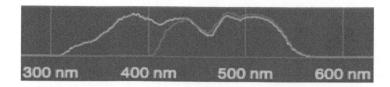

FIGURE 12.22 Spectrometer output of sparkling orange drink (left, thick line) and Fanta (right, thin line).

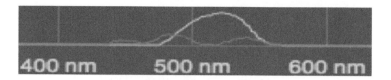

FIGURE 12.23 Spectrometer output of grape juice (top, thick line) and Crush Grape (bottom, thin line).

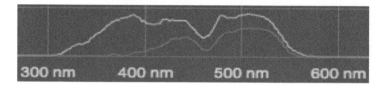

FIGURE 12.24 Spectrometer output of sweetened tea (top, thick line) and Coca-Cola (bottom, thin line).

12.8   DIAGNOSTIC APPLICATIONS

Pulse Oximeter

Our tissues are actually semitransparent to certain light wavelengths. If we put a finger in front of a tungsten bulb, we can see the transmission spectrum of approximately 1 cm of tissue. The spectrometer can be used to make blood oxygenation measurements by recording differences in absorption in the finger in two wavelengths: red and infrared (Figure 12.25).

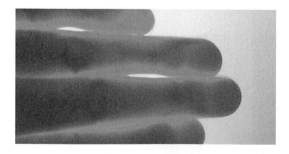

FIGURE 12.25 Determination of the blood compound by a transmission measurement at the fingertip.

There are two challenges for making a pulse oximetry: First, the thickness of fingers can vary considerably. Second, a fingertip is not homogenous. There are unknown quantities of skin, bone, muscle, various blood types, and so on in the light path between the light and the camera. Pulse oximetry overcomes these obstacles by using the technique where the relative sizes of the pulsatile signals generated by the red and infrared sources are differentiated, allowing specific analysis of arterial blood (Figure 12.26).

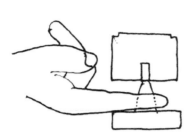 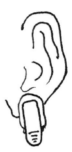

FIGURE 12.26   Determination of the blood compound by a transmission measurement at the fingertip (left) and eardrum (right). (From K. Sugiura. Pulse oximeter probe. U.S. Patent 5551423, 1996, http://www.google.com/patents/US5551423; and L. R. Hill and S. E. Titcomb. Ear lope clip with heart beat sensor. U.S. Patent 4334544, 1982, http://www.google.com/patents/US4334544.)

Blood Glucose Monitoring

For many years, glucose monitoring has been an invasive process. Can we take a needleless measurement of blood glucose? Optical spectral analysis provides alternatives for this. There are several light sources to be considered: visible, infrared, and ultraviolet (UV) wavelengths.

A spectrometer can be potentially used as a noninvasive alternative, using a halogen lamp as a light source. For example, by analyzing the transmitted (wavelengths in the range 600 to 1,700 nm) and reflected light from the skin surface (spectral region 400 to 1,000 nm), the concentration of hemoglobin and the water content can be calculated.

Sustained high levels of sugars in the blood ultimately cause proteins to stick together, thereby damaging the function of the proteins. These damaged proteins are called advanced glycation end products (AGEs).[251] AGEs show fluorescence with an excitation wavelength of 360 nm (in the UV wavelength) and an emission wavelength of 430 nm (in visible wavelength). Using the light sources of a high-power UV-LED (light-emitting diode) (wavelength 365 nm) and a high-power neutrally white LED, the fluorescence and reflecting qualities of the skin surface can be measured with an optical reflection sensor. The approximate concentration of AGEs can be estimated from the skin fluorescence spectra.

---

[251] http://www.diabetesincontrol.com/articles/64-feature-writer-article/632

Although both methods discussed can be used for the development of a quick and affordable diagnostic screening system, the LED light is more practical because it is much smaller than a halogen lamp, enabling a more compact, energy-saving solution.

Optical Therapy

Optical therapy systems contain a combination of the photosensitizer and the light system. Normally, the photosensitizers from different manufacturers have different absorption characteristics and different therapeutic agents also have different emission qualities. To optimize the biological efficiency of the optical therapy procedure, we can use spectrometry to measure the optical properties of the light sources that are well adapted to the optical absorption qualities of the photosensitizer.

Cancer Detection

Studies have shown that cancerous tumors can be distinguished from surrounding healthy tissue by their increased autofluorescence and different diffuse properties.[252,253,254,255] Currently, most endoscopes use white light or narrow-bandwidth light such as blue and green to differentiate normal and tumor tissues. If we can miniaturize the spectrometer so that it can be mounted on the tip of the endoscope, then it is possible to transmit light of a specific spectra through the fiber-optical waveguide in the scope.[256,257,258,259]

12.9   SUMMARY

A spectrometer provides an analytical method to measure the absorbance of a material under a light source. It is a powerful tool for ambient diagnosis. Beer's law teaches us that absorbance is proportional to the length, the concentration, and the constant value for each kind of chemical. Diffusion grating creates constructive and destructive interference waves and can be used as a prism. CDs, DVDs, and the grating film are affordable materials for building personal spectrometers. An improvised spectrometer can be made by adding simple and inexpensive attachments to a standard mobile phone or a webcam. We covered a simple algorithm for calculating the spectrum curve for RGB images. Through some initial experiments, we found potential applications in ambient diagnoses, for example:

---

[252] N. Thekkek and R. Richards-Kortum. Optical imaging for cervical cancer detection: solutions for a continuing global problem. *Nature Reviews Cancer* 8:725–731, 2008.

[253] Brancaleon et al., In vivo fluorescence spectroscopy

[254] Bargo et al. In vivo determination of optical properties

[255] B. Lin, S. Urayama, R. M. G. Saroufeem, D. L. Matthews, and S. G. Demos. Characterizing the origin of autofluorescence in human esophageal epithelium under ultraviolet excitation. *Optics Express* 18:21074–21082, 2010.

[256] Thekkek and Richards-Kortum, Optical imaging for cervical cancer detection

[257] Brancaleon et al., In vivo fluorescence spectroscopy.

[258] Bargo et al., In vivo determination of optical properties

[259] Lin et al., Characterizing the origin of autofluorescence

- Pulse oximeters
- Glucose meters
- Optical therapy
- Tumor detection

PROBLEMS

1. Use your cell phone to improvise a light sensor. Design an experiment to investigate Beer's law. Note that you do not have to use beer to do the experiment.
2. Test a diffraction pattern with a laser and a CD disk, shown in Figure 12.8. Calculate the diffraction distance from the center.
3. Test a diffraction pattern with a laser and a DVD disk, shown in Figure 12.8. Calculate the diffraction distance from the center. Compare with the CD results.
4. Equation 12.8 is used to mix RGB channels in the way of human perception. Find reasons behind the three weights or define your own with citations. Compare your results with regular RGB to grayscale conversion results.
5. Follow the instructions on Public Lab (http://www.publiclab.org) to build a mobile phone-based spectrometer with a CD or DVD disk and cardboard. Calibrate your spectrometer with the app from Public Lab and upload your calibrated images to the Public Lab website.
6. Follow the instructions on Public Lab (http://www.publiclab.org) to build a webcam-based spectrometer with a CD or DVD disk and cardboard. Calibrate your spectrometer with the app from Public Lab and upload your calibrated images to the Public Lab website.
7. Use your DIY spectrometer to test the samples of skim milk, 2% milk, and whole milk. Discuss the results with a graph.
8. Use your DIY spectrometer to analyze the contents in your detergent. Compare your results with the database on Public Lab and discuss with other users online. Summarize your findings in the report.
9. Study the spectrometer sample database on Public Lab and analyze the usability of the crowdsourcing data. Write suggestions for improvements.
10. Compare the functions and usability of the pulse oximeter in this chapter with the heart sound-based pulse meter in Chapter 4 and the webcam-based pulse meter in Chapter 7. Summarize your findings in a report.

Section 4

Crowdsourcing

13 Remote Sensing

> The whole point of seeing through something is to see something through it.
>
> —C. S. Lewis

13.1 INTRODUCTION

In the last four chapters, we studied personalized ambient diagnostic systems. Starting this chapter, we explore how to obtain health information from public spaces, including surveillance cameras, thermal imaging systems, and even the microwave-based full-body scanner systems at airports. We use digital human models and high-frequency electrical magnetic field simulators to study the human-machine system so that we can optimize sensitivity and specificity of the system before it is ever built. In particular, we explore

- Remote sensing in public spaces
- Digital human models
- Proportional models
- Microwave imaging and simulation
- Extracting the biometric data from three-dimensional (3D) point clouds

13.2 REMOTE SENSING IN PUBLIC SPACE

Remote sensing devices such as surveillance cameras, thermal imaging, and microwave imaging systems in public places can capture a pedestrian's physiological data, such as body temperature, body mass index (BMI), and other health indices, from a distance without interrupting the pedestrian. This enables public health entities to survey health measurements, such as obesity, in an open space or identify individual people who have epidemic symptoms. For example, thermal imaging equipment was used to scan passengers at the airport terminals in Australia and China for the influenza A (H1N1) virus, commonly referred to as swine flu. In 2009, the Australian government ordered mandatory thermal scans of all incoming international passengers as a measure against the influenza A virus. Figure 13.1 shows a thermal imaging system of passengers' temperatures on their heads.

The rapidly growing 3D holographic imaging systems in airports have created significant potential in ambient diagnostics. Current devices operate using a millimeter wave transceiver to reflect the signal of the human body.[260] The scanner creates a 3D point cloud around the body. As the millimeter wave signal cannot penetrate the skin,

---

[260] Joseph Laws, Nathaniel Bauernfeind, and Yang Cai. Feature hiding in 3D human body scans. *Information Visualization* 5(4): 271–278(8), 2006.

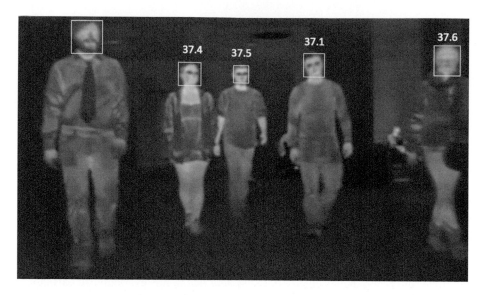

FIGURE 13.1 Thermal imaging systems can sense body temperature remotely, which enables screening a flow of pedestrians without a traffic jam.

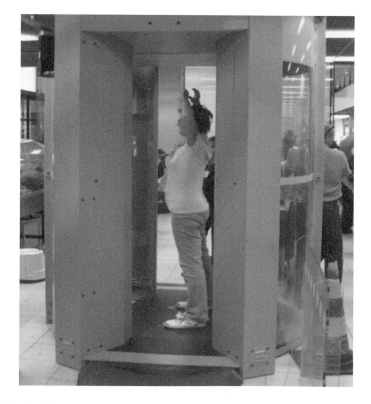

FIGURE 13.2 Microwave imaging system in Amsterdam airport.

a 3D human surface can be generated. Figure 13.2 shows the scanner in operation at the Amsterdam Airport.

How can we automatically analyze the scanned images? Can we develop dual-use technologies for health diagnoses? For example, as an option, the microwave imaging system at the airport can print out a passenger's BMI on his or her travel ticket without additional cost. In this chapter, we discuss how to extract soft biometric data, such as BMI and waist measurements, from the 3D human scan data and how to model the medical diagnosis based on the soft biometrics. In addition, the digital human modeling technique for soft biometrics studies is introduced.

13.3   HUMAN BODY SEGMENTATION

To reduce the feature search space, we need to segment the 3D scan data into certain body areas that contain possible targets. Since the human subjects are assumed to be in a standing pose, the 3D point cloud can be segmented into to two-dimensional (2D) slices horizontally. Then, we search for the region of target slices. Examining each slice from top to bottom is a rather computationally expensive process. Here, we present a novel approach to reduce the search space by making use of intrinsic proportions.

Automatic segmentation of the human body has been studied before extensively.[261,262,263,264,265,266] Unfortunately, there are limitations in the existing algorithms, such as coordinate dependency, robustness, and speed. Some algorithms only work within small bounding boxes that do not result in an acceptable performance since the boxes need to be detected prior to the execution of the algorithm, and they are not noise resistant.[267] In this Chapter, we explore a new approach based on our knowledge of human anatomic proportion, which is a relative measurement that uses an object in the scene to measure other objects.

Proportions of Human Bodies

Intrinsic proportion measurements have been used in architecture and art for thousands of years. Artists use analogous measurements that are invariant to coordinate

[261] Naoufel Werghi. Segmentation and modeling of full human body shape from 3-D scan data: a survey. *IEEE Transactions on Systems* 37(6):1122–1136, 2007.

[262] J. H. Nurre, Locating landmarks on human body scan data. In *Proceedings of the International Conference Recent Advances in 3-D Digital Imaging Model*, Ottawa, ON, Canada, 1997, pp. 289–295.

[263] J. H. Nurre, J. Connor, E. Lewark, and J. Collier. On segmenting the three-dimensional scan data of human body. *IEEE Transactions on Medical Imaging* 18(8):787–797, 2000.

[264] L. Dekker, I. Douros, B. F. Buxton, and P. C. Treleaven. Building symbolic information for 3-D human body modeling from range data. In *Proceedings of the International Conference on Recent Advances in 3-D Digital Imaging Model*, Ottawa, ON, Canada, 1999, pp. 388–389.

[265] L. Dekker, S. Khan, E. West, B. Buxton, and P. Treleaven. Models for understanding the 3-D human body form. In *Proceedings of the IEEE Workshop on Model-Based 3-D Image Analysis*, Mumbai, India, 1998, pp. 65–74.

[266] C. L. Wang, T. K. Chang, and M. Yuen. From laser-scanned to feature human model: a system based on fuzzy logic concept. *CAD* 35:241–253, 2003.

[267] C. A. M. Suikerbuik, J. W. H. Tangelder, H. A. M. Daanen, and A. J. K. Oudenhuijzen. Automatic feature detection in 3D human body scans. In *Proceedings of the Conference: SAE Digital Human Modelling for Design and Engineering*, 2004.

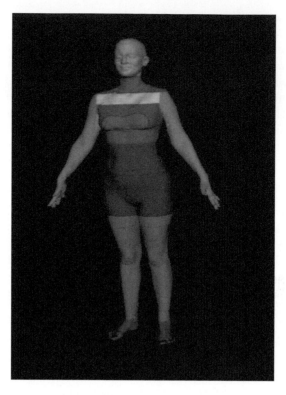

FIGURE 13.3   Segment body parts with proportions and locations (in different shades).

systems. For example, artists often use the head to measure the height and width of
a human body and use an eye to measure the height and width of a face. Figure 13.3
shows a sample of the vertical proportion in a typical art book and the actual distribution of head-to-body proportions calculated from the CAESAR (Civilian American
and European Anthropometry Resource) project dataset. The results show that, on
average, a human is between six and eight heads tall. Based on our observations
from 100 3D scan datasets of adults from sixteen to sixty-five years old, including
subjects from North America, Europe, and Asia, we found that the length of one
and a half head units from the bottom of the head is enough to cover the chest area.
In addition, the chest width is about three heads wide. Figure 13.3 shows an output
of the feature segmentation based on the intrinsic proportion from a sample in the
CAESAR database.

Using the proportion-based approach, we can use the object inside an image as a
reference to measure the rest of the objects within the same image. Instead of measuring absolute values, we can measure the relative proportions between objects,
increasing robustness of the measurement without intensive calibrations.

We can also develop a formal representation of the proportions by creating a
graph in which nodes represent regions and are connected to each other by edges
and where the weight is defined as the distance between the nodes in proportion to
the height of the head. Initially, we stretch the graph such that it overlays the entire

body. We then create a link between each node and its respective counterpart. We link the head, shoulders, arms, elbows, hands, neck, breasts, waist, legs, knees, and

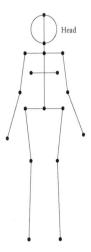

FIGURE 13.4 Analogia graph of a human figure with the length of the head used to measure the rest of the body (e.g., this figure is seven heads tall).

feet to their respective regions.

Analogia Graph

An analogia (from Greek means "proportion") graph is an abstraction of a proportion-preserving mapping of a shape. Assume that in a connected nonrigid graph G there is an edge with a length u. The rest of edges in G can be normalized as $p_i = v_i/u$. Let X and Y be metric spaces d_X and d_Y. A map $f: X \rightarrow Y$ is called an analogia graph if for any $x, y \in X$ one has

$$d_y\big(f(x), f(y)\big)/u = d_x(x, y)/u \qquad (13.1)$$

Analogia graphs are common in the fine arts. Instead of using absolute measurements of distances and sizes, artists often use intrinsic landmarks inside the scene to estimate the relationships. For example, an artist might use a number of heads to estimate the height of a person and a number of eyes to measure the length of a nose. Figure 13.4 is an analogia graph of a human body.

We can reduce the search space of the 3D body scans with an analogia graph. Here, we assume that the body is standing with the arms hanging to the sides in a nonconcealing way. If the arms are too close to the body, then the holograph imager cannot produce an accurate representation of the body. In that case, items on the side of the body could be completely missed because the area between the arm and the body would not be clearly defined. We start by dividing the 3D data points into 2D slices. The points are "snapped" to the nearest planes, enabling us to convert a 3D problem to a 2D one. Examining each slice from top to bottom is rather an expensive process. Here, we present a novel approach to reduce the search space by making use of intrinsic proportions. It is a relative measurement that uses an object in the scene to measure other objects.

Verification with the CAESAR Dataset

To collect the human anatomic proportion knowledge, we can select 100 samples of 3D human scans from the CAESAR anthropology database, which contains landmarks and the ground truths of physical measurements. The dataset consists of adults from sixteen to sixty-five years old, including subjects from North America, Europe, and Asia. Figure 13.5 shows an output of the ratio of navel height to full height. Then, we use the ratio of the navel to decide the concerned ratio range, based on the samples from the CAESAR database. Figure 13.5 shows the mean value of the navel ratio is about 0.594.

We further assume the distribution of the ratio is normal. We need the calculation to cover the probability value of 97.5%. Therefore, the estimated interval of the ratio is 0.566 to 0.622. After this, we calculate each circumference from the height ratio 0.566 to 0.622 with the step of 0.002. Then, we need to determine the proper ratio of the waist circumference to the mean value.

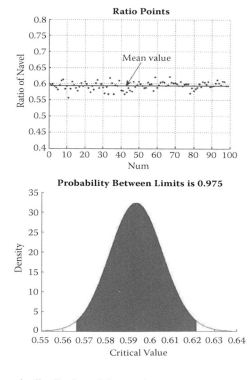

FIGURE 13.5   The ratio distribution of the navel.

The waist contour is extracted by the intersection of the 3D human body model and a level plane with a proper height ratio. The result is the points that constitute the surface of body. Figure 13.6 illuminates the sketch map of a 3D scan body model. The cutting is processed by the intersection of a 3D human body model and a level plane with a proper height ratio. The result is the contour that is constituted by surface points of body.

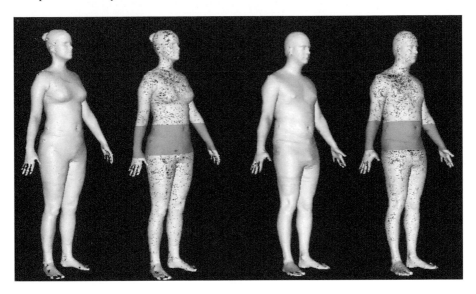

FIGURE 13.6   Samples of segmented target areas.

13.4   WAIST PERIMETER AND BODY MASS CALCULATIONS

From a health perspective, the waist perimeter has a strong relation with high cholesterol, diabetes II, hypertension and heart disease, and so on. Sunyer suggested that a number of cross-sectional studies have associated central fat distribution with risk factors for cardiovascular disease (CVD).[268] Most have used the waist/hip (W/H) ratio as a measure of central fat. Despre et al.[269] suggested that waist perimeter is a better surrogate marker of deep abdominal adipose tissue accumulation than W/H. This effect is independent of BMI and, in some studies, is a stronger predictor of diseases.[270]

In 2000, the body volume index (BVI) was devised as a computer-based measurement of the human body for obesity and an alternative to the BMI. BVI is currently

[268] F. X. Pi Sunyer. The epidemiology of central fat distribution in relation to disease. *Nutrition Research* 62:S120–S126, 2004.
[269] J. P. Despre, D. Prud'homme, M. C. Pouliot, et al. Estimation of deep abdominal adipose-tissue accumulation from simple anthropometric measurements in men. *American Journal of Clinic Nutrition* 54:471–477, 1991.
[270] F. X. Pi-Sunyer. Medical hazards of obesity. *Annals of Internal Medicine* 119:655–660, 1993.

undergoing clinical trials in the United States and Europe.[271] BVI is calculated by using 3D body data to determine volume or weight distribution. BVI makes an inference regarding the body's distribution of fat and weight using complex and detailed body composition data.[272] Measuring BVI requires special 3D scanner equipment that cannot be used in everyday healthcare because it is too expensive.

Each graph resulting from the cutting is constituted by a series of discrete points. It is formed by three parts, including two arms and the trunk contour. Typical data is shown in the left of Figure 13.7. There may be several gaps in the trunk contour, which would increase the hardship of perimeter computing.

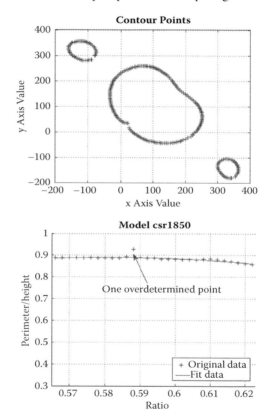

FIGURE 13.7 Typical contour points and data filter to reduce the influence of over-determined value.

[271] A. Romero-Corral, V. K. Somers, J. Sierra-Johnson, R. J. Thomas, M. L. Collazo-Clavell, J. Korinek, T. G. Allison, J. A. Batsis, F. H. Sert-Kuniyoshi, and F. Lopez-Jimenez. Accuracy of body mass index in diagnosing obesity in the adult general population. *International Journal of Obesity* 32(6):959–956, 2008. doi:10.1038/ijo.2008.11. PMID 18283284.

[272] Abd Tahrani, Kristien Boelaert, Richard Barnes, Suzanne Palin, Annmarie Field, Helen Redmayne, Lisa Aytok, and Asad Rahim. Body volume index: time to replace body mass index? *Endocrine Abstracts (Society for Endocrinology, British Endocrine Societies)* 15:104, 2008.

After finding the perimeter, we have to calculate the perimeter of the trunk contour with those cutting points, and we must be careful not to mix up the points of the two arm contours. Since those points were arranged randomly, we cannot just use any method.

Basically, the k-means cluster algorithm can be introduced first. However, the result of this method is not perfect because the selection of initial points is typically random. This results in the mixing up of the arms with some parts of the trunk. There is one more problem. When the arms of the model were lifted at some height, the cutting points do not exist in the arm contours anymore. This problem does not happen often, but we do have to confront it, as we have to consider the instance of handicapped people.

The perimeter was calculated by the principle of integrals. Assume the contours have a series of points. Each point has pairwise axis values. Then, the approximate perimeter can be calculated by the sum of Euclidian distances of the sequenced points. The method processes the input points from the contours. Because the input data is constituted mainly by discrete random arranged points, we can find the neighbor points first and then calculate the perimeter.

The pseudocode for the algorithm is as follows:

1. Set initial values, including:
    Number of neighbor points
    Max neighbor distance
2. Select the point that has the minimum distance to the center point as the start point.
3. Repeat:
    3.1   Find N neighbors to the current point.
    3.2   Find unused closest neighbor, add distance to perimeter;
          Set the flag as used;
          Set the closest neighbor as the current point.
        3.2.1   If N neighbor points have been used, and the distance to start point exceeds max neighbor distance, find more neighbor points and repeat to 3.2, until the neighbors' number exceeds an initial set value.
        3.2.2   If the neighbor's number exceeds an initial set value, the points must be too sparse to calculate. Stop repeating and give the warning.
4. Until all neighbors have been used and the distance to the start point is less than the max neighbor distance, add the distance to perimeter.

Experiments show that the proper value of the initial neighbor number is eight. When points are very sparse and the distance is very uneven, the value may be set to ten or more. The max neighbor distance must be set carefully. If the value exceeds too much, the point contour may include the points of arms in error. The number forty is suitable in most situations. This method can also be used in the distance calculation of a closed curve formed by discrete points.

After the calculation of the perimeter of each cutting ratio, we obtain a vector Y, which is expressed by the equation $Y = [y_1, y_2, \ldots, y_n]^T$. Each y_i is the perimeter at the ith cutting ratio. The model may contain a few overdetermined data that came from the error of calculation or the singularity part in the 3D model. So not to influence the last computation, we may use an exponential function to fit the data and successfully filtered out the errors. Consider the exponential function:

$$y = a_0 + a_1 e^{-t} + a_2 t e^{-t} \tag{13.2}$$

The unknown coefficients are computed by performing a least squares fit. The set of simultaneous equations was constructed and solved by forming the regression matrix X:

$$X = \left[\begin{pmatrix} 1 & \exp(-t_1) & t * \exp(-t_1) \\ \vdots & \vdots & \vdots \\ 1 & \exp(-t_n) & t * \exp(-t_n) \end{pmatrix} \right] \tag{13.3}$$

The coefficients were solved for by multiplying X by the inverse matrix of Y:

$$A = XY^{-1} \tag{13.4}$$

Here, the series ratio of cutting plane to height formed the vector t in Equation 13.2. Then, we obtained the regression matrix X from Equation 13.3. The corresponding perimeter to each ratio formed the vector Y in Equation 13.4. We could obtain the coefficients by solving Equation 13.4. With those results, the fit data could be calculated by Equation 13.2. Figure 13.7 shows the result of the filter process. It efficiently reduced the influence of overdetermined points.

To validate the correction of the waist perimeter, we can collect the waist pant's size code from model files. Comparing with the waist perimeter, the average error is 10.24%. Think about how errors come from the pant's size code; this error is acceptable in this extent. More detailed information can be seen in Table 13.1.

Other biometrics, such as the body volume, can also be calculated from 3D scans. So, we can also obtain the approximate value of the weight. Commonly, the body volume was directly influenced by the weight. There is also a common equation between the body volume and weight:

$$\text{Volume} = 1.01 * \text{Weight} - 4.937 \tag{13.5}$$

The volume calculation is also inspired by the principle of integrals. We cut the 3D body into enough interval distance slices. Then, when we add the product of every slice area with the interval, we obtain the approximate volume of the 3D human body. From the volume weight equation, we could obtain the calculation weight. Figure 13.8 shows the comparison to the reported weight. Table 13.1 shows the error rate. From the weight calculated, we can obtain the BMI of a human body.

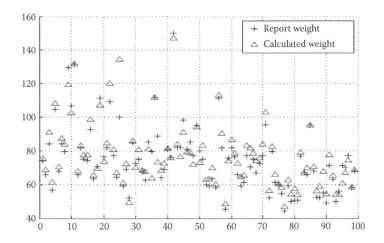

FIGURE 13.8   The weight comparison of reported and calculated values.

TABLE 13.1 Waist and Weight Error Comparison (%)

	Average Error	Max Error	Min Error
Waist	10.24	22.49	−3.9
Weight	5.84	24.35	−0.63

13.5   FUZZY DIAGNOSTIC HEURISTICS

Many clinical diagnoses are based on verbal expressions that can be modeled by fuzzy logic.[273]

A fuzzy diagnosis set F on the feature space $\Re^n$ is defined by a membership mapping function $\mu_F : \Re^n \to [0,1]$. For any feature vector $f \in \Re^n$, the value of $\mu_F(f)$ is called the degree of membership of f to the fuzzy diagnosis set F. For a fuzzy set F, there is a smooth transition for the degree of membership to F besides the hard cases $f \in F\big(\mu_F(f)=1\big)$ and $f \notin F\big(\mu_F(f)=0\big)$. We introduced fuzzy inference to evaluate the health index with the input of waist perimeter and height (Figure 13.9). The input is formed as

$$\mu_w(\text{Waist}) \text{ where } W = \{Slender, Moderate, Fat, SeriouslyFat\}$$

$$\mu_h(\text{Height}) \text{ where } H = \{Low, Normal, Tall, VeryTall\}$$

---

[273]   R. Zhang, Z. M. Zhang, and S. Khanzode. A data mining approach to modeling relationships among categories in image collection. In *Proceedings of ACM KDD 2004*, pp. 749–754, 2004.

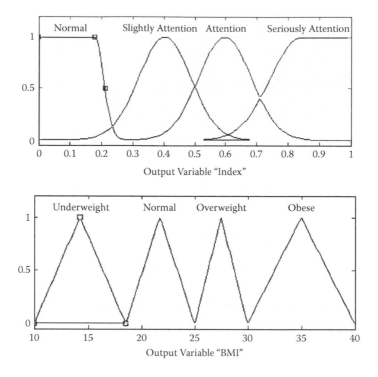

FIGURE 13.9   The fuzzy logic of health conditions and BMI.

Four intervals were used to ascertain the criticality of disease mentioned, so the output and the BMI output can be denoted as:

$$\mu_o(\text{Health}) \text{ where } O = \{Normal, SlightlyAttention, Attention, SeriouslyAttention\}$$

$$\mu_o(\text{BMI}) \text{ where } O = \{Underweight, Normal, Overweight, Obese\}$$

For implementation, the Gaussian curve membership function can be used:

$$A(x) = \exp\left(-\frac{(x-c)^2}{2\sigma^2}\right) \tag{13.6}$$

where c is the center and σ is the variance of the Gaussian curve.

We can calculate the waist perimeter/height ratio through the fuzzy system and compare it with the BMI value, which is the ratio of body weight over height.[274] The results are shown in Figure 13.10.

The method of waist perimeter calculation and fitting was tested on 100 datasets from the CAESAR database. Compared with the personal information in the 3D

274 http://www.cdc.gov/nccdphp/dnpa/healthyweight/assessing/bmi/adult_BMI/about_adult_BMI.htm

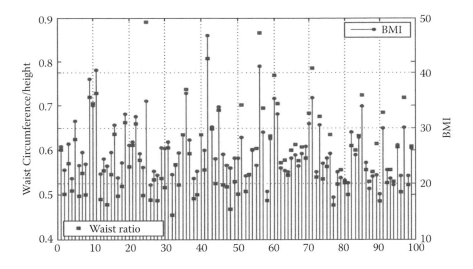

FIGURE 13.10   Waist perimeter/height ratio and BMI.

model datasets, the calculation of waist perimeter was accurate. Visual inspection showed that the fuzzy inference results matched the appearance of the 3D scanned models. Figure 13.11 is the interface of our demonstration system. The right bar contains several pieces of information calculated with methods mentioned.

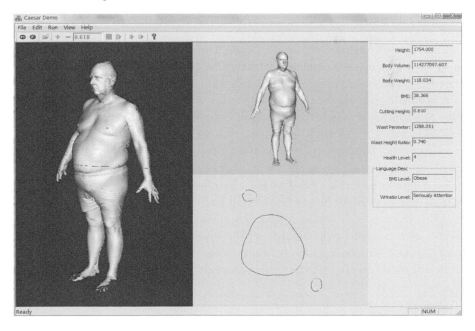

FIGURE 13.11   Screenshot of male BMI.

13.6   DIGITAL HUMAN MODELING

The advantage of human modeling is to enable designers to evaluate new technologies, such as microwave imaging system, before a physical system is ever built. This forward-thinking approach intends to transform the development of diagnostic technologies from being device specific and proprietary to being device independent and open source. It also transforms biomedical research into a systematic design process, which requires multidisciplinary innovations in digital human modeling, computer vision, and information visualization.

The following problems warrant our scientific investigations: given the available databases of anthropological models and the physical parameters of human imaging systems, how can we simulate the scanning imagery data to be used as an open source for broader research communities? How can we develop effective algorithms to find the human surface features from the 3D scanning data? Also, how can we distinguish foreign objects from the human body? Figure 13.12 shows an illustration of the framework.

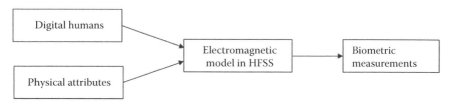

FIGURE 13.12   The framework of the multidisciplinary modeling process that merges computer simulation, computer vision, and bioinformatics.

The *physically augmented virtual human model* is the central idea in the study. In the world of medical research and development, scientists often use so-called phantoms to calibrate a new medical instrument.

Affordable phantom databases and artifacts, such as MathWorks' MRI (magnetic resonance imaging) brain phantom images,[275] National Library of Medicine's Visible Humans,[276] and DARPA's Digital Soldier,[277] significantly reduce development cycles and increase opportunities for interdisciplinary collaboration and education. In this chapter, we explore how to develop digital human models that not only contain finite surface elements but also physical properties, for example, the reflection of microwave beams on the skin and concealed objects beneath clothing. This requires high-fidelity modeling within a high-frequency (900 MHz to 33 GHz) electromagnetic field simulation. The tasks include mapping the imperfect laser-scanning surface data to the finite element material data, formulating the electromagnetic exciting sources, and calibrating the simulated model.

[275]   MathWorks MRI Phantom. http://www.mathworks.com/matlabcentral/fileexchange/loadFile.do?obj ectId=1759&objectType=file

[276]   NLM, Visible Human Project. http://www.nlm.nih.gov/research/visible/visible_human.html

[277]   DARPA Virtual Soldier. http://www.wired.com/news/medtech/0,1286,60016,00.html

The algorithm for detecting human surface features is designed to segment the human body and reduce the search space for anomalous objects. Many machine learning algorithms are coordinate dependent and limited by the training data space (e.g., artificial neural networks).[278] Some algorithms only work within small bounding boxes that do not warrant acceptable performance. For example, if a feature detection algorithm takes one hour to process, then it is not useful for a real-time-screening system.[279,280] Here we want to develop a model that is invariant to poses and coordinates. From a computer vision point of view, detecting features from 3D body scan data is nontrivial because human bodies are quite diverse. The technical methodology of function fitting has been used for extracting special landmarks, such as ankle joints, from 3D body scan data. This process is similar to the method for extracting landmarks from terrain.[281,282] Curvature calculation is also introduced from other fields, such as the sequence-dependent curvature structure of DNA and nude figures.[283,284] These curvature calculations use methods such as chain code,[285] circle fit, ratio of end-to-end distance to contour length, ratio of moments of inertia, and cumulative and successive bending angles. Curvature values can be calculated from the data by fitting a quadratic surface over a square window and then calculating the directional derivatives of this surface. Sensitivity to data noise is a major problem in both the function fitting and curvature calculation methods because typical 3D scanning data is very noisy. Template matching appears to be a promising method because it is invariant to the coordinate system. However, defining a template and where to match the template are challenging issues because they are unique to each particular feature.

13.7   PHYSICALLY AUGMENTED VIRTUAL HUMAN MODEL

The full-scale virtual human models can be built from the digital surface-scanning data, such as the CAESAR database (with the necessary license agreement), which contains 5,000 males and 5,000 females aged sixteen to sixty-five, where 5,000 of them are North American, 2,400 are Asian, and 2,600 are from the European survey of Italy, the Netherlands, and other countries. As we know, all models in the database have feature landmarks that are important anthropomorphic measurements. We may keep them in our test bed. However, all of the models wore tight-fitting underwear.

[278] P. Keller, L. McMkin, D. Sheen, A. McKinnon, and A. J. Summet. Privacy algorithm for cylindrical holographic weapons surveillance systems. *Proceedings SPIE. Applications and Science of Computational Intelligence III*, 4055:476–483, 2000.

[279] C. A. M. Suikerbuik. Automatic feature detection in 3D human body scans. Master's thesis INF/SCR-02-23, Institute of Information and Computer Sciences, Utrecht University, the Netherlands, 2002.

[280] Suikerbuik et al., Automatic feature detection.

[281] P. J. Besl and R. C. Jain. Three-dimensional object recognition. *ACM Computing Surveys* 17(1):75–145, 1985.

[282] M. Brady, J. Ponce, A. Yuille, and H. Asada. Describing surfaces. *Computer Vision, Graphics, Image Processing* 32:1–28, 1985.

[283] D. A. Forsyth and M. M. Fleck. Body plans. In Proceedings CVPR 1997, 1997, pp. 678–683.

[284] D. A. Forsyth and M. M. Fleck. Identifying nude pictures. In *Proceeding of Third IEEE Workshop on Applications of Computer Vision*, 1996, pp. 103–108.

[285] M. Sonka et al. *Image processing, analysis and machine vision.* PWS Publishing, Boston, 1999.

Therefore, we have to remove that by applying a low-pass filter. Besides, we may also use a laser 3D scanner[286] to collect additional samples as references. For these scanned models, we can manually annotate the human landmarks. Figure 13.13 shows a sample of 3D human body-scanning data, and Figure 13.14 shows the output of the microwave imaging simulation from the High Frequency Structure Simulator (HFSS),[287] a powerful tool for numerical simulations of electromagnetic standing waves in 3D systems with spatially varying material properties based on the finite element method.

Here we input the human scan model to HFSS and then assign the electromagnetic material properties to the 3D objects. We can simplify the computing problem through the use of frequency snapshots instead of a full broadband frequency sweep and by modeling portion of the body instead of the whole.

13.8   SURFACE ANALYSIS

There are many 3D surface analysis methods: bump-hunting, voxel intensity based, curvature-based and spatial density-based clustering, and so on.[288,289,290,291,292,293,294,295] Here, we introduce two models: the intensity-based method and the surface-based method.

Intensity-Based Method

For the intensity-based method, we can use HFSS to simulate the scattered radio waves from the objects and human body. A typical human scanner's wave range is between 500 MHz and 33 GHz, which makes it a great challenge to simulate the whole body imaging at the resolution of 1 mm with the existing computing resources. To simplify the problem, we crop the 3D human model to a solid $1 \times 1 \times 0.5$ ft^3 slab with a metal object on the skin. With this simplification, the problem can be solved in less than 64 GB of main system memory using a direct solver.

---

[286] http://www.3d3solutions.com.

[287] http://www.ansoft.com/products/hf/hfss/.

[288] D. B. Neill and A. W. Moore. Anomalous spatial cluster detection. In *Proceedings KDD 2005 Workshop on Data Mining Methods for Anomaly Detection*, 2005, pp. 41–44.

[289] D. B. Neill and A. W. Moore. Rapid detection of significant spatial clusters. In *Proceedings 10th ACM SIGKDD Conference on Knowledge Discovery and Data Mining*, 2004, pp. 256–265.

[290] M.-L. Shyu, S.-C. Chen, K. Sarinnapakorn, and L.-W. Chang. A novel anomaly detection scheme based on principal component classifier. In *Proceedings of the IEEE Foundations and New Directions of Data Mining Workshop*, 2003.

[291] J. Zhang and M. Zulkernine. Anomaly based network intrusion detection with unsupervised outlier detection. In *Symposium on Network Security and Information Assurance—Proceedings of the IEEE International Conference on Communications (ICC)*, Istanbul, Turkey, June 2006.

[292] Shyu et al., A novel anomaly detection scheme.

[293] J. Gomez, F. Gonzalez, and D. Dasgupta. An immuno-fuzzy approach to anomaly detection. *Proceedings of the 12th IEEE International Conference on Fuzzy Systems (FUZZIEEE)*, 2:1219–1224, 2003.

[294] K. Burbeck and S. Nadjm-Tehrani. ADWICE: anomaly detection with real-time incremental clustering. In C.-S. Park and S. Chee (eds.), *ICISC 2004*. LNCS, vol. 3506. Springer, Heidelberg, 2005.

[295] J. A. Wise, J. J. Thomas, K. Pennock, D. Lantrip, M. Pottier, A. Schur, and V. Crow. Visualizing the non-visual: spatial analysis and interaction with information from text documents. In *Proceedings of the 1995 IEEE Symposium on Information Visualization*, Atlanta, GA, October 30–31, 1995, p. 51.

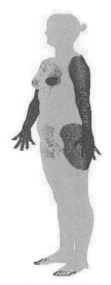

FIGURE 13.13 Sample of the human surface mesh data.

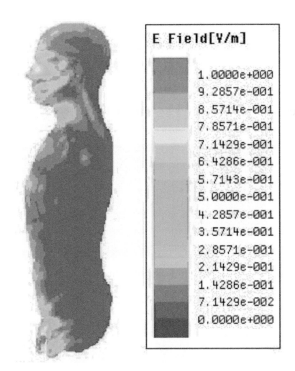

FIGURE 13.14 HFSS simulation of the wave-intensive image of the human body at 22 GHz.

We can use the material property for the body with a permittivity and conductivity matching that of seawater ($\varepsilon_r = 81$ and conductivity = 4 S/m). Human muscle is characterized up to 6 GHz ($\varepsilon_r \approx 50$, conductivity ≈ 6 S/m), so we can use seawater and would not expect a significant difference for the qualitative purposes of this simulation. Figure 13.14 shows the result for the scattered electric field due to a 1-V/m incident plane wave propagating perpendicular to the body's front surface.

Figure 13.14 is the plot of the complex magnitude of the electric field. If instead we plotted for a sequence of phases between 0 and 180 degrees, we would see the field magnitude propagate across the body.

Surface-Based Method

For the surface-based method, the curvature is defined as the rate of change of slope. In our case, the discrete space, the curvature description must be slightly modified to overcome difficulties resulting from violation of curve smoothness.

We can start by slicing the digital model horizontally. We average the points between the slices. The curvature scalar descriptor here finds the ratio between the total number of boundary pixels (length) and the number of boundary pixels where the boundary direction changes significantly. The fewer the number of direction changes, the straighter the boundary is. In this case, we map the points on the slice to a polar coordinate system because the body is in a round shape. Then, we use a function of the radius and angles of the points to calculate the anomalous features. Figures 13.15 and 13.16 show the final detection results.

Fusion of the intensity-based modeling and surface-based modeling methods would improve the surface analysis accuracy and reduce the noise. However, because we have heterogeneous human models with different resolution and different orientations and sizes, model registration appears to be a challenge. For the actual human-scanning systems, this is not a problem because the coordinates of the point clouds are known to the designers.

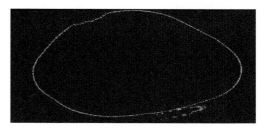

FIGURE 13.15   Slice-based feature representation (the abnormal curve is at the bottom right corner.

13.9   SUMMARY

This chapter explored new ways of conducting health diagnoses in public spaces with a focus on microwave imaging devices in airports.

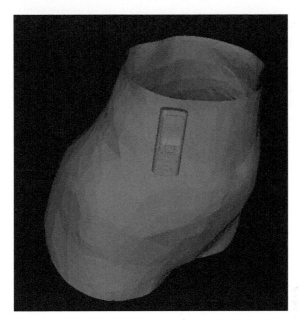

FIGURE 13.16   Segmentation of a mobile phone from the skin.

Virtual human models can be used for designing and evaluating soft biometric technologies before a physical system is built. Given the available databases of anthropological models from CAESAR, 3D scanners, and the physical parameters of human imaging systems, we are able to simulate the scanning imagery data with the HFSS.

This forward-thinking approach intends to transform the development of ambient diagnostic technologies from being device specific and proprietary to being device independent and open source. It also advances ambient diagnostics toward a systematic design process, enabling multidisciplinary innovations in digital human modeling, computer vision, information visualization, and computational aesthetics. The results of this study would benefit public health and custom-fit products that are designed for personal 3D scanning data.

PROBLEMS

1. Bring five friends to a location to take a few photos. Estimate each individual's height based on the knowledge about the objects in the scene (e.g., an elevator's height as a unit) to measure people's height. Compare the estimated values with the ground truths. Summarize the results in a report.
2. Find twenty online images that contain adult men and women in standing positions. Crop ten males and ten females from the images. Measure their heights with the length of the person's head as a unit. For example, a man's height is 7.5 heads. Plot the height distributions among men and women. Calculate the average heights for men and women in head units.

3. List average proportions for everyday objects, such as humans, dogs, and cars, assuming a bounding box around the objects. Use the height-to-width ratio as the proportional measurement.

4. Find a live webcam such as EarthCam.[296] Extract pedestrians from footage using background subtraction, assuming the webcam is stationary.

5. Count the pedestrians from the same webcam used in Problem 4.

6. Estimate the heights of the pedestrians from the same webcam used in Problem 4, using the landmarks in the scene.

7. Estimate the pedestrians' BMI from the webcam used in Problem 4, using landmarks in the scene.

8. Use the Kinect to scan human body surfaces to estimate waist measurements. Compare the results between the single view scan and multiview scan. Analyze the accuracy by comparing with the ground truth.

9. Survey devices at the local airport and discuss the "dual-use" potentials of the security systems for ambient diagnosis.

10. Assume you are asked to design a thermal imaging system for checking pedestrians' temperature. You want to simulate the thermal imaging system with digital human models so that you may test the system virtually before it is made. Explore the off-the-shelf products and databases. Write a proposal for building the simulator with diagrams, descriptions, vendor lists, and cost estimations.

---

[296] http://www.earthcam.com/

14 Games for Diagnoses

> Nothing is particularly hard if you divide it into small jobs.
>
> —Henry Ford

14.1 INTRODUCTION

It is estimated that three billion hours per week are spent playing video games world-wide.[297] Video games are about dynamic interaction with a system or other players with rules, creating windows for ambient diagnoses in an exciting, ubiquitous, and affordable process. Widely available mobile platforms and new tools have enabled game design, production, and distribution through smartphones, over the web, and via downloadable services. Now, it is possible for individuals to conceive, develop, and publish their own games. This chapter explores how to design video games for diagnostic purposes. In particular,

- Trend of games for diagnosis
- Elements of a game engine
- Networked games
- Finite-state machine (FSM)
- Motion capture and control
- Game displays
- Game development tool kits

14.2 EMERGING GAMES FOR DIAGNOSIS

There are many categories of video games. Here, we only focus on three categories: perception–action processes, social interactions, and crowdsourcing.

Perception–Action Games

Most video games are related to perception–action processes: they require real-time input, processing, and display. Examples of these types of games include the pinball machine, driving simulations, and sports games. Perception–action games can be used for observing a user's physical well-being, including his or her visual saccade, gestures, reaction time, and most important, eye-hand coordination. In the early days, a user's actions would be input into the computer through a mouse or keyboard. Today, a user's actions can be sensed by Wii, Kinect, web camera, and mobile phone

---

[297] M. Griffiths. Video games and health. *British Medical Journal* 331(7509):122–123, 2005.

sensor such as gyroscopes, accelerometers, near-field communication (NFC), and compasses.

Figure 14.1 shows a Kinect-based tennis game for evaluating eye-hand coordination after recovering from a stroke. In the game, the Kinect sensor detects the position of a hand that controls the tennis racket. Based on the swiping speed of the racket, the ball lands inside or outside the targeted area, following the law of physics. The play is comparable to common video games. However, it has subtle differences. For example, the challenge levels and the scoring system are designed to be proportional to the eye-hand coordination evaluation scale: from no coordination (0) to perfect coordination (10). The game can also record gestures over time, allowing therapists or patients to zoom in to particular moments.

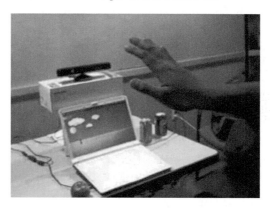

FIGURE 14.1 The gesture-controlled tennis game is designed for evaluating eye-hand coordination. The hand-tracking sensor above the laptop is Microsoft Kinect.

Social Interaction Games

Online games provide not only a virtual world for social interactions but also a window for ambient diagnoses of special groups of users, such as autistic people, who often find it challenging to engage in face-to-face social interaction in the real world.

Advanced online game engines such as Second Life™ provide useful social interaction tools for users with special needs. Digital avatars allow autistic users to communicate anonymously. Some use the editor to make an avatar that mimics the real self. Others select from prefabricated avatars, reflecting the player's self-image.

Autistic users can also meet in the virtual world to share common interests. A user group called Autistic Liberation Front was formed to meet regularly to address their rights. Some autistic users use text-to-voice interfaces that enable them to chat with others freely without hesitation. Online games provide useful information and knowledge about autistic patients that otherwise could have been missed by regular diagnostic methods. For example, the Second Life[298] game enables autistic users to

---

[298] http://www.secondlife.com

interact with others in dance, music, and chat naturally. Some users openly claim they are autistic, and they often help researchers to have a better understanding of their world and noninvasively evaluate their social skills, interaction preferences, interaction intensity, and self-confidence. Many online conversations during the game in fact have research and clinical values (e.g., the cognitive process of patients with autism). Temple Grandin, a professor with autism, described her thinking as often in pictures or videos.[299] But in the game, autistic players were able to disclose that they personally did not think in pictures, and autistic people have different types of thinking processes. However, many autistic people do share common issues, such as oversensitivity to touch and sound.

Figure 14.2 is a screenshot of an autistic user who danced in Second Life. Similar to the real world, Second Life is also diversified. Behind the digital avatars, real people often talk openly, even more than in the real world, given a comfort level of the Second Life social interaction environments. The greatest part of online game platforms is its user-created content, including personalized avatars, outfits, gestures, furniture, animals, houses, landscapes, music, languages, privacy, and players' viewpoints.

Still, it is important to note that online gaming is a double-edged sword. Online communities create a bond and competition. Addiction to online games can become a problem for some users.

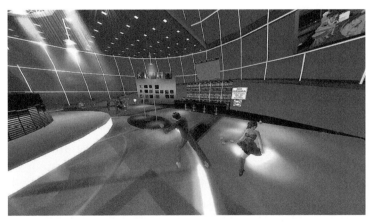

FIGURE 14.2   The autistic user on the right danced in the social interaction game Second Life, where she interacted with others. The game allowed the user to customize her appearance and chat in voice or text messages.

Crowdsourcing Puzzle Games

It was estimated that over 300 million Rubik's cubes have been sold since 1977. Today, sales continue to be over 500,000 cubes worldwide each year. Online games also consume roughly 200 million minutes of human attention each day, which is a

[299] Temple Grandin. *Thinking in pictures: my life with autism.* Vintage Books, New York, 1995.

lot of cognitive surplus. Crowdsourcing is a process that connects many volunteers to solve a complex problem. An example of crowdsourcing is dividing a puzzle into many small pieces and letting thousands of online users work together to solve it. Crowdsourcing is used in gaming platforms so that users are not only entertained but also trained or educated. In addition, crowdsourced games can serve as a resource for scientific research. "Gamification" of certain tasks makes users more motivated and engaged in the problem at hand.[300,301,302,303]

The feasibility of a crowdsourced approach has been tested in a game-based malaria image analysis. In particular, this approach investigated whether anonymous volunteers with no prior experience would be able to count malaria parasites in digitized images of thick blood smears by playing a web-based game (Figure 14.3).[304,305] Game players begin with a short tutorial to first learn the characteristics of an infected blood cell. Then, they are presented with a six-by-eight grid of blood cells. The player's task is to click on the parasites. When a player found all of the parasites present in one image within a limited amount of time, the player has completed a "level," and the game continues by presenting a new image. Otherwise, the game is over.[306]

Meanwhile, all of the players' clicks were registered in a database. After one month, all the collected data were preprocessed to group all the clicks that players placed around the different objects in the image: parasites, white blood cells (leukocytes), and background noise.

Analyzing blood samples is a time-consuming process. Where doctors are scarce, diagnosis can take even longer. Having many nonprofessional gamers do the labor-intensive work not only speeds things up but also improves the accuracy of the results. For example, a single person's response may inevitably have some mistakes. However, if we combine ten to twenty, maybe even fifty, nonexpert gamers, we can improve the overall accuracy greatly in terms of analysis. According to a recent publication,[307] recruited nonprofessional volunteers diagnosed malarial blood cells almost as accurately as a trained pathologist.

Phylo is another two-dimensional (2D) puzzle game that uses crowdsourcing techniques to solve the multiple sequence alignment (MSA) problem, which is to arrange multiple sequences of DNA or RNA to identify regions of similarity and

---

[300] B. Good and A. Su. Games with a scientific purpose. *Genome Biology* 12:135, 2011.

[301] M. Nielsen. *Reinventing discovery: the new era of networked science*. Princeton University Press, Princeton, NJ, 2011.

[302] J. McGonigal. *Realty is broken: why games make us better and how they can change the world*. Penguin (Nos-Classics), New York, 2011.

[303] M. Swan. Crowdsourced health research studies: an important emerging complement to clinical trials in the public health research ecosystem. *Journal of Medical Internet Research* 14(2):e46, 2012.

[304] http://malariaspot.org/ accessed February 14, 2013; the original paper is at http://www.jmir.org/2012/6/e167/

[305] http://www.theatlantic.com/health/archive/2012/05/a-video-game-where-players-help-real-doctors-diagnose-malaria/256759/

[306] http://www.theatlantic.com/health/archive/2012/05/a-video-game-where-players-help-real-doctors-diagnose-malaria/256759/

[307] M. A. Luengo-Oroz, A. Arranz, and J. Frean. Crowdsourcing malaria parasite quantification: an online game for analyzing images of infected thick blood smears. *Journal of Medical Internet Research* 14(6):e167, 2012.

trace the source of certain genetic diseases. The key idea of Phylo is to convert the MSA problem into a casual game that can be played by ordinary web users with minimal prior knowledge of the biological context.[308]

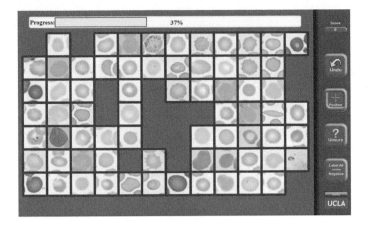

FIGURE 14.3 Crowdsourcing for blood cell pattern recognition (Courtesy of the open source journal *PLoS ONE.*)

Phylo has a simple 2D graphical user interface that allows users to move multiple sequences of DNA or RNA back and forth horizontally (Figure 14.4). Each letter in a sequence is coded with a color. The goal of the game is to match as many colors as possible. Human vision is good at spotting the misalignment of colors and shapes. The creators of Phylo expect that a large amount of human alignment input may help to solve the computationally expensive MSA problem.

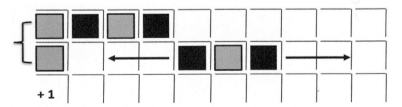

FIGURE 14.4 Phylo game for DNA sequence matching.

Since the launch of Phylo in November 2010, the system received more than 350,000 solutions submitted from more than 12,000 registered users. Results show that solutions submitted contributed to improving the accuracy of up to 70% of the alignment blocks considered.[309]

---

[308] http://phylo.cs.mcgill.ca/
[309] http://www.plosone.org/article/info:doi/10.1371/journal.pone.0031362

Foldit is a more sophisticated crowdsourcing game for three-dimensional (3D) protein folding. As we know, proteins can be involved in diseases in many different ways, such as in AIDS, cancers, and Alzheimer's disease. The more we know about how certain proteins fold to a compact shape, the better we can design new proteins to combat the disease-related proteins and cure the diseases. However, a small protein can consist of a long chain of 100 to 1,000 amino acids. The number of different ways even a small protein can fold is astronomical because there are so many degrees of freedom (Figure 14.5).

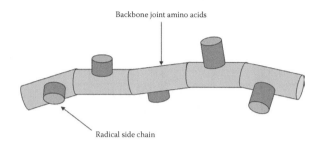

FIGURE 14.5   A protein consists of a polypeptide backbone with attached radical side chains. The different side chains make each protein distinct.

In Foldit, the players manipulate different lengths of side chains and backbones until they fit into the smallest volume possible. The challenge is that every piece moved affects every other piece. Game scores are awarded by how much energy would be needed to hold a protein in the shape the player has created. The real challenge comes from competing against other players to make the highest-point version of a specific protein.

So far, more than 100,000 people have downloaded Foldit, turning the game into a massive multiplayer competition. Remarkably, the highest score record holder was a teenager who turned into a folding expert in Foldit. The recent paper published in *Nature* included Foldit players as coauthors. [310]

Design Trade-Offs

Growing social games are moving away from device-centric rich graphics toward network-centric simple graphics for average phone platforms. On the other hand, social games for smartphones are moving from simple graphics toward richer graphics for both device-centric casual games or network-centric multiplayer games such as Second Life (Figure 14.6). We need to study design trade-offs between rich graphics versus simple graphics and server-centric versus client-centric alternatives. The following sections explore the essentials of game engines and publically available game development tool kits.

---

[310]   S. Cooper, F.Khatib, A.Treuille,J. Barbero, J.Lee, M.Beenen, A.Leaver-Fay, D.Baker, Z.Popvic, and FoldIt players. Predicting protein structures with a multiplayer online game. *Nature,* 466, 756-760, August 5, 2010. Also see FoldIt web site: http://fold.it/portal/

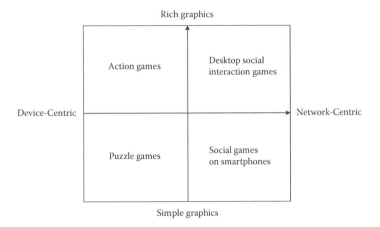

FIGURE 14.6   Design trade-offs between rich graphics versus simple graphics and server-centric versus client-centric.

14.3   ANATOMY OF GAME ENGINES

In the early days of computer programming, games were typically written in an assembly language for a particular hardware, and little software could be reused between games. The term *game engine* arose in the mid-1990s, in parallel with the growing 3D games, enabling developers to take advantage of software frameworks for graphics, physics, databases, and interfaces. Figure 14.7 illustrates a basic diagram of the typical structure of a game engine. The reusable game modules significantly increase productivity and reduce difficulties to novices.

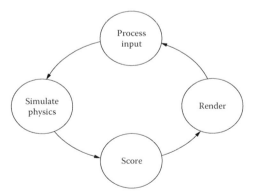

FIGURE 14.7   A typical game engine consists of input processing, game world simulation, and 2D or 3D rendering.

A video game is a real-time database that continuously updates key variables. The core functionality provided by a game engine includes input process, rendering engine (render) for 2D or 3D graphics, and a physical engine for simulating the game world. Like an operating system, a game loop needs to be initialized at the start to assign values to the essential parameters, and the game has an orderly shutdown procedure for saving game object statuses and clearing up temporary data files. Besides, a game engine also includes sound, scripting, animation, networking, streaming, memory management, multiple threading, localization support, and a scene graph.

Process Input

The game engine continuously monitors a user's input, which can be represented as a vector or a message. It is contains critical data, such as the duration of command, view angles, forward, sideways, and upward movements, and button fields. The duration of the command field corresponds to the number of milliseconds of simulation to which the command corresponds. The view angles field is a vector representing the direction the player was looking during the frame. The forward, sideways, and upward move fields are the impulses determined by examining the keyboard, mouse, and joystick to see if any movement keys were held down. Finally, the buttons field is simply a bit field with one or more bits set for each button that is held down.

A game engine can also receive user input from sensors such as Kinects, gyroscopes, accelerometers, compasses, orientation sensors, cameras, GPSs, and NFC interfaces.

No matter what the input device is, a game engine needs to extract a user's input and convert it into a control signal (Figure 14.8). In a simplified version, for example, say we have a hand position of $x = 100$, assuming the hand is moving in one dimension. The game engine then draws a moving pad with its center at $x = 100$. At the next sampling interval, the hand position is sensed at $x = 110$. The game engine processes it again and moves the pad to the right. This process continues indefinitely. A moving object in game design is often called a "sprite." In a 2D situation, a sprite is a bitmap with a control point, normally the centroid. The bitmap is alpha rendered so that its shape can be blended into the background smoothly.

A video game is an event-driven program. An event is simply some intended user input, like a button push or a mouse click. A game must specifically define what actions players can perform and what events those actions should trigger. Unless specifically coded somewhere else, such as the default action resulting from pressing the Home button, a developer must specifically tell the program which events

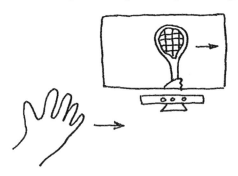

FIGURE 14.8   User's hand position sensing and input processing.

(user actions) to wait for and what to do in response to each type of event. When a user performs some input to which the game is attuned, that triggers some action response from the program.

For video games, an event can be expressed as a message. Game clients collect local events and send them to the server. The server updates its real-time event database and broadcasts events to related clients. To minimize the event-handling workload, the game engine usually defines an effective zone for an event. For example, an avatar's walking event might be relevant to the residents on the same island as the avatar but have no impact on other islands in the virtual world. This localization helps to reduce the processing load.

Physics Engine

A physics engine has the sole purpose of moving objects around in a simulated physical world. Physics engines take into consideration the physics properties of objects, such as their mass, shape, material, and current trajectory, and then calculate a new position and state for those objects. In general, a game engine feeds initial state data to the physics engine and then responds to the physics engine's feedback. For example, the game engine loads a level and tells the physics engine that there are ten objects in the scene at certain positions. The physics engine then processes updates of those objects' states as the game engine asks the physics engine to update the objects and report on their changes. Graphics data is often synced to changes from the physics engine, so that changes made by the physics engine show up on the player's screen.

The most importation function of a physics engine is collision detection. Collision detection is an essential part of 3D games. It ensures that the game physics are relatively realistic, so that a man will walk on the road instead of under the road, and he will walk along the wall instead of walking through the wall. How well a game can detect collisions is an integral part of the believability and enjoyment of the game.

One way to detect a collision in a 3D world is the sphere-plane detection method.[311] We can use this technique to detect if the user has bumped into an object. The sphere-plane method is relatively easy to compute since not every polygon of a more complex model has to be compared to the environment to see if a collision has occurred. The viewer or camera can be thought of as one solid entity, such as a ball, instead of a human with several limbs.

Detecting collisions with a sphere tends to be easier to calculate because of the symmetry of the object. The entire surface of a sphere is the same distance from the center, so it is easy to determine whether an object has intersected with a sphere. If the distance from the center of the sphere to an object is less than or equal to the sphere's radius, then a collision has occurred.

Depending on which side of the plane the sphere is on, the distance value can be either positive or negative. If the distance becomes zero, then the sphere is intersecting the plane. The game program will first check if a collision will result when the object moves in the desired direction (Figure 14.9). If there is a collision, then the program will respond appropriately, such as by refusing to move in the desired direction.

---

[311] http://www.edenwaith.com/products/pige/tutorials/collision.php

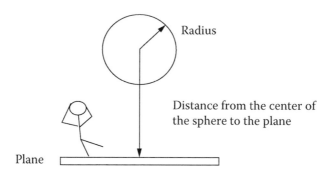

FIGURE 14.9 Collision detection.

A game engine usually embeds collision detection as a material property that designers or users can turn on or off. Collision detection is computationally intensive and is only assigned to key objects that are near the viewer. Collision detection may also be set in different resolutions (e.g., broad or narrow) (Figure 14.10). At the broad level, the detection is based on bounding boxes. At the narrow level, the detection is based on actual polygon contours. The broad level is much faster than the narrow level.

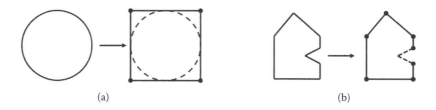

(a)   (b)

FIGURE 14.10 Broad versus narrow collision detection. Collision detection. (a) Boxes surround objects when coarse resolution is sufficient. (b) Polygons are used for higher resolution, but the outline of an object may only be convex.

Score

Score or bonus systems are essential to video games. The score could come from the simulation of physics, such as the number of balls hit, the number of letters in the DNA sequences that are aligned, or the energy of the protein folding. The game server usually keeps track of players' scores and updates global score ranks.

The award for high scores is normally peer recognition as many players are volunteers. However, some social games do have virtual currencies. For example, Second Life has the currency "Linden dollars," which has a dynamic exchange rate of roughly US$1 to 300–400 Linden dollars. The virtual money actually has market value and can be converted to real-world currencies according to the exchange rate at that time.

Render

Rendering engines generate 2D or 3D computer graphics in real time. Similar to the work of physics engines, rendering is computationally intensive. In many cases, we prefer to use 2D graphics instead of 3D graphics.

In 2D cases, how to display moving objects (sprites) that blend into the background is important. Those sprite shapes can be generated by adding an alpha mask using software such as Photoshop™ (Figure 14.11). The alpha channel is an additional channel that can be added to an image. It contains transparency information about the image, and depending on the type of alpha, it can contain various levels of transparency. The alpha channel basically controls the transparency of all the other channels. By adding the alpha channel to an image, you control the transparency of the red, green, and blue channels.

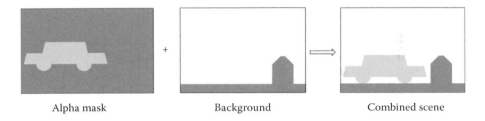

| Alpha mask | Background | Combined scene |

FIGURE 14.11   Alpha channel created by Photoshop for transparent sprite shape contour.

The largest benefit of using alpha channels is visual appeal. Without alpha channels, images layered over one another would not be antialiased and therefore would have blocky jagged edges.[312] This is not at all attractive. Another benefit of alpha channels is speed. When the game saves an image with the alpha channel, all of the opacity levels are saved with it. One can then place that image over anything one likes, and the image will still maintain its appearance. This saves time because one can place the image directly over a background without the need to save that image in exactly the right spot over that exact background.

For 3D graphics, a game engine usually includes a library of rendering algorithms, mostly originating from OpenGL, an open source 3D graphics library. 3D graphics often use the number of polygons to measure the complexity or size of the rendering problem. The more polygons there are, the longer the rendering time will be. Game engines have optimized 3D rendering by rendering the visible area only. All of the obscured objects or the back of an object will not be rendered in 3D. In many games, 2D instead of 3D images are used for distant objects. For mobile games, more 2D moving sprites are used than 3D rendered objects to reach the fast speed with minimal computing resources.

---

[312] http://www.icongalore.com/xp-icon-articles/alpha-channel-explained.htm

14.4 NETWORKING

Most action games played on the network today are client-server games. In these games, there is a single, authoritative server that is responsible for running the global logic. One or more clients are connected to this. Figure 14.12 is a diagram of the client-server architecture.

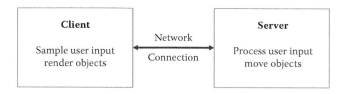

FIGURE 14.12   Client-server game architecture.

The clients normally cannot communicate directly with each other; this is not a peer-to-peer connection (Figure 14.13). The server controls the global map, and the players update local activities. For example, Player 1 tells the server: "I have moved one step to the left, and my screen shows I am walking to the left." The server would respond: "I received your data, and I am updating your position on the global map; I am going to tell other players that you have moved to a new position."

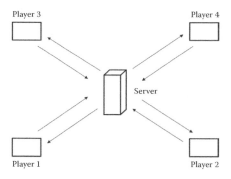

FIGURE 14.13   Multiple players interact with each other through a server.

14.5 FINITE-STATE MACHINE

Finite-state machines have been broadly used in video game designs. Each machine has a set of states that follow a certain path. A state has transitions to other states, which are caused by events or actions within a state. For example, we can define a simple behavior model for an animated avatar in three states: standing, walking, and sleeping. For each state, there is an animation sequence associated with it. The avatar's state can be changed when an event happens; for example, the avatar's state changes from walking to standing when the avatar collides with a wall or changes from walking to sleeping when the avatar arrives at a bed.

FSMs simplify game design for avatars and objects by specifying finite states. For many game engines, FSMs allow developers to attach a script to a specific state, providing a framework for behavioral descriptions. Figure 14.14 illustrates an example of the three states of an avatar.

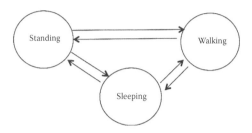

FIGURE 14.14   Finite-state machine of an avatar: standing, walking, and sleeping.

FSMs do not cover concurrent behaviors such as walking and sleeping. They do not scale up very well for logic programming as the number of states increases. However, they are still useful models for designing small or midsize games.

14.6   WORLD MODELING

A world model is the stage on which a game occurs. A world model is usually divided into several scenes. In each scene, actors come and go. Many game engines provide an editor for world models, typically a 3D modeling tool including camera position and orientation and lights (Figure 14.15). In addition, developers can add sound tracks, Internet radio channels, background images, and ambient lights for time of the day.

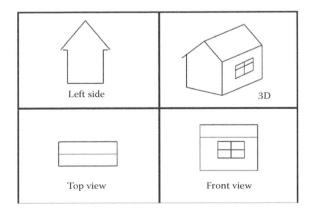

FIGURE 14.15   A world editor screen of Game Studio 3D with multiple camera views: top, front, side, and 3D shaded view.

14.7 MOTION CAPTURE AND CONTROL

Motion capture ("mocap") is a process by which to record people's movement. In motion capture sessions, movements of one or more actors are sampled many times per second. Early techniques used images from multiple cameras and calculated 3D positions, but motion capture records only the movements of the actor, not his or her visual appearance. This animation data is often mapped to a 3D model so that the model performs the same actions as the actor.

The infrared marker-based mocap method has been widely used in the video game industry (Figure 14.16). It is often used for scripting avatar's gestures. Placing infrared reflecting markers on a model's joints and key points, the multiple infrared cameras track the markers in a 3D space. The advantage of the method is its accuracy. However, it is inconvenient to put on the special mocap suit, and the mocap system is expensive.

The Wii sensor is also a marker-based motion capture device. The infrared sensor can sense a player's motion through triangulation of the infrared signals. Currently, a hacked Wii device can work directly with computers, providing an alternative for game development.

Glove sensors can capture finger movements. These gloves have channels of magnetic gel that change their output when the fingers move.

Force sensors are more accurate motion capture devices. The robotic actuator can sense a player's force on the stick or a tube (endoscope) and also provide force feedback to the player as well.

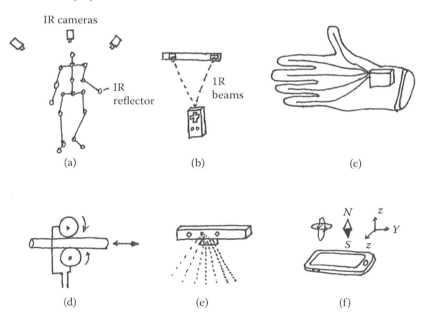

FIGURE 14.16 Motion capture and control devices: (a) infrared (IR) motion capture system, (b) Wii, (c) motion control glove, (d) force feedback; (e) Kinect 3D sensor, and (f) motion sensors on a smartphone.

The growing marker-less mocap methods such as Kinect provide an alternative to traditional mocap technologies. Kinect's Skeleton application programming interface (API) enables real-time key point tracking for up to two people and position tracking for up to four people. Taking tennis game design, for example, we can use a Kinect to sense the player's hand position and use the live position to control the tennis racket (see Figure 14.8).

Webcams can also be used for marker-less motion tracking, using background subtraction or optical flow. However, their resolution is not as high as that in Kinect or marker-based methods. Webcams can be used for approximate motion sensing though, such as hand or head tracking.

Micro electromechanical system (MEMS) sensors on a mobile phone provide a variety of sensory devices, such as accelerometers and gyroscopes. Accelerometers are sensitive to translational motions, while gyroscopes are more sensitive to orientation changes. For example, gyroscope input can be used for game design; the gyroscope senses the angles of the tilted phone and controls the object's moving direction accordingly.

14.8   GAME DISPLAYS

High-definition display technologies for monitors and phones have significantly improved visual effects. This is also good news for ambient diagnoses. For example, vision tests with Retina Display provide a high pixel density so that the human eye is unable to notice pixilation at a typical viewing distance.

Head-Mounted Display

Head-mounted displays (HMDs) enable the viewer to have an immersive visual experience while moving the head freely. HMDs also shield the player from distracting environments. Combined with motion sensors, HMDs are able to track head orientation and movement, creating a first-person viewing experience that a regular flat screen cannot (Figure 14.17). Besides, new HMDs such as Google Glass

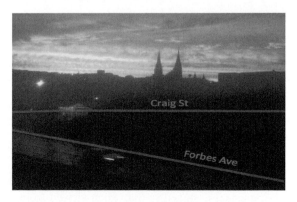

FIGURE 14.17   An HMD view of the augmented reality map for navigation, where the street names are superimposed on the live video.

devices are able to overlay a graphical model on top of real-world scenes, creating a so-called augmented reality. Video game images can be projected onto real-world images through holographic media on the lenses of glasses or can be merged in the processor and projected to HMD screens.

Stereoscopic Display

Stereoscopic displays are widely used in eye exams, such as tests for lazy eye, which doctors use to find out whether a patient's two eyes are moving together. Stereoscopic displays are also used for depth perception tests, which reveal vision defects.

HMDs can be used for personal stereo displays. HMDs create two perfect separate viewing channels for stereoscopic vision. As many video games contain 3D models, we can calculate stereo-pair images with the depth cue of disparity, which affords more accurate 3D percepts than conventional displays.

Stereoscopic video games can be projected onto a large screen with two regular data projectors with horizontal and vertical polarized filters in front of the lens. A typical stereoscopic projection screen needs a special coating film to reflect polarized lights, and such a film is expensive. An affordable alternative is to spray a metallic silver paint on any flat surface to turn it into a projection screen. To view the projected stereoscopic images, the players need to wear polarized 3D glasses, similar to the kind movie theaters provide.

Autostereoscopy is a method of displaying stereoscopic images without the use of special glasses (Figure 14.18); it is also called glasses-free 3D display. Autostereoscopic displays include parallax barriers, lenticular lenses, and volumetric displays such as swept-volume displays.

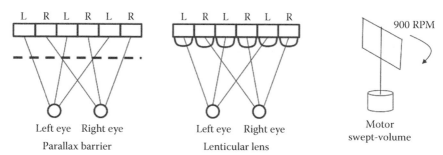

FIGURE 14.18 Autostereoscopic displays: parallax barrier LCD, lenticular lens, and swept-volume display.

A parallax barrier is a grid with a series of precision slits placed in front of the normal LED (light-emitting diodes) screen, allowing each eye to see a different set of pixels and creating a sense of depth through the parallax effect. A lenticular lens is an array of magnifying lenses designed so that when viewed from slightly different angles, different images are magnified, giving the illusion of depth. A disadvantage of this technology is that the viewer must be positioned in a well-defined spot to experience the 3D effect. Another disadvantage is that the effective horizontal pixel count viewable by each eye is reduced by one-half.

Swept-surface or swept-volume displays are volumetric displays that use a z-axis rotating screen. When the screen is rotating at 900 rpm, we can perceive a volumetric scene. The content of the display synchronizes with the rotating angle of the screen so that the viewer can even see the back of a sculpture if the viewer walks around the display.

14.9   GAME DEVELOPMENT TOOL KITS

Following are samples of game development tool kits. Note that simple 2D games are more useful in ambient diagnostics than photorealistic 3D games, especially on mobile platforms, for which graphical processor and networking resources are very limited.

Image Tagging

Image tagging is a key function for ambient diagnostics, especially in crowdsourcing. It provides annotations that both humans and machines can understand. Tags are words or phrases meant to act as keywords. They are searchable within the site and can show popular topics. They also improve search relevance.

Many social media sites already have provided image-tagging utilities, such as Facebook, where the user can tag an image by placing a box on a specific spot on a photograph and give it a name and a location. This enables users to identify objects by visual inspection or by matching the list of contained objects with their tag displays. Another capability incorporates the site's concept of "friends." If the section of the photograph tagged is identified as a friend on the site, the person's name will link to the person's profile. In addition, the site will count this image in the "photos of" feature on the person's profile, allowing the inclusion of photos added by other users.

Tags are metadata and can be embedded directly into image files for portability. Tags can be written in XML (Extensible Markup Language) in general, but there are many dialects, such as FotoNotes, a data format for annotating images. Adobe Systems also created a metadata framework for images called XMP (Extensible Metadata Platform), a subset of XML. Other image metadata include the MPEG-7 standards for the multimedia content description interface, allowing embedded game objects onto videos and vice versa. There are many tools for creating image tags. For example, Thing Link is a tool for image tagging,[313] and Photo Tagger is an iPhone application for tagging photos.[314]

---

[313] http://www.thinglink.com/
[314] https://itunes.apple.com/us/app/photo-tagging-tool/id576451336?mt=8

Flash Game Engines

Flash game engines are a tool for building browser-based 2D games.[315] Here, we introduce two Flash game engines: Flixel and FlashPunk.

Flixel can turn an idea from a sketch to a playable game quickly. It works on image pixels directly instead of on vector drawings. In many cases, this can be faster than letting Flash handle the drawing itself, making it a good choice for graphically intense games. The rest of Flixel's features include tile maps, collisions, particles, and a debugger. Flixel is ideal for rapidly prototyping a game.

FlashPunk has a unique animation library, allowing developers to apply programmatic motion to in-game objects. It includes collision detection (i.e., checking for object overlap). However, there are no physics libraries featured out of the box, leaving developers to build their own or plug-in an existing physics library. Built-in physics means faster development, but external libraries mean more freedom and control. The idea of control is evident across the FlashPunk project, with space left for developers to substitute their own code or other libraries for many of the core features.

JavaScript Game Engine

The JavaScript game engine can be embedded into any web page and will run for everyone on desktops, netbooks, game consoles, and handheld devices, giving developers the largest user base of any platform. A JavaScript code usually resides on the server machine, or cloud. It runs on the client's side when the user opens the web page. Therefore, a JavaScript-based game code is normally simple and short.

jsGameSoup[316] is a game engine class in JavaScript. It has a cross-browser event-handling class, game entity and sprite management classes, collision detection, sound effects playback with audio class, FMS, and URL and query string parsing classes.

Second Life

Second Life is perhaps the most innovative online virtual world ever developed, enabled by a number of free client programs so that real-world users can interact with each other through avatars, or residents. Residents can explore the online world, known as the "grid," meet other residents, socialize, participate in individual and group activities, and create and trade virtual property and services with one another.

Rich in high-quality 3D content, contributed mainly by online users, Second Life is a user-centric social medium. Unlike a traditional computer game, Second Life does not have a designated objective or traditional game play mechanics or rules. Second Life is a multiuser virtual world because the virtual world is centered around interaction between multiple users. As it does not have any stipulated goals, it is irrelevant to talk about winning or losing in relation to Second Life. Likewise, unlike a

---

[315] http://www.netmagazine.com/features/top-three-flash-game-engines
[316] http://jsgamesoup.net/

traditional game, Second Life contains an extensive world that can be explored and interacted with, and it can be used purely as a creative tool set.

Second Life is not a typical online action game such as World of Warcraft, but rather more or less a virtual "piazza" where people can meet from different parts of the world. Potential applications of online virtual worlds are attracting the interest of many researchers around the world. In 2007, Second Life released sources for its client application under the GPL (General Public License), allowing anyone to extend it by building a modified client. Because of avatars' anonymity – one user may have up to five avatars and versatile social interaction scenarios (e.g., living, playing, talking, texting, or building together), Second Life has been a virtual psychology lab for many doctoral students from fields like clinical psychology and the social sciences.

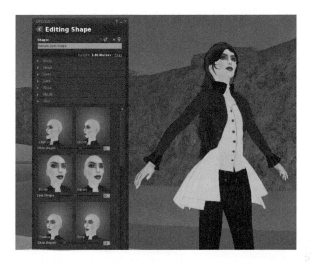

FIGURE 14.19 Avatar appearance editing toolbox in Second Life.

Second Life is a platform for a non-programmer to prototype a social interaction game, given built-in utilities, such as a 3D modeling tool and the scripting language (Figure 14.19). The 3D modeling tool contains appearance editing tools and simple geometric shapes that allow residents to build virtual objects. A user can change the appearance of an avatar, such as the shape of the eyes, nose, mouth, and body.

There is also a procedural scripting language, Linden Scripting Language, which can be used to add interactivity to objects. Sculpted prims (basic shapes), mesh, textures for clothing or other objects, animators, and gestures can be created using external software or imported by simple dragging and dropping of the scripts to objects in real time. It is an innovation in software engineering—an object can "wear" a code like a cloth. For example, a user can drag a gesture script for walking like a fashion model or like a gangster. The user may also transform the avatar from a human to a different being, such as a cockroach like in Kafka's novel, by dragging the new appearance script.

Second Life allows researchers to build and test cognitive experiments at an extremely low cost. The collaborative platform of Second Life enables developers to work together from different parts of the world. Figure 14.20 is a screenshot of an online game experiment, Hanoi Tower, developed by an author in the United States and a student in Australia. Hanoi Tower is a famous cognitive game about problem-solving strategy. It has three pegs for holding multiple disks. The goal is to move the disks from the starting peg to the end peg one disk a time. Smaller disks must always be on top of larger ones. The avatar in the black cloth is the American author, and the avatar with a gray tail on the right is the Australian student. The game design contains three rings and three pegs, edited with a 3D modeling tool. The script describes the moving rules and event handling. Second Life handles the physics automatically that detect the collisions between the rings, pegs, and the base, ensuring the rings will not drop into the earth or fly away. As it turns out, the game was successfully created by the Australian author and tested by many online users. It allows multiple users to play from different locations, and it allows users to simulate real-world physical movements like picking an object up, moving it, and dropping it. However, the simulation also creates unexpected effects, such as perceptual illusions; for example, the ring may sometimes seem to be on the top of a peg due to the depth illusion caused by the 3D model. A stereo display system can correct the depth problem, but it would increase the complexity of the model.

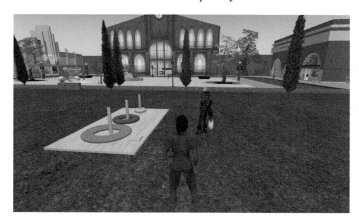

FIGURE 14.20 The Hanoi Tower game was developed remotely in Second Life. The man wearing the leather jacket was the author. The man wearing the wolf tail was the Australian student.

Second Life is a model of real life. The borderline between the two is blurring. Some interfaces are extended to the real world and beyond; for example, voice chat incorporates physical properties such as the distance between the speakers. "Wearable" translators enable users to read translated text messages as they are typing.

Researchers may push the envelope of the virtual world to its limit and discover new problems and find new solutions along the way. For example, social interaction in online virtual worlds occurs through text messaging, audio, and visual modalities, as for almost any other current digital entertainment system. Tactile-based inter-action has not yet been explored. A haptic interface has been developed to help visually impaired people navigate and explore the simulated 3D environment by exploiting the force feedback capabilities of these devices.[317]

OpenSim

OpenSim or OpenSimulator is a clone of Second Life in open source. It is a server platform for hosting virtual worlds that are compatible with the client for Second Life, although it can host alternative worlds with different features with multiple protocols. Compared to Second Life, OpenSim has much smaller online communities. However, the open source platform gives developers ultimate freedom to write modules at any level in C# or through the use of plug-in modules. OpenSim can operate in one of two modes: stand-alone or grid mode. In stand-alone mode, a single process handles the entire simulation. In grid mode, various aspects of the simulation are separated among multiple processes, which can exist on different machines. Stand-alone mode is simpler to configure but is limited to a smaller number of users, such as a research group. Grid mode has the potential to scale up as the number of users grows.[318]

Game Studio 3D

Game Studio is a rapid game-authoring system for interactive 3D applications (Figure 14.21), including physics engines, avatar modelers, and world artwork editors. It is a commercial game engine at an affordable price range. It offers three levels of access. Beginners can click together 3D racing or action games from preas-sembled game templates. A simple action or car-racing game can be built in a few hours this way. Advanced developers can create commercial-quality applications with the lite-C scripting language. They can use the included level and model editors to create the avatars and world artwork. For professional-level developers, the Game Studio A8 can be programmed in C++ or C# and interfaced with high-end editors such as 3DS MAX™ or MAYA™.

Unreal

Unreal Engine 3 is a professional game engine developed by Epic Games. The Unreal Development Kit (UDK) is free for noncommercial and educational use. UDK has been used in game development, architectural visualization, mobile game develop-ment, 3D rendering, and digital films. Developers can share code and experiences through the Unreal Developer Network[319] that connects peers in the world.

[317] Maurizio de Pascale, Sara Mulatto, and Domenico Prattichizzo. Bringing haptics to Second Life for visually impaired people. In M. Ferre (ed.), *EuroHaptics 2008*, LNCS 5024. Springer-Verlag, New York, 2008, pp. 896–905.

[318] http://en.wikipedia.org/wiki/IBM_Virtual_Universe_Community

[319] http://udn.epicgames.com/Main/WebHome.html

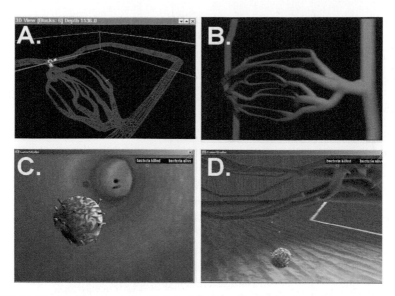

FIGURE 14.21   BioSim game developed with Game Studio 3D A1. World model and biological characters implemented in the game. (a) Wireframe model of the vascular system world model; (b) 3D photorealistic model showing arteries and capillaries; (c) the macrophage (white blood cell) is inside the bloodstream with red blood cells; (d) after actively moving out of the bloodstream, the macrophage approaches bacteria that infected human body tissue.

UnrealScript (UScript) is the script language of the Unreal Engine and is used for authoring 3D game code and game play events. UnrealScript is very similar to C/C++ and Java. However, it differs widely from these traditional languages in that UnrealScript addresses issues that these other languages do not. One of the major features of UnrealScript is that it enables scripted artificial intelligence (AI) behavior (e.g., having avatars follow predefined actions rather than choosing them dynamically).[320] With the scripted AI behavior, it is much faster to execute by applying a simple rule rather than running a complex physical simulation model, and it is easier to write, understand, and modify. The game-specific scripting language allows non-programmers to create or modify the game behavior. For example,

```
if glucose = low and in-take = no
        weak …
        fall …
else
        run …
return
```

However, scripted AI behavior will need many scripted rules whose actions are difficult to predict. It may cause complex debugging problems. Also, scripted AI behavior may limit players' creativity; for example, players would try things that are

---

[320] http://web.cs.wpi.edu/~rich/courses/imgd4000-d09/lectures/C-Scripting.pdf

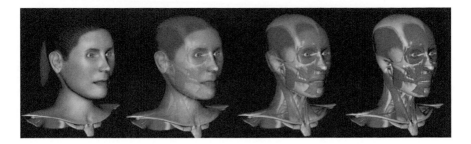

FIGURE 14.22   Anomalous Medical animated sequence of normal chewing, based on OGRE 3D.

supposed to work, and they would be disappointed when they do not. Players will learn the limits of the scripts and exploit them.

OGRE 3D

OGRE (Object-Oriented Graphics Rendering Engine) is a 3D game engine specializing in real-time hardware-accelerated 3D graphics. Since 2001, OGRE has grown to become one of the most popular open source graphics-rending engines. It has been used in a large number of production projects outside of games, simulators, scientific visualization, and educational software, such as the nongaming application 3D medical simulation called Anomalous Medical, a medical framework based around the human head. It offers a detailed and anatomically correct model of the human head that one can move around, look into, and examine in various other ways. This enables developers to create a wide variety of applications, covering dental issues, nerve blocks, certain muscle areas, and so on that can be loaded in to deal with specific medical situations and defects. Figure 14.22 shows an animation of a normal chewing sequence. This app is a great tool for visualizing how the anatomy functions during normal chewing.

14.10   SUMMARY

In this chapter, we studied the emerging uses of video games for diagnoses, mainly in three categories: observing perception–action processes, observing social interactions, and crowdsourcing. The following were discussed:

- A typical game engine consists of input processes, a physics engine (i.e., collision detection), score calculation, and rendering algorithms. However, for diagnostic or scientific discovery purposes, it is not necessary to have all of the elements, such as a physics engine and photorealistic 3D rendering. In many cases, a simple graphical user interface is enough.
- Client-server networking enables multiple users to play online games. To resolve the network delay issues, we can predict an avatar's motion by extrapolating or interpolating methods.
- An FSM is an essential modeling tool for designing an avatar's finite states. However, it does not cover the concurrent behaviors.

- World modeling is a basic platform for designing the stage where avatars show up. It contains multiple views in multiple windows.
- Motion capture and control devices enable developers or users to input the gesture data for controlling the game. New devices such as Kinect create new opportunities for markerless motion capture and real-time gesture-based control.
- State-of-the-art game display technologies such as Retina Display, HMD, and stereoscopic display devices enable users to have surrealistic visual experiences.
- Finally, we presented a variety of open source game development tool kits, from low-end image-tagging tools such as Flash game engines and JavaScript game engines, to high-end development tool kits such as Second Life, OpenSim, Game Studio 3D, Unreal, and OGRE 3D.

PROBLEMS

1. Download the game Second Life and select your avatar. Edit the avatar with Second Life editing utilities, such as profile, facial, body, and outfit features. Observe the population on the island. Observe the languages and social interactions in the virtual world.
2. Build a 3D ball in Second Life's sandbox area (it is free to test your objects). Save your objects in your account. Test the physics engine inside Second Life, for example, testing collision detection by walking into a tree and observe whether the tree has a collision detection border or not (the avatar can pass through the tree). Record the video and analyze the results in the report.
3. Test what would happen to the avatar if there were no collision detection on the ground.
4. Teleport your avatar to a party event and observe the social interactions on the island and network latency. Summarize your observations in a report.
5. Draw an FSM for your avatar behavior. Define the states when the avatar is idle without input from the user or the updates from the server.
6. Observe your avatar's interaction modes (chat, voice, dance, idle, move together, etc.) and the personal spaces (distance between avatars).
7. Use the Kinect to develop a video game to evaluate a user's hand coordination by drawing air graffiti on the screen. Discuss the potential for diagnoses.
8. Select a game from an online store that can be used for ambient diagnoses, such as tremor evaluation or measuring the effectiveness of a physical therapy.
9. Use JavaScript to develop a 2D image-mching game (e.g., matching images with words). Make a demo on a web page. Discuss the potential in crowd-sourcing for acquiring diagnostic knowledge.

15 Social Media

Objects are gathered by attributes.

—Chinese Proverb

15.1 INTRODUCTION

Social media enable network citizens to share health information and search for information about rare diseases that local doctors may not be able to help them with. The keywords used in each search inquiry can also be a crowdsourcing resource for the monitoring of epidemic diseases such as the swine flu. Social media are powerful tools for ambient diagnoses. They save lives. This chapter explores

- How to analyze the relevancy of the content of social media
- How to analyze the reputation of a social media site
- How to visualize a social network
- How to analyze correlation of variables
- What are the tools for designing and analyzing social media?

15.2 THE PREGNANT MAN

A man found a pregnancy test kit in the medicine cabinet where his ex-girlfriend had left it.[321] As a joke, he urinated on it, and much to his surprise, the kit showed a positive symbol. A friend of the man thought the situation funny enough to create a "rage comic" about it and post it on the social media website Reddit (Figure 15.1).[322]

The very first person to comment on the post was a user named goxilo, who wrote, "If this is true, you should check yourself for testicular cancer. Seriously. Google it." Goxilo turned out to be correct: The man visited the doctor and was found to have testicular cancer. The hormone hCG (human chorionic gonadotropin) is also produced by the tumors in a very rare type of testicular cancer, choriocarcinoma. Choriocarcinoma is dangerous and aggressive; it can spread throughout the body before the patient is even aware of its existence.

Luckily, the Reddit user's friend saw the doctor early enough to make treatment possible. After the diagnosis, the man's friend posted another rage comic to Reddit with an update.[323] The comic drew more than 1,300 comments from concerned strangers in three days.[324]

---

[321] http://www.forbes.com/sites/daviddisalvo/2012/11/10/how-a-pregnancy-test-told-a-man-that-he-has-testicular-cancer/
[322] http://imgur.com/Xt6B5
[323] http://imgur.com/oG492
[324] http://www.reddit.com/r/fffffffuuuuuuuuuuuu/comments/12kihx/pregnant_man_rage/c6wyitw

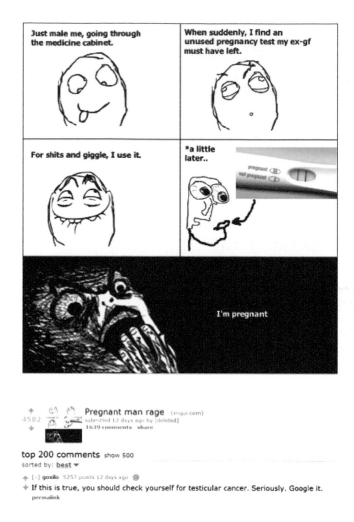

FIGURE 15.1 The original "pregnant man" post on the social media site Reddit and the key response from a user. (Courtesy of imgur.com for image use.)

Testicular cancer is a very rare disease, and it is hard to detect at the early stages. Social media helped this particular patient receive timely advice. Now, let us reengineer this story to find out what the patient did right to trigger the avalanche of responses online.

15.3 RELEVANCY ANALYSIS

First, let us look at the social media site Reddit that the man used. Reddit is a popular website for young and energetic users.[325] Content on Reddit is ranked based on users' ratings, so the most highly voted new links and comments end up at the top and are

---

[325] http://www.reddit.com/

most easily viewed by users. Reddit as a whole has 400 million unique viewers, 43 million users, and 37 billion page views.[326]

Reddit provides a platform for social networking, mainly within topic groups. The relevancy of a post to the theme of the topic group is critical, or the post is ignored. Also, there really is no substitute for lots of good content. Web surfers normally have very short attention spans. Only topics that are interesting in some way, such as by being humorous, controversial, or newsworthy, can attract the glimpse of a large number of users. That a woman is pregnant will not be big news to the people outside her group of friends. However, a man who claims to be pregnant is newsworthy, comical, and controversial. Reddit has cleverly designed top-level themes for posting, such as "pics," "funny," "gaming," "IamA," "today I learned," and "WTF" (Figure 15.2). When comparing these topics to, for example, ABC News' themes like "world," "politics," "investigative," "health," and "money," it is easy to see that Reddit has targeted more diverse, young, and energetic web surfers.

For each subject, Reddit has five classifications for users to browse posts: "hot," "new," "rising," "controversial," and "top." Posts are sorted into these categories by user votes. What can one learn from Reddit? The top ten most popular genres can be grouped into three categories: fun (funny and gaming), visual (pics and video), and new (WTF, world news, politics, IAmA, Today I Learned, and Ask Reddit) (Figure 15.3).

The pregnant man message was posted on the funny group, which attracted massive attention. The post was also packaged in a comic style that stood out from the majority of the text posts on Reddit.

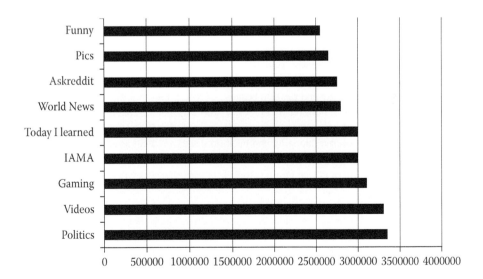

FIGURE 15.2   Chart of Reddit top-level themes.

---

[326] Craig Smith. How many people use the top social media, apps and services? *Digital Marketing Ramblings* April 3, 2013. Accessed April 6, 2013.

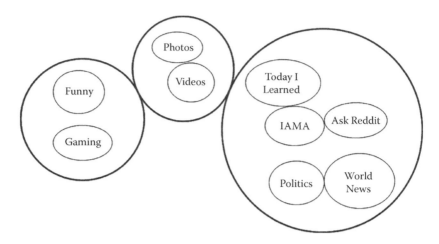

FIGURE 15.3   Cluster of Reddit top-level themes: I see, I learn, and I have fun.

Katamari Effect

Katamari Damacy is a puzzle-action video game in which things start small but build up gradually. Much like in the game, a small niche subject on Reddit might generate a large volume of follow-up posts and external link juice. The following are a portion of the posts about the pregnant man on Reddit gathered at the time of writing. As you can see, within one month, the follow-ups moved from gastro-intestinal symptoms to other symptoms.

- If this is true, you should check yourself for testicular cancer. Seriously. Google it. [5,487 points]
- Reminds me of a guy who posted a picture of his feet and someone commented telling him he has a serious back issue and he can tell by looking at his feet. Turns out he did and got help because of reddit. [560 points]
- On my phone now, but I recall a redditor who commented that his poop that morning looked like coffee grounds. Because of Reddit, he found out that was a sign of internal bleeding and he should seek medical attention immediately. [360 points]
- I've never heard of coffee ground stool. I thought that was called Starbucks. [242 points]
- Correct. Coffee ground emesis (vomiting) is a sign of upper gi bleeding. If he had upper gi bleeding the stool would look dark, black like tar by the time he passed his rectum. Smells really bad and is sometimes purplish. Lower gi bleeding is mostly redish, dark red, or sometimes clots. That's the general answer, but shit changes. I've never heard of coffee ground stool. [101 points]
- Maybe it was vomiting? [83 points]
- And if you ever piss blood get yourself to the ER yesterday. A friend of mine was kicked in the stomach during a rugby game at college and came into class to tell us he'd pissed blood. He was being manly man about it, but it scared the shit out of me for some reason. I took him to ER, speeding all the way, and the doctors told me I'd saved his life by speeding. [75 points]

- Supposedly a disgruntled employee shat in the coffee machine at a McDonalds once. Nobody noticed because, well, McDonalds coffee. [31 point]

Figure 15.4 shows the path of thinking from the pregnant man to testicular cancer. Using analogical thinking, the second post *recalled* the photo of the foot that led to back injury issues. Furthermore, the third post recalled the case of black stool that is a sign of internal bleeding. This analogical thinking seems illogical but created a symptom–diagnosis knowledge base of the kind people have used for thousands of years.

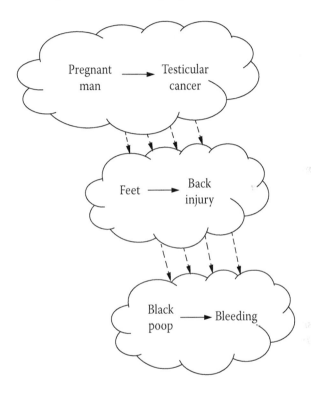

FIGURE 15.4   Topic-shifting dynamics by analogical thinking.

Sprout Branches

Social networks are dynamic in nature. They are born; they grow, transform, and merge; and often, they die. In graph theories, network expansions have been abstractly measured as the growth rate of random nodes. In social networks, those expansions are not random. Instead, they grow or decline in interconnected clusters that carry the original DNA with allowable mutation. The ratio of the increased number of nodes versus the original branch of nodes is called the sprout rate (Figure 15.5).

Growing special interest groups is a strategy in social networking. For example, Reddit is a website that is made up of a large number of different communities, called subreddits. There are currently 10,000 active subreddits out of over 100,000

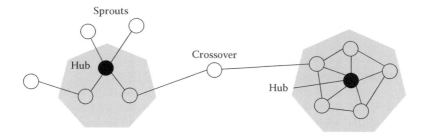

FIGURE 15.5   Sprout, crossover, and hub patterns.

total,[327] each made up of users who together form an individual community with its own topics, goals, and standards. Subreddits drive Reddit's growth, as more focused communities continue to branch off popular posting topics.

Social networks are also volunteer networks. User-based moderators in Reddit create new communities or are added to subreddits that already exist. Moderators can add or remove other moderators, remove spam or inappropriate posts from their subreddits, respond to requests and feedback, and adjust the visual appearance of their subreddits.

Similarly, Facebook encourages users to create their own pages with special interests. Successful pages such as the series "I Fucking Love XYZ" ("I Fucking Love Science," "I Fucking Love Biology," "I Fucking Love Archeology") and other nearly professional pages ("Interesting Engineering," "Designer," and "Evolution") have attracted millions of readers. Many are actually made by professional organizations, such as museums and universities. Pages have the same style and format as the rest of the Facebook site, but they are normally hosted and updated by individual page creators.

Crossover Groups

Crossover is common in genetic algorithms; a number of genes cross over to other groups. In social networks, crossover is also a valuable mechanism for a user to access information from other groups. Many social networks in fact encourage crossover posting by embedding links from other sites. For example, Facebook can play videos posted on YouTube or Vimeo. Furthermore, a friend's friend may have different interests or be linked to special interest groups with different "genes." Here, we define the number of crossover interactions over the total interaction as the crossover rate.

Privacy

Today, social networks have prioritized users' privacy significantly. When we talk about privacy, it is normally associated with identity: passwords, date of birth, home

---

[327] John Herrman. Reddit general manager explains why he won't ban creepy. *BuzzFeed* October 11, 2012. Accessed April 6, 2013.

address, family details, travels and activities, and so on. These are necessary measures for security purposes (e.g., for preventing online identity theft). As a result, users select privacy options to *divide* their social networks. For example, a user might choose to make his or her profile or content open to the public, open to friends but not friends' friends, or open to a few close friends. These segmentations create borderlines for interactions, either one way or two ways. We can call this the privacy rate, ranging from 0 (all public) to 100 (all private).

Intimacy is associated with privacy. However, when *anonymity* is possible, users sometimes post intimate details publicly, such as details about personal health conditions, marital status, depression, surgeries, and personal images and videos. For example, the pregnant man posted his private experiment to the public on Reddit, which has over three million possible viewers.

Intimacy is not only physical but also psychological. It is the act of connecting with someone deeply. Wherever social networks exist, there is intimate content posted in public anonymously. We evaluate the level of intimacy using the "intimacy rate," ranging from 0 to 100 (very personally, physically, and psychologically revealing). Amazingly, those who post with a high intimacy rate often receive lots of unexpected help. Their lives may even be saved.

Visual Effects

Facebook, like Reddit, is also a popular social media site. It is more image-oriented and historically was something like an electronic yearbook for students, so it still retains its visual roots. An interesting photo is usually more attractive to users than a plain text message. Even many quotes and scientific stories are embedded into pictures, leaving words as captions.

Over 90% of the daily information we encounter is visually based. Visual interaction enables an instinctive response indicating whether a picture is interesting, boring, disgusting, or anything else. However, as more and more Facebook members use mobile applications to access the site, the resolutions and sizes of images become problematic. For example, the default image orientation on many phones is either landscape or square. Some phones may automatically crop a portrait-oriented image to a square image.

15.4   REPUTATION ANALYSIS

Interaction Frequency

How often a user interacts on a social medium is an important measurement for ambient diagnosis. The interaction frequency (IF) can be defined as the number of a type of interaction per duration (e.g., the number of log-ins to the Facebook site per week). Although there is no definite minimal IF value, by using common sense, a person normally can tell where the threshold is. If the IF on a site is too low below a threshold, then no one would revisit the site. If Sergey Brin, one of the cofounders of Google, only posted two blog posts on his site in a year, then perhaps no one would revisit his website. We call the lowest IF a survival IF (SIF) value. It is critical for a site designer to know the expected IF (EIF), maximal IF (MIF), and SIF. The SIF may also be used as a measurement for filtering out weak links.

Facebook does a good job monitoring interaction frequencies. For example, it has an activity log database to track the timeline of interaction details. This, of course, can be used for monitoring users' online behaviors, habits, and preferences.

IF may also be used for ambient diagnostics (Figure 15.6). Assume an elderly person who lives alone has "normal" frequencies of checking e-mails and logging on to Facebook daily. If there is no sign of interaction for a few days, it might be time to check on the person. The following section on visualization discusses how to present the interaction patterns visually.

	Like	Share	Comments	Post
1	2		2	1
2				
3	9	2		
4	1		1	
5	1			
6	6	3	4	
7				
8				
9				
10	6	3	1	
11	2			
12	1		1	
13	6	1		
14				
15				
16				
17	1			
18				
19				
20				
21				
22				
23				
24				

FIGURE 15.6   Interaction histogram of 24-hour activity log data from Facebook.

The Power Law

Not everything in a social network is equal; and not every social network site is equal. It is sometimes the case that a small number of savvy users have massive groups of friends or fans and frequent posts, but the rest of the network members have much fewer friends or few posts. Some users just read posts but do not leave comments or post their own content, engaging in one-way interaction. We call those center-of-attention sites or savvy users "hubs" or "gateways." Through hubs, users can easily access different groups. Without hubs, a social network has the potential to die quickly.

This unique property of a social network is called the scale-free network; the position of the individuals is irrelevant for forming connections. Individuals with high numbers of contacts can be represented by the *power law*, in which the fraction $P(k)$ of nodes in the network having k connections to other nodes goes for large values of k as

$$P = c \cdot k^{-\gamma} \tag{15.1}$$

where c is the constant, and γ is a parameter whose value is typically in the range $2 < \gamma < 3.5$, although occasionally it may lie outside these bounds.

The power law is also called Zipf's law, which usually refers to the "size" of an occurrence of an event relative to its rank. It was named after George Kingsley Zipf, a Harvard linguistics professor, who discovered that a very small group of words makes up the most frequently used words in the English language. The majority of words are not used often at all.

In science and engineering, we often use log-log plots (logarithmic scales on both the horizontal and vertical axes) to reveal the so-called monomial of the form $p = c \cdot k^m$, which appears as a straight line in a log-log plot, with the power and constant term corresponding to the slope and intercept of the line (Figure 15.7). Thus, the plot is useful for recognizing the power law relationship and estimating parameters (Figure 15.8). Any base can be used for the logarithm, although the most common are 10, e, and 2.

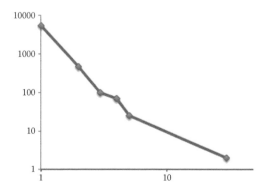

FIGURE 15.7 Power law of hub effect of Reddit points and number of posters in log-log scales.

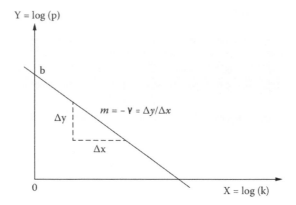

FIGURE 15.8   Log-log plot for estimating parameters of a power law relationship.

Given a monomial equation $p = c \cdot k^m$, taking the logarithm of the equation with any base yields

$$\log(p) = m \log(k) + \log(c) \tag{15.2}$$

Setting $X = \log(k)$ and $Y = \log(p)$, which corresponds to using a log-log plot, yields the equation

$$Y = m \cdot X + b \tag{15.3}$$

where $m = -\gamma$ is the slope of the line (gradient), and $b = \log(c)$ is the intercept on the $\log(p)$ axis, meaning where $\log(k) = 0$, c is the p value corresponding to $k = 1$.

PageRank

To create a successful website or page, the contents need to be interesting (relevant) and important (reputable). How can one attract incoming links to a website? The number and value of sites that link to a page is often referred to as the page's "link juice" or "Google juice."

Google uses a "crawler" or "spider" called the "Googlebot" to automatically index pages on the web. Google usually takes an average of six to eight weeks to index a newly submitted site. When a user submits the site URL to Google, Googlebot goes through each link on each page. It reads through all the site pages to pick up keywords, then saves and indexes the pages in its catalog cache. Thus, it is important to make sure that all the pages of a site link to each other so that Googlebot has easy access to all of the relevant pages. Another way to make sure this is done is to have a site map for all the pages.

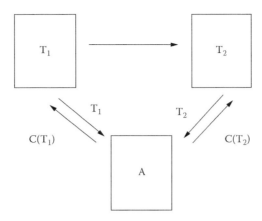

FIGURE 15.9   Illustration of PageRank algorithm.

Being indexed by Googlebot is just the first step to being ranked on Google, so one should not expect pages to show up in searches immediately. One must give it some time and work on optimizing the web pages.

PageRank[328] (PR) is an algorithm that determines how important a page is compared to the other pages on the web (Figure 15.9). In the algorithm, a link to a page counts as a vote of support. PR does not take into consideration anchor text, whether sites are related, spam, and other factors. PR just shows link popularity. It is useful in determining whether a site is working properly or to see if a site has been penalized, for instance. However, over time, this metric has fallen by the wayside a bit and is mostly useful now only in general ways.

Assume page A has pages $T_1 \ldots T_n$ that point to it (i.e., are citations). The parameter d is a damping factor that can be set between 0 and 1. We usually set d to 0.85. Also, $C(A)$ is defined as the number of links going out of page A. The PR of a page A is given as follows:

$$PR(A) = (1-d) + d \cdot \sum_{i=1}^{n} \frac{PR(T_i)}{C(T_i)} \qquad (15.4)$$

Note that the PRs form a probability distribution over web pages, so the sum of all web pages' PRs will be one. PR or PR(A) can be calculated using a simple iterative algorithm and corresponds to the principal eigenvector of the normalized link matrix of the web. Also, a PR for 26 million web pages can be computed in a few hours on a medium-size workstation. There is also a MATLAB code for demonstrating how the PR works.[329]

The Google toolbar (http://toolbar.google.com/) actually displays PR on the toolbar of web browsers. The toolbar PR goes from 0 to 10 in a logarithmic scale.

---

[328] Lawrence Page, US Patent 6,285,999 B1. http://www.google.com/patents?vid=6285999
[329] http://en.wikipedia.org/wiki/PageRank

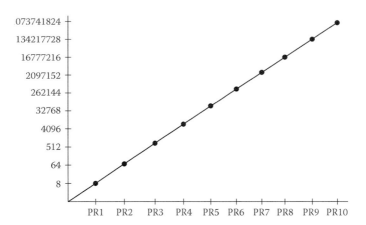

FIGURE 15.10   Relationship between PageRank and external backlinks.

The mechanics of PR are logarithmic (Figure 15.10). If we want to see a higher PR, it is not the volume of links alone that matters. We must consider and seek out higher-rank pages for obtaining links. For example, according to a recent report from checkpagerank.net,[330] the website Reddit's PR is strong (8/10), with 438,345,253 external backlinks. The results also showed that the site has over 915,404 referring domains. Amazingly enough, the survey tool also uses backlinks from .edu and .gov sites as a measurement of reputation (e.g., 587,511 .edu backlinks and 804,161 .gov backlinks). Checkpagerank.net also reports the history of the website: for Reddit, seven years and fourteen days for false PR detection.

The superstar website cnn.com's PR is very strong (9/10) with 144,094,945 external backlinks, 781,413 referring domains, 302,014 .edu backlinks, and 60,795 .gov backlinks. As we can see here, CNN has a stronger PR than Reddit with fewer external backlinks. What principles can be learned from this? Good places for a page to be linked to by an external site might include a page where no "no follow" tags are used, a relevant page to the website being linked to, a page with a higher PR, and by a link that is not used for other purposes like redirecting.

The Google Toolbar's PR is an important index for ranking popularity, and it is updated on Google infrequently, usually in quarters. Google does have an internal and more sophisticated version of PR that is updated much more frequently. If the designed website is relatively new (e.g., less than a year old) and has dynamic parts, the PR will probably be outdated by the time one actually sees it.

15.5   VISUALIZING SOCIAL NETWORKS

Force-Directed Graph

The force-directed graph[331] is an algorithm that not only can aesthetically visualize the layout of a network but also can project approximate feature vector distances to a

---

[330] http://www.checkpagerank.net/
[331] http://bl.ocks.org/benzguo/4370043

two-dimensional (2D) or three-dimensional (3D) space. The algorithm is a simulation of a mass-spring physics, where each graph node is connected by a spring. The system consists of repulsive forces between all graph nodes and attractive forces between adjacent nodes. The force models considered correspond to Hooke's law (repulsion forces) and Coulomb's law (attraction forces). The algorithm iteratively tries to reduce stress between each graph node and dynamically plot the graph until the equilibrium is reached. An overview of the force-directed graph is available.[332] Figure 15.11 shows scenarios of attraction and repulsion forces when the two graph nodes are too close or too far apart, similar to one pressing or pulling a spring with two hands.

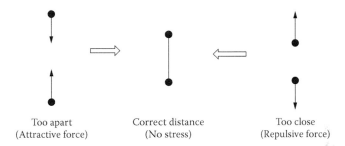

Too apart	Correct distance	Too close
(Attractive force)	(No stress)	(Repulsive force)

FIGURE 15.11   Using attraction force or repulsion force to make the distance correct.

To solve the multi-body mass-string model is a nontrivial problem. Fortunately, we can set some concurrent constraints; for example, the node should stay within a bounding box, and the distance between any two nodes should be within a fixed number (i.e., $\| x_2 - x_1 \| \leq 100$ pixels).

The pseudocode for the algorithm is as follows:

1.   Initialize the node positions.
2.   Do iteratively:
3.   Calculate repulsive forces.
4.   Calculate attractive forces.
5.   Rearrange positions to fit the canvas.
6.   Stop when the node distance criterion is met.

For more explanation of the pseudocode, a link is available.[333] Open source code can be found in a few places online. There are sites with JavaScript code with examples.[334,335]

Figure 15.12 shows an example of the force-directed graph of the interaction (co-occurrence) between characters in Victor Hugo's *Les Misérables* in each scene. In the graph, all the characters are divided into eight groups and coded in different colors. The force-directed graph places related characters in closer proximity, while unrelated characters are farther apart, but not too far away.

---

[332] http://cs.brown.edu/~rt/gdhandbook/chapters/force-directed.pdf
[333] http://web.archive.org/web/20080410171619/http://www.teknikus.dk/tj/gdc2001.htm
[334] http://philogb.github.io/blog/2009/09/30/force-directed-layouts/
[335] http://blog.ivank.net/force-based-graph-drawing-in-as3.html

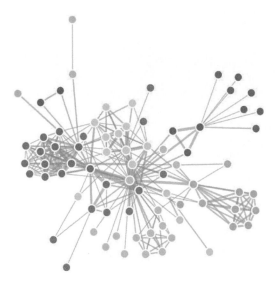

FIGURE 15.12 The force-directed graph of the interaction (co-occurrence) between characters in Victor Hugo's *Les Misérables* at each scene. Users can drag the nodes to move the graph dynamically.

There are also editing tools for building force-directed graphs; for example, Force Editor includes pan and zoom functions, based on another open source, D3.js. Force Editor enables the user to drag from an existing node to add a new node or link (Figure 15.13).

The force-directed graph is simple, intuitive, and aesthetically pleasing. However, it is computationally expansive. It would be slow to visualize large network problems, such as millions of nodes. In addition, the algorithm may run into local optima.

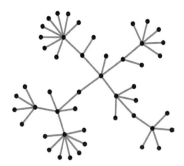

FIGURE 15.13 Force Editor enables users to add and delete nodes on the force-directed graph.

To avoid the problem, we can randomize the initial starting positions and run a few times to obtain better results.

15.6   CORRELATION ANALYSIS

Correlation analysis is a holy grail for data mining from social media. The word *correlation* is made of *co-* (meaning "together") and *relation*. Given two data sets, correlation analysis aims to find out whether the two sets are strongly linked together or not. If so, they are said to have a high correlation. Correlation can have a value, which shows how good the correlation is and if it is positive or negative.

Correlation is positive when the values in the two datasets increase together. For example, the sale of ice cream is correlated with the temperature in summer. The hotter it is, the more sales there are. A perfect positive correlation value is 1.

Correlation is negative when one value decreases as the other increases. For example, leather jacket sales are negatively correlated with the temperature. The hotter the weather is, the fewer sales there are. A perfect negative correlation value is −1.

No correlation means the two are not linked (e.g., the number of dust storms on Mars and number of likes on Facebook per month). The correlation value here is 0.

Scatter Plot

A scatter plot is a basic tool to begin to discover correlations with simple visualizations. Scatter plots are possible to make in Excel. Under the Chart menu in Excel, we can enter the two sets of data, for example, $\{x_i, y_i, i = 1, 2, \ldots, n\}$. Figures 15.14 and 15.15 show positive- and negative-correlation examples, respectively. To have a high correlation, we expect that the data points are as close to the straight line as possible.

However, more often the real-world data is complex. For example, the two sets of data can have no connection. In some other some cases, the relationship can be nonlinear. For example, when the temperature is too hot outside, people may not want to leave their air-conditioned homes for ice cream, so the sales will drop instead of going up. This phenomenon is also true in the relationship between physical performance and stress. When stress is low, the performance is worse. Increasing stress

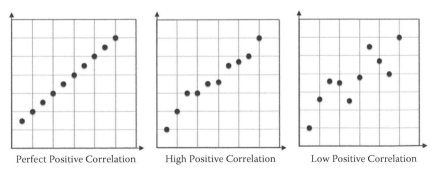

Perfect Positive Correlation   High Positive Correlation   Low Positive Correlation

FIGURE 15.14   Positive correlation examples.

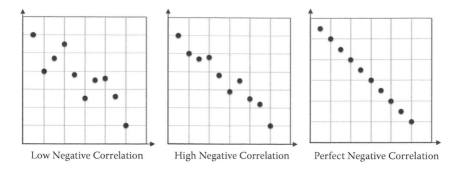

Low Negative Correlation   High Negative Correlation   Perfect Negative Correlation

FIGURE 15.15   Negative correlation examples.

can make an impression on the performance, but if we increase too much, the performance will become worse. For this kind of nonlinear correlation, we can linearize the problem by splitting the data into two or more linear segments. For example, in the ice cream case, we can divide the data according to "not too hot" and "too hot" segments. In the performance case, we can divide the data into "not too stressed" and "too stressed" segments.

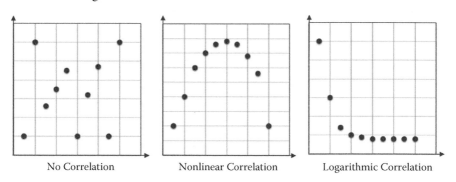

No Correlation   Nonlinear Correlation   Logarithmic Correlation

FIGURE 15.16   No correlation, nonlinear correlation, and logarithmic correlation.

As we discussed in a previous section, many online data shows logarithmic relationships (e.g., number of Facebook posts vs. number of users). In this case, we can try to plot $\log(X)$ and $\log(Y)$ to see if this helps to linearize the relationship. Figure 15.16 shows three scenarios: no correlation, nonlinear, and logarithmic correlations.

Pearson's Correlation Coefficient

In the 1880s, Karl Pearson developed a measure of the strength of linear correlation between two variables, giving a value between +1 and −1 inclusive. The value zero means no correlation. Assume x_i and y_i are two variables. $\bar{x}$ and $\bar{y}$ are their respective means.

$$r_{xy} = \frac{\sum\limits_{i=1}^{n}(x_i - \bar{x})(y_i - \bar{y})}{\sqrt{\sum\limits_{i=1}^{n}(x_i - \bar{x})^2 \sum\limits_{i=1}^{n}(y_i - \bar{y})^2}} \qquad (15.5)$$

The Pearson coefficient of correlation has been widely used in scientific analysis, including data mining from social media. The calculation is intuitive and can be done on a calculator or in Excel. Table 15.1 shows a typical range of Pearson coefficients of correlation.

TABLE 15.1 Correlation Coefficient Range

Correlation Coefficient	Relationship
$R > 0.8$	Very strong
$0.6 < R < 0.8$	Moderately strong
$0.3 < R < 0.5$	Fair
< 0.3	Poor

It is worth noting that *correlation is not causation*. When a correlation exists, it does not mean that one thing causes the other. For example, whenever the city of Pittsburgh has the Three Rivers Art Festival, it always rains and thunderstorms. It seems there is a correlation between the festival and rain. In fact, there is no direct causation between the two. However, both are correlated with a common variable: time of year. Normally, the festival is hosted in early June, when it is a rainy season in the Pittsburgh region.

Furthermore, a high correlation coefficient value may not be statistically significant (e.g., too few data points to justify). To validate the analysis, the Student *t* test is recommended. For more information, please refer to statistic textbooks or online materials.[336]

There are also approximate methods of calculating the coefficient, based on rank correlation, for example. That is reviewed in the following section.

Spearman's Rank Correlation

In 1904, Charles Spearman published a paper about a nonparametric measure of statistical dependence between two variables. It measures how well the correlation between two variables is using a monotonic function. A perfect Spearman correlation of +1 or −1 occurs when each of the variables is a perfect monotone function of the other without any repeated values.

---

[336] W. Mendenhall. *Introduction to probability and statistics*. Duxbury Press, Pacific Grove, CA, 1979.

Spearman's correlation uses ordinal scales (i.e., scores, orders, or ranks), in which we can only care about ranks instead of absolute values. Assume we study n types of cancers and we obtain the ranks from Google based on number of searches per type of cancer x_i and the ranks from the National Cancer Institute's (NCI's) annual report based on new cases per y_i. We can list the data as in Table 15.2.

TABLE 15.2 Ranking Data

Type	Google Rank (x_i)	NCI Rank (y_i)
Skin cancer	2	3
Colon cancer	1	2
Stomach cancer	3	4

Charles Spearman's rank coefficient is[337]

$$r_s = \frac{\sum_{i=1}^{n} (x_i - \overline{x})(y_i - \overline{y})}{\sqrt{\sum_{i=1}^{n} (x_i - \overline{x})^2 \sum_{i=1}^{n} (y_i - \overline{y})^2}} \tag{5.6}$$

where $\overline{x}$ and $\overline{y}$ are means.

When there are no ties in either the x observations or the y observations, the Equation 5.6 can be simplified to

$$r_s = 1 - \frac{6 \sum_{i=1}^{n} d_i^2}{n(n^2 - 1)} \qquad \text{where } d_i = x_i - y_i \tag{5.7}$$

As you can see, Spearman's rank coefficient is a nonparametric test that only preserves the ordinal relationship in the data. In contrast, Pearson's coefficient is a parametric test, which has more resolution than Spearman's.

Like Pearson's method, Spearman's coefficient calculation needs to pass the statistical significance test as well. There is a table designed for Spearman's test.[338] One important hint from the test is that the number of the ranks should be at least eight. Therefore, the rank data for the rudimentary problem is not enough.

---

[337] C. Spearman. The proof and measurement of association between two things. *American Journal of Psychology* 15:72–101, 1904.
[338] Mendenhall, *Introduction to probability and statistics*, 6th edition, PWS Publishers, 1983

15.7   SUMMARY

Emerging cases have proven that social media can be used for ambient diagnostics. The relevancy of posted content on social media sites is important in attracting the right viewers and obtaining relevant responses, building from small and then growing gradually—the Katamari effect. Groups branching out, cross posting, anonymity for intimate posting, and visual effects help users find the right viewers in social networks. A site's reputation and popularity also play a key role in attracting viewers. Interaction histograms show how often a particular interaction takes place. PR measures how much connection a page has to reputable sites. The power law explains the fact that only a small number of sites, groups, or individuals can generate a large amount of traffic in social media.

A force-directed graph is a physics-inspired tool for visualizing a social network. It can be used to analyze the co-occurrence of events and network dynamics. However, a force-directed graph does not have a scalable performance when the size of a social network is large (e.g., city size), and it may have local optima problems.

Finally, the massive social media data brings us the renaissance of correlation analytical methods. Pearson's coefficient is for checking the linearity, based on absolute values, but Spearman's coefficient is for checking the monotony based on ordinal ranks. Both have great potential in discovering hidden correlations for ambient diagnoses.

PROBLEMS

1. Prove that Pearson's coefficient of correlation is equivalent to cosine angle similarity. You may derive the equations between the two or use experiments to test the hypothesis. Discuss the conditions.
2. Compare force-directed graphs with the multiple dimension scaling (MDS) method. Discuss the similarities and differences. At what conditions are they are identical? Use a simple example to support your point.
3. Find the top ten words from the Internet. Use a log-log plot to see if they fit a power law. Estimate the values for the parameters.
4. Use the Google PR tool to find the PR of a web domain page you are interested in. Discuss how to increase the PR.
5. Plot an IF histogram of your one-week interactions with social media.
6. Use the Google Keyword Tool to search the keyword *elderly*. (A) Discuss the top ten topics related to elderly issues. (B) Discuss the differences between the local searches and national searches.
7. Research additional new data for Table 15.2, including more cancer types and search counts from Google and the NCI annual survey about related cases. Calculate Pearson's coefficient of correlation and plot of the scatter chart. Write a report about your findings and analysis.
8. Research additional new data for Table 15.2, including more cancer types and search counts from Google and the NCI annual survey about related cases. Calculate Spearman's coefficient and plot the scatter chart. Write a report about your findings and analysis.
9. Based on the results from Problems 7 and 8, compare the two methods.

10. Use the open source Rage Comic to write a story and post it on Reddit. Discuss the feedback from the posted group. Cluster the comments you received based on the attributes you select.

11. Use a force-directed graph to plot the co-occurrence of your friends in a one-week timeframe. Discuss the results in your report.

12. Study the Kawasaki disease case.[339] Discuss the strategies one might use to find diagnostic information about rare diseases on social networking sites.

13. Study the case study of the vitamin B_{12} deficiency posts on Facebook's Evolution page. You will need to log in to Facebook and search for the Evolution page. Write a report covering the following:

    A. Complete a relevancy analysis about the posts.
    B. Complete a reputation analysis for the Evolution page.
    C. Read the posts and summarize the related topics.
    D. Read all the posts and then plot the relationship between the number of individuals and number of posts they posted (e.g., three users posted two comments; five users posted one comment; one user posted twenty comments; and so on).
    E. Discuss whether the curve fits the power law and why.
    F. Plot the number of likes, posts, and shares over time to show the dynamics of the page.

---

[339] Deborah Kogan. How Facebook saved my son's life. *Slate* July 13, 2011, n.p. Accessed February 25, 2013.

Section 5

Appendices

A Sample Code

CHAPTER 2 DATA TRANSFORMATION

DCT compression in gray scale in MATLAB

```
function dctc(imageName, threshold)
    RGB = imread(imageName);           % read image
    I = rgb2gray(RGB);                 % convert to gray
    J = dct2(I);                       % DCT coefficients
    J(abs(J) < threshold) = 0;         % set small coefficients to 0
    K = idct2(J);                      % inverse DCT
    imshow(I), figure, imshow(K,[0 255])
end
```

Wavelet compression in gray scale in MATLAB

```
function wavelet2(imageName, percent)
    I = imread(imageName);                    % read image
    I = rgb2gray(I);                          % convert to gray
    A = double(I);                            % convert to 16-bit
    N = ceil(log2(length(A)));                % round up
    [C,S] = wavedec2(A,N,'haar');             % get coefficients
    DIM = floor(length(C)*(percent*0.01));    % energy retention DIM
    C(DIM+1:end) = 0;                         % compress coefficients
    E = waverec2(C,S,'haar');                 % reconstruct image
    IR = uint8(E);                            % convert to unsigned 8-bit
    imshow(IR);                               % show and save output
end
```

Wavelet compression in color in MATLAB

```
% Wavelet Compression Demo Function
% imageName:  input image name (e.g. 'saturn.png')
% percent:    energy retention percent (e.g. 50)
%
function wavelet1(imageName, percent)
    I = imread(imageName);                % read image
    I = double(I);                        % convert to 16-bit
    R = I(:,:,1); G=I(:,:,2); B=I(:,:,3); % get R,G,B values
    N = ceil(log2(length(R)));            % round up
    [RC, RS] = wavedec2(R, N, 'haar');    % get coefficients for R
    [GC, GS] = wavedec2(G, N, 'haar');    % get coefficients for G
```

```matlab
[BC, BS] = wavedec2(B, N, 'haar');        % get coefficients for B
DIM = floor(length(RC)*(percent*0.01));   % energy retention DIM
RC(DIM+1:end) = 0;                         % compress for R
GC(DIM+1:end) = 0;                         % comrpess for G
BC(DIM+1:end) = 0;                         % comrpess for B
RR = waverec2(RC, RS, 'haar');             % reconstruct for R
GR = waverec2(GC, GS, 'haar');             % reconstruct for G
BR = waverec2(BC, BS, 'haar');             % reconstruct for B
IR = cat(3, RR, GR, BR);                   % put back to RGB matrix
IR = uint8(IR);                            % convert to unsigned 8-bit
imshow(IR);                                % show and save output
imwrite(IR, sprintf('a%02d.JPG', percent), 'JPG');
end
```

CHAPTER 7. VIDEO ANALYSIS

Read and write frames in MATLAB

```matlab
% Input frames with VideoReader
inputObj = VideoReader('test.avi')
nFrames = inputObj.NumberOfFrames;

% Set up output video with VideoWriter
workingDir = pwd
outputVideo = VideoWriter(fullfile(workingDir,'output2.avi'));
outputVideo.FrameRate = inputObj.FrameRate;
open(outputVideo);

% Display and write frames
for k = 1 : nFrames
    my_rgb_frame = read(inputObj, k);
    figure(1), imshow(my_rgb_frame)
    writeVideo(outputVideo, my_rgb_frame);
end
close(outputVideo);
```

CHAPTER 9. MOBILE SENSORS.

Simple sensor log in Java

```java
package com.aravind.sensors;

import java.io.File;
import java.io.FileNotFoundException;
import java.io.FileWriter;
import java.io.IOException;
import java.net.InetAddress;
import java.net.NetworkInterface;
```

```java
import java.net.SocketException;
import java.text.SimpleDateFormat;
import java.util.Date;
import java.util.Enumeration;

import com.aravind.sensors.R;

import android.annotation.SuppressLint;
import android.app.Activity;
import android.app.AlertDialog;
import android.content.Context;
import android.os.Bundle;
import android.os.Environment;
import android.text.format.Formatter;
import android.util.Log;
import android.view.View;
import android.widget.Button;
import android.widget.TextView;
import android.graphics.Color;
import android.hardware.Sensor;
import android.hardware.SensorEvent;
import android.hardware.SensorEventListener;
import android.hardware.SensorManager;
import android.hardware.SensorListener;

public class SimpleSensorLog extends Activity implements SensorListener {

final String tag = "Simple Sensor Readings";
String logStringA, logStringO;
SensorManager sm = null;
SensorManager smAux = null;
 SensorManager mySensorManager;
 Sensor myProximitySensor;
boolean logging  = false;
TextView xViewA = null;
TextView yViewA = null;
TextView zViewA = null;
TextView xViewO = null;
TextView yViewO = null;
TextView zViewO = null;
TextView proximity0 = null;
TextView lp = null;
Button button1 = null;
File backupPath1;
File backupPath2;
String Ans = null;

/** Called when the activity is first created. */
@SuppressLint("NewApi")
@Override
public void onCreate(Bundle savedInstanceState) {
```

```
super.onCreate(savedInstanceState);

sm = (SensorManager) getSystemService(SENSOR_SERVICE);
smAux = (SensorManager) getSystemService(SENSOR_SERVICE);
setContentView(R.layout.main);
xViewA = (TextView) findViewById(R.id.xbox);
yViewA = (TextView) findViewById(R.id.ybox);
zViewA = (TextView) findViewById(R.id.zbox);
xViewO = (TextView) findViewById(R.id.xboxo);
yViewO = (TextView) findViewById(R.id.yboxo);
zViewO = (TextView) findViewById(R.id.zboxo);
proximity0 = (TextView) findViewById(R.id.proxo);
Ip  = (TextView) findViewById(R.id.ip);
button1 = (Button) findViewById(R.id.button1);
button1.setBackgroundColor(Color.GREEN);

Thread t = new Thread();
t.start();

button1.setOnClickListener(new View.OnClickListener() {


    public void onClick(View v) {
            logging = !logging;
            if (logging == true) {
                    button1.setBackgroundColor(Color.RED);
                    button1.setText("Click to stop logging");
            }
            else {
                    button1.setBackgroundColor(Color.GREEN);
                    button1.setText("Click to start logging");

            }
                    SimpleDateFormat formatter = new
                    SimpleDateFormat("yyyy_MM_dd_HH_mm_ss");
            Date now = new Date();
            final String fileName = formatter.format(now) + ".txt";
            Runnable runnable = new Runnable() {

    public void run() {
            while (true) {
                    if (logging == true) {
                            Log.d(tag, "sai");
                            FilebackupPath=Environment.getExternalStorageDirectory();
            backupPath = new File(backupPath.getPath() + "/Android/data/aravind/
files");

            if(!backupPath.exists()){
              backupPath.mkdirs();
            }
            FileWriter fos;
```

```
                        try {
                          fos = new FileWriter(backupPath.getPath() + "/" + fileName, true);

                          fos.write((logStringA  + logStringO + "\n"));
                          fos.close();
                        } catch (FileNotFoundException e) {
                          e.printStackTrace();
                        } catch (IOException e) {
                          e.printStackTrace();
                        }
                            }
                            else
                                  Log.d(tag, "ram");
                      }
                  }
            };

        Thread mythread = new Thread(runnable);
        mythread.start()
            }
      });
    }


@SuppressLint("NewApi")
public void onSensorChanged(int sensor, float[] values) {
      synchronized (this) {
          Log.d(tag, "onSensorChanged: " + sensor + ", x: " + values[0] +
                        ", y: " + values[1] + ", z: " + values[2]);
          if (sensor == SensorManager.SENSOR_ORIENTATION) {
                  xViewO.setText("Orientation X: " + values[0]);
                  yViewO.setText("Orientation Y: " + values[1]);
                  zViewO.setText("Orientation Z: " + values[2]);
                  logStringO = values[0] + ", " + values[1] + ", " + values[2];
          }
          if (sensor == SensorManager.SENSOR_ACCELEROMETER) {
                  xViewA.setText("Accel X: " + values[0]);
                  yViewA.setText("Accel Y: " + values[1]);
                  zViewA.setText("Accel Z: " + values[2]);
                  logStringA =  values[0] + ",  " + values[1] + ", " + values[2];

          }
          if (sensor == SensorManager.SENSOR_MAGNETIC_FIELD) {
                  proximity0.setText("Magnetic Field:" + values[0]);
          }
          try {
                      for (Enumeration<NetworkInterface>  en  =  NetworkInterface.
      getNetworkInterfaces();
          en.hasMoreElements();) {
                            NetworkInterface intf = en.nextElement();
                for (Enumeration<InetAddress> enumIpAddr = intf.getInetAddresses();
                      enumIpAddr.hasMoreElements();) {
                  InetAddress inetAddress = enumIpAddr.nextElement();
```

```java
                if (!inetAddress.isLoopbackAddress()) {
                    String ip = Formatter.formatIpAddress(inetAddress.hashCode());
                    Log.i(tag, "***** IP="+ ip);
                    Ip.setText(" IP address is " + ip);
                }
            }
        }
    } catch (SocketException ex) {
        Log.e(tag, ex.toString());
    }
    }
}

public void onAccuracyChanged(int sensor, int accuracy) {
    Log.d(tag,"onAccuracyChanged: " + sensor + ", accuracy: " + accuracy);
    }


@Override
protected void onResume() {
    super.onResume();
    sm.registerListener(this,
                SensorManager.SENSOR_ORIENTATION |
                SensorManager.SENSOR_ACCELEROMETER |
                SensorManager.SENSOR_MAGNETIC_FIELD,
                SensorManager.SENSOR_DELAY_NORMAL);

    }

@Override
protected void onStop() {
    sm.unregisterListener(this);
    smAux.unregisterListener(this);
    super.onStop();
    }
}
```

Android manifest for sensor log in XML

```xml
<?xml version="1.0" encoding="utf-8"?>
<manifest xmlns:android="http://schemas.android.com/apk/res/android"
    package="com.aravind.sensors"
    android:versionCode="1"
    android:versionName="1.0.0">
    <uses-permission android:name="android.permission.INTERNET" />
  <application android:icon="@drawable/icon" android:label="Simple Sensors">
    <activity android:name="com.aravind.sensors.SimpleSensorLog"
            android:label="Simple sensors app">
      <intent-filter>
        <action android:name="android.intent.action.MAIN" />
        <category android:name="android.intent.category.LAUNCHER" />
```

```
        </intent-filter>
      </activity>
    </application>
</manifest>
```

Android layout for sensor log in XML

```xml
<?xml version="1.0" encoding="utf-8"?>
<LinearLayout xmlns:android="http://schemas.android.com/apk/res/android"
    android:layout_width="fill_parent"
    android:layout_height="fill_parent"
    android:layout_gravity="center"
    android:orientation="vertical" >

    <TextView
        android:layout_width="fill_parent"
        android:layout_height="wrap_content"
        android:layout_gravity="center"
        android:text="Simple Sensor Log" />

    <TextView
        android:layout_width="fill_parent"
        android:layout_height="wrap_content"
        android:text="Accelerometer" />

    <TextView
        android:id="@+id/xbox"
        android:layout_width="fill_parent"
        android:layout_height="wrap_content"
        android:layout_gravity="center"
        android:text="X Value" />

    <TextView
        android:id="@+id/ybox"
        android:layout_width="fill_parent"
        android:layout_height="wrap_content"
        android:text="Y Value" />

    <TextView
        android:id="@+id/zbox"
        android:layout_width="fill_parent"
        android:layout_height="wrap_content"
        android:text="Z Value" />

    <TextView
        android:layout_width="fill_parent"
        android:layout_height="wrap_content"
        android:text="Orientation" />

    <TextView
        android:id="@+id/xboxo"
```

```
        android:layout_width="fill_parent"
        android:layout_height="wrap_content"
        android:text="X Value" />
  <TextView
        android:id="@+id/yboxo"
        android:layout_width="fill_parent"
        android:layout_height="wrap_content"
        android:text="Y Value" />

  <TextView
        android:id="@+id/zboxo"
        android:layout_width="fill_parent"
        android:layout_height="wrap_content"
        android:text="Z Value" />

  <TextView
        android:id="@+id/proxo"
        android:layout_width="fill_parent"
        android:layout_height="wrap_content"
        android:text="Proximity" />

  <TextView
        android:id="@+id/ip"
        android:layout_width="wrap_content"
        android:layout_height="wrap_content"
        android:text="IP Address" />

  <Button
        android:id="@+id/button1"
        android:layout_width="117dp"
        android:layout_height="wrap_content"
        android:layout_gravity="bottom"
        android:scrollHorizontally="false"
        android:text="Click to Start logging" />
</LinearLayout>
```

CHAPTER 11. POCKET MICROSCOPES

Blob labeling in MATLAB

```
% the function vislabel(L) that can be downloaded from Mathworks website.
clear all;
A = imread('rice.png');              % read image
B = edge(A, 'canny');                % edge detection
se = strel('disk', 1);               % set brush shape as disk with 1 iteration
B2 = imclose(B, se);                 % dilate and then erode blobs
```

```
B3 = imfill(B2,'holes');              % fill interior gaps
B4 = bwlabel(B3);                     % labeling
L = bwperim(B4);                      % draw outlines around cells
vislabels(L)                          % call function VisLabel(L) and write labels
```

CHAPTER 12. PERSONAL SPECTROMETER

Spectrum from RGB images in MATLAB

```
I = imread('image.jpg');                        % read image
IR = I(:,:,1);  IG=I(:,:,2);  IB=I(:,:,3);      % split into RGB channels

% convert to a gray-scale based on human perception
Y = 0.29900*IR+0.58700*IG+0.11400*IB;

% Select a narrow strip (10 pixels) along the center from the image
% Determine the average for each wavelength
[n,m]=size(Y);
mid=floor(n/2);
E = mean(Y(mid-5:mid+5,:),1);
Wavelength = linspace(350,750,m);               % visible wavelength
figure
subplot(211)
image(I)
set(gca,'XTick',[ ],'YTick',[ ])
title('Original Image','FontWeight','bold')
subplot(212)
plot(Wavelength,E)
set(gca, 'yTick', [0 25 50 75 100]);
title('Spectrometer')
xlabel('Wavelength [nm]')
ylabel('Color intensity (0 – 100%)')
ylim([0 100])
grid on
```

B Further Readings

CHAPTER 1 INTRODUCTION

1. Cai, Y. (ed.) *Digital Human Modeling*. LNAI 4650. Springer. 2008
2. CLIPS Open Source link: http://clipsrules.sourceforge.net/
3. Ginsberg, J., M.H. Mohebbi, R.S. Patel,L.Brammer, M.S.Smolinski, L.Brilliant. Detecting influenza epidemics using search engine query data. *Nature*. Vol. 457. No. 19. Feb. 2009 http://www.springer.com/computer/ai/book/978-3-540-89429-2
4. Lindsay, Robert K., Bruce G. Buchanan, E. A. Feigenbaum, and Joshua Lederberg. DENDRAL: A Case Study of the First Expert System for Scientific Hypothesis Formation. *Artificial Intelligence*. 61, 2 (1993): 209-261.
5. Moore, G. E. Cramming more components onto integrated circuits" (PDF), 1965. *Electronics Magazine*. p. 4. http://www.cs.utexas.edu/~fussell/courses/cs352h/papers/moore.pdf
6. Pearl, J. *Probabilistic reasoning in intelligent systems*. Morgan Kaufmann, Inc. 1988
7. PROLOG Open Source link: http://gprolog.univ-paris.fr/
8. Simon, H.A. *The science of artificial*. The MIT Press. 1980
9. Suslick, K. S. Synesthesia in Science and Technology: More than Making the Unseen Visible. *Current Opinion in Chemical Biology*. Bio. 2012, 16, 557-563.
10. WikiPedia on MYCIN: http://en.wikipedia.org/wiki/Mycin, captured on November 19, 2013
11. Witten, I. and E. Frank. *Data mining*. Morgan Kaufmann Publishers, Inc. 2000

CHAPTER 2 DATA TRANSFORMATION

12. Chernoff, H., & Rizvi, M. H. (1975). Effect on classification error or random permutations of features in representing multivariate data by faces. *Journal of American Statistical Association*, 70, 548-554.
13. Intal, OpenCV, Intel, 2013, http://opencv.org/
14. Mathworks. Image Processing Toolbox for using with MATLAB. User Guide. http://amath.colorado.edu/computing/Matlab/OldTechDocs/images_tb.pdf
15. Phillipou, G., Geographical display of capillary blood glucose data using Chernoff Faces. Diabestic Medicine. Vol. 9. No.3. pp.293-294. April 1992.
16. .Sonka, M., V. Hlavac, R. Boyle. *Image Processing Analysis, and Machine Vision*. PWS Publishing. 3rd Edition, 2007

CHAPTER 3 PATTERN RECOGNITION

17. Burges, C. A Tutorial on Support Vector Machines for Pattern Recognition, *Data Mining and Knowledge Discovery*. 2:121–167, 1998

18. George, R.M. and Charles, C. *Facial Geometry – Graphic facial analysis for forensic artists.* Thomas Publisher, 2007
19. MacQueen, J.B. Some Methods for classification and Analysis of Multivariate Observations, Proceedings of 5-th Berkeley Symposium on Mathematical Statistics and Probability, Berkeley, University of California Press, 1:281-297, 1967
20. Witten, I. and E. Frank. *Data mining.* Morgan Kaufmann Publishers, Inc. 2000

CHAPTER 4 SOUND RECOGNITION

21. Anderson, K., Qiu, Y., Whittaker, A.R., Lucas, Margaret: Breath sounds, asthma, and the mobile phone. *Lancet.* 358:1343-44 (2001)
22. Angier, N.: In Mammals, a Complex Journey. New York Times, October 13, 2009
23. Ariel Roguin, Rene Theophile Hyacinthe Laënnec (1781–1826): The Man Behind the Stethoscope, *Clinic Medicine Research*: 4(3): 230-235
24. Ben J. Shannon, Kuldip K. Paliwal, A Comparative Study of Filter Bank Spacing for Speech Recognition, Microelectronic Engineering Research Conference 2003
25. Breebaart, J. and M. McKinney, Features for Audio Classification, Philips Research Laboratories, 2008
26. Cai, Y. and Abascal, J.: *Ambient intelligence in everyday life.* Lecture Notes in Artificial Intelligence, LNAI 3864, Springer. (2006)
27. Clendening L. *Source book of medical history.* 1st ed. New York, NY: Harper & Brothers; 1942. 313–330.
28. Davies MK, Hollman A. Rene Theophile-Hyacinthe Laënnec (1781–1826) *Heart.* 1996;76:196.
29. Donald Blaufox, *Ear to the chest: an illustrated history of the evolution of the stethoscope*, The Parthenon Publishing Group, 2002, ISBN: 1-85070-278-0
30. Elisabeth Bennion, *Antique medical instruments*, University of California Press, 1979, ISBN: 0-85667-052-9
31. FFmpeg, http://ffmpeg.org
32. Foote, J., Content-based retrieval of music and audio. *Multimedia Storage and Archiving Systems II*, 1997 138-147
33. Hearing Central LLC, How the Human Ear Works, http://www.hearingaidscentral.com/howtheearworks.asp, 10/25/2010
34. Hewitt, R. Seeing with OpenCV, Part 4: Face Recognition with Eigenface, 2007.
35. Jacaly Duffin, *To see with a better eye: a life of R.T.H. Laennec*, Princeton University Press, 1998, ISBN: 0-691-03708-6
36. Jay V. The legacy of Laënnec. *Archives of Pathology and Laboratory Medicine.* 2000;124:1420–1421.
37. Ji, Q., Luo, Z.X., Zhang, X.L., Yuan, C.X., Xu, L.: Evolutionary Development of the Middle Ear in Mesozoic Therian Mammals. *Science* 9, October 2009: Vol. 326, No. 5950, pp. 278-281
38. Leonardo Alfredo et al., Classification of Voice Aging Using Parameters Extracted from the Glottal Signal. *Lecture Notes in Computer Science*, 2010, Volume 6354/2010, 149-156
39. Lindsay I Smith, A tutorial on Principal Components Analysis, 2002
40. Logan. B. et al., Mel Frequency Cepstral Coefficients for Music Modelling, Cambridge Research Laboratory, 2000

41. Martin, T. and Ruf, I.: On the Mammalian Ear. *Science*, 9 October 2009: Vol. 326, No. 5950, pp. 243-244

42. MathWorks, Manual of Neural Network Toolkit, 2013: http://www.mathworks. com/help/pdf_doc/nnet/nnet_ug.pdf

43. Moore, A. Tutorials for Machine Learning: http://www.autonlab.org/tutorials/ kmeans11.pdf

44. Murphy, R., S. Holford, and W. Knowler Visual lung-sound characterization by time-expanded wave-form analysis, *New England Journal of Medicine*, 296:968-971, April 28, 1977.

45. Marian, P. Cardiophone, http://electroschematics.com/502/cardiophone/

46. Par, R.T.H. Launnec, De l'Auscultation Médiate ou Traité du Diagnostic des Maladies des Poumons et du Cœur (On Mediate Auscultation or Treatise on the Diagnosis of the Diseases of the Lungs and Heart) published in Paris in 1819

47. Pasterkamp, H., Kraman, S.S., Wodicka,G.R.: Respiratory sounds: advances beyond the stethoscope. *American Journal of Respiratory Critical Care Medicine*. 156:974-87 (1997)

48. Peter, G., Cukierman, D., Anthony, C., and Schwartz, M.: Online music search by tapping, in Cai, Y. and Abascal, J. (eds): *Lecture Notes in Artificial Intelligence*, LNAI 3864, Springer, 2006

49. Pfeiffer, S. and S. Fischer, Effelsberg,W.: Automatic audio content analysis, Tech. Rep. No. 96-008, University of Mannheim, 1996.

50. Siegel, M. et al, Vehicle Sound Signature Recognition by Frequency Vector Principal Component Analysis. *IEEE Trans. on Instrumentation And Measurement*, vol. 48, no. 5, October 1999

51. Sigurdur Sigurdsson at al., *Mel Frequency Cepstral Coefficients: An Evaluation of Robustness of MP3 Encoded Music*, Technical University of Denmark, 2006

52. WikiPedia. Spectrogram, http://en.wikipedia.org/wiki/Spectrogram, retrieved on 07/30/2010

53. Spiteri, M.A., Cook, D.G, Clark, S.W: Reliability of eliciting physical signs in examination of the chest. *Lancet*. 2:873-75. (1988)

54. Turk, M. and Pentland, A. Eigenface for Recognition. *Journal of Cognitive Neuroscience*, Vol. 3, No. 1, 1991. http://www.face-rec.org/algorithms/PCA/ jcn.pdf

55. Tutorial,2009.http://onionesquereality.wordpress.com/tag/mahalanobis-distance/

56. Tzanetakis, G. and P. Cook: Musical genre classification of audio signals. *IEEE Transaction on Speech Audio Processing*, vol. 10, pp. 293–301, 2002.

57. Wen-Hung Liao and Yu-Kai Lin: Classification of Non-Speech Human Sounds: Feature Selection and Snoring Sound Analysis, *Proceedings of the 2009 IEEE International Conference on Systems, Man and Cybernetics*

58. Windowing Function, http://en.wikipedia.org/wiki/Window_function, retrieved on 07/30/2010

CHAPTER 5 COLOR VISION

59. Carey, J. R.; Suslick, K. S.; Hulkower, K. I.; Imlay, J. A.; Imlay, K. R. C.; Ingison, C. K.; Ponder, J. B.; Sen, A.; Wittrig, A. E. Rapid Identification of Bacteria with a Disposable Colorimetric Sensor Array. *Journal of American Chemical Society*. 2011, 133, 7571-7576.

60. Lim, S. H.; Feng, L.; Kemling, J. W.; Musto, C. J.; Suslick, K. S. An Optoelectronic Nose for Detection of Toxic Gases. *Nature Chemistry*, 2009, 1, 562-567.

61. Lin, H.; Jang, M.; Suslick, K. S. Preoxidation for Colorimetric Sensor Array Detection of VOCs. *Journal of American Chemical Society*. 2011, 133, 16786–16789.
62. Suslick, K. S. Synesthesia in Science and Technology: More than Making the Unseen Visible. *Current Opinion in Chemical Biology*. 2012, 16, 557-563.

CHAPTER 6 KINECT SENSORS

63. Besl, P. J. and N.D. McKay (1992). A Method for Registration of 3-D Shapes. *IEEE Transactions on Pattern Analysis and Machine Intelligence* (Los Alamitos, CA, USA: IEEE Computer Society) 14 (2): 239–256. doi:10.1109/34.121791
64. Borenstein, G. Making Things See: 3D vision with Kinect, Processing, Arduino and MakerBot, *Make*, February 2012, ISBN: 978-1449307073
65. Borenstein, G. *Making Things See*. O'Reilly. 2012
66. Elena Tsiporkova, Dynamic Time Warping Algorithm for Gene Expression Time Sequences.
67. Jaron Blackburn and Eraldo Ribeiro, Human Motion Recognition Using Isomap and Dynamics Time Warping, *Lecture Notes in Computer Science*, 4814: 295-298, 2007
68. Kinect for Windows SDK beta, Skeletal Viewer Walkthrough: C++/C#
69. Melgar, E. R. and C.C. Diez, Ardiono and Kinect Projects, Apress, 2012
70. Prime Sensor™. NITE Controls User Guide. Copyright 2011. PrimeSense Inc.

CHAPTER 7 VIDEO ANALYSIS

71. Demand, K., A. Oliver, N. Oostendorp, K, Scott, *Practical Computer Vision with SimpleCV: The Simple Way to Make Technology*, July 2012, ISBN: 978-1449320362, O'Reilly Media
72. Laganiere, R. *Open CV2 Computer Vision Application Programming Cookbook*, May 2011, ISBN: 978-1849513241, Publisher: Packt Publishing
73. Linda G. Shapiro, George C. Stockman, *Computer Vision*, Prentice Hall, 2001
74. Murat A. Tekalp, Digital Video Processing, Prentice Hall, 1996
75. Novik, A. *The Essential Guide to Video Processing*, Elsevier, 2009
76. Yunqian Ma and Gang Qian (eds), *Intelligent Video Surveillance: Systems and Technology*, CRC Press, 2010

CHAPTER 8 FATIGURE DETECTION

77. Duchowski, A. *Eye tracking methodology*. Springer, 2nd edition. 2007
78. Grace, R. et al. A drowsy driver detection system for heavy vehicles, Technical Report, Robotics Institute, 2001: http://www.ri.cmu.edu/pub_files/pub2/grace_richard_2001_1/grace_richard_2001_1.pdf
79. Milborrow, S. Active shape models with STASM, May 28, 2013: http://www.milbo.users.sonic.net/stasm/
80. Viola, P. and Jones, M. Robust real-time face detection. *International Journal of Computer Vision*, Vol. 57, No.2, pp.137-154, 2004. http://www.vision.caltech.edu/html-files/EE148-2005-Spring/pprs/viola04ijcv.pdf
81. WikiPedia. Mackworth Clock, 2013

CHAPTER 9 MOBILE SENSORS

82. Jackson, T.W. *Android Apps for Absolute Beginners*, ISBN: 978-1430234463, Apress
83. Mednieks, Z., L. Dornin, G. Blake Meike, M. Nakamura, *Programming Android*, ISBN: 978-1449389697, O'Reilly Media
84. TinyOS: http://www.tinyos.net/

CHAPTER 10 BODY MEDIA

85. Holmes, J. System for analyzing thermal data based on breast surface temperature to determine suspect conditions. US 20100056946 A1, May 27, 2010
86. MC10 Inc. http://www.mc10inc.com/, captured in 2013
87. PillCam. http://givenimaging.com/, captured in 2013
88. Emotiv. http://emotiv.com/, captured in 2013

CHAPTER 11 POCKET MICROSCOPES

89. Mudanyali O, Oztoprak C, Tseng D, Erlinger A, Ozcan A (2010) Detection of waterborne parasites using field-portable and cost-effective lensfree microscopy. *Lab Chip* 10: 2419–2423. http://www.medgadget.com/2013/03/iphone-microscope-helps-detect-parasitic-worm-eggs.html
90. RANSAC, WikiPedia: http://en.wikipedia.org/wiki/RANSAC
91. Rowe, D. Demo software: SIFT Keypoint detector, captured in December 2013 http://www.cs.ubc.ca/~lowe/keypoints/
92. Rowe, D. U.S. Patent 6,711,293, Method and apparatus for identifying scale invariant features in an image and use of same for locating an object in an image. March 23, 2004
93. Smith, D. et al. Cell-Phone-Based Platform for Biomedical Device Development and Education Applications. *PLOS One*, March 02, 2011 http://www.plosone.org/article/info%3Adoi%2F10.1371%2Fjournal.pone.0017150

CHAPTER 12 PERSONAL SPECTROMETER

94. Public Lab: http://publiclab.org/
95. Smith, D. et al. Cell-Phone-Based Platform for Biomedical Device Development and Education Applications. *PLOS One*, March 02, 2011. http://www.plosone.org/article/info%3Adoi%2F10.1371%2Fjournal.pone.0017150

CHAPTER 13 REMOTE SENSING

96. Cai, Y. (Ed.) *Digital Human Modeling*, LNAI 4650, Springer, 2008
97. Laws, J. and Y. Cai, A privacy algorithm for 3D human body scans, ICCS'06 Vol. IV, pp. 870-877, 2006, ACM Digital Lib: http://dl.acm.org/citation.cfm?id=2107390

CHAPTER 14 GAMING FOR DIAGNOSIS

98. FoldIt: http://fold.it/portal/
99. Keorner, B.I. New Videogame Lets Amateur Researchers Mess With RNA by Wired. July 5, 2012
100. Lee, J., S. Yoon, W. Kladwang, A. Treuille, M.L. Rhiju Das, D. Cantu, EteRNA participants. RNA Design Rules from a Massive Open Laboratory by (in submission)

CHAPTER 15 SOCIAL MEDIA

101. Barabási, Albert-László (2003). Linked: How everything is connected to everything else and what it means for business, science, and everyday life. Plum. ISBN 978-0-452-28439-5.
102. Mendenhall, W. Introduction to probability and statistics. Duxbury Press. 1979
103. Page, L. US Patent 6,285,999, September 4, 2001. Method for node ranking in a linked database.

Index